ORIENTAL MEDICINE

– *A Modern Interpretation*

by Hun Young Cho

Translated and Revised by
Kihyon Kim, OMD, Ph.D.

Yuin University Press
No. 12

This book does not replace the services of a licensed health care provider in the diagnosis or treatment of illness or disease. The information presented here should not be used for treatment or prevention of disease without the advice of an Oriental medical physician or other medical authority.

Published by Yuin University Press
2007 E. Compton Blvd.
Compton, CA 90221

ISBN 0-915649-00-4

Printed in the United States of America
Book & Cover Design by Choong Chan Lee

First Edition
July 1996

10 9 8 7 6 5 4 3 2 1

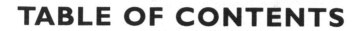

TABLE OF CONTENTS

TRANSLATOR'S
PREFACE

$\mathcal{O}$riental medicine, as defined by the book *World Medicine*, is one of the six major healing systems of the world and is currently enjoying high popularity in the United States. According to a survey done by the World Health Organization, more than one–third of the world's population is being treated with Oriental medicine (acupuncture). Dating back some 5,000 years, Oriental medicine has been practiced systematically, rationally and consistently by the people of China, Korea, Japan and southeast Asian countries. European countries began using it when the Jesuits and Dutch merchant traders brought back the information from China in the 16th century.

Unlike Western medicine, Oriental medicine is holistic in its approach to diagnosis and treatment of disease. Transcending the dichotomy of mind and body, it treats the root cause of an illness rather than its manifestation. Oriental medicine emphasizes the cultivation of health rather than treatment and cure of disease; it treats the person rather than the disease. It is for these reasons that many people worldwide use Oriental medicine to manage their health.

This book, *Oriental Medicine – A Modern Interpretation*, was originally written in 1934 by Mr. Hun Young Cho, who was a Congressman in Korea. At that time, the status of Oriental medicine had deteriorated significantly due to the growing popularity of Western medicine. Explaining the impetus for the book, Mr. Cho wrote the following in the original preface: "I found it regrettable and disconcerting that Oriental medicine, which had made the most contribution and had such a great effect on public medicine, was deteriorating daily."

Mr. Cho was well ahead of his time; I believe that he was the first person to explain Oriental medicine in scientific terms, particularly in comparing Oriental medicine to "hormone regulating medicine." Mr. Cho uses the language of western anatomy and physiology to provide a rational and scientific explanation of the Five Element Theory, allowing the layman to easily understand this important Oriental medical theory. His comparison of differing characteristics of Oriental medicine and Western medicine is direct and lucid. He wanted to make use of the best points of both medicines for the improvement of humankind. Oriental and Western medicine are complementary healing methods much like the two wings of a bird. Mr. Cho believed that both medicines must co–exist and support one another.

I have translated this book because I feel that anyone can benefit from the author's originality, in–depth knowledge and foresight in explaining Oriental medicine. English speaking countries have not been exposed to many of the ideas presented in this book. I believe this book facilitates the understanding of Oriental medicine from a different viewpoint, particularly by using everyday examples to illustrate difficult concepts.

In addition to discussing some of his clinical cases, which further demonstrate his profound insight in his approach to diagnosis and treatment, Mr. Cho addresses more intangible concerns, such as the correct attitude a doctor should take, the role medicine should play, the reverence for life and its true meaning.

I have tried to stay true to the original text as much as possible, but because certain nuances can be lost in translation, I have revised some passages to make them more readable. It is my belief that all English–speaking readers will benefit from this book – students and practitioners of Oriental Medicine as well as layman, in their quest for better health – and for more harmonious, balanced and peaceful lives.

Kihyon Kim
Los Angeles
Spring 1994

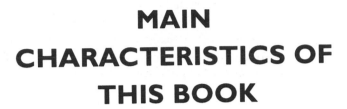

MAIN CHARACTERISTICS OF THIS BOOK

■ **Make the Fundamentals of Oriental Medicine Understandable**

In an Oriental medical treatment, there is neither a fixed "wonder drug" according to the name of a disease nor a fixed "disease" for one medicine. Even though the name of the disease is the same, medicines will differ according to the constitution and symptoms of the patient. By knowing the fundamentals of Oriental medicine, medicines can be applied freely and easily.

The research method of Western medicine is that of identifying the "principal disease" and the "principal medicine," thus its position differs from Oriental medicine. Describing Oriental medicine entirely from the holistic viewpoint is the distinctive characteristic of this book.

■ **Present Poetic Oriental Medical Concepts in a Logical Scientific Manner**

Traditional Oriental medicine contains sections of legends and myths in its contents, and is written in Chinese characters with difficult phrases and unscientific explanations, thus having many difficult points for the general public to understand. In this book, however, the explanations are logical and the compositions have been simplified.

■ **Provide Examples that Illustrates Oriental Concepts Best**

Examples were chosen entirely from the things anyone can experience in daily life.

■ **Compare the Different Oriental Medical Schools of Thought**

Generally, people seem to think that Oriental medicines are all identical, but there are actually different sects and conflicting theories even in Oriental medicine. Studying Oriental medicine without knowing this would be futile. The special feature of this book is that it comments, one by one, on the doctrines of those different perspectives.

■ **Base Instruction on Clinical Experience**

The theories of predecessors were not followed without criticisms. They have been affirmed through actual experience and their authenticity has been confirmed personally by the author.

■ Compare Oriental and Western Medicine

Until now there has been neither connection nor harmony between Oriental and Western medicine. This is because their theoretical viewpoints have been too far apart. While it is true that most consider these two disciplines to be at odds with each other, this is an erroneous understanding. Since Oriental and Western medicine each have distinctive features, their contributing fields and branches are different. Where they are similar is their goal to protect and improve the quality of life for humankind. As long as the subjects of their research are not outside the human body, disease or medicine, there must naturally be concurring points and harmonizing characteristics. For this reason, effort was put into identifying those points in this book.

■ Demystify Oriental Medicine

Attention was made to enable anyone to simply, safely and effectively use the treatment methods of Oriental medicine in a practical manner.

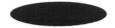

ACKNOWLEDGMENTS

I would like to thank following people for the kind help they have given me:

My sincere thanks goes to Sally Gallwey and Marie Katherine Toulet for going over entire manuscript for initial reviewing and editing. To doctors, David Wells and John Lamont for reviewing the manuscript. To doctors, Jun Sik Park, Sung Hwan Lee, Jung Min Kim and Hyuk Kyu Kim for helping me with some of the difficult passages in the original text. I am also indebted to professor Jae Yong Shin for his constant encouragement and with the help on researching some of the missing information in the original text. I would also like to thank the students at the Emperor's College of Traditional Oriental Medicine, especially Al Stone and Eric Wu for reading and editing the final draft of the manuscript and giving me much needed advice. Though I cannot name all of them here due to space limitation, much appreciation goes to all the friends and colleagues and also to students at both Emperor's College and Yuin University for encouragement and support. Most of all, I would like to thank my parents for all the support and love they have given me over the years.

NOTICE
– Usage of medical terminology

$\mathcal{W}$ords having different meanings in Oriental and Western medicines will be capitalized when referring to their meaning in Oriental medicine. The Oriental meanings are generally hypothetical constructs referring to physiological processes rather than anatomical entities. Examples of such words are "Heart," "Liver," "Spleen," "Triple Burner," "Blood," etc. Terms that are taken from the Oriental language are italicized and capitalized. Examples of these terms include *Qi*, *Yin*, *Yang*, *Zang Fu*, *Taiyang*, etc.

INTRODUCTION

I. THE DUTY OF ORIENTAL AND WESTERN MEDICINE

There is a worldwide trend towards Oriental medicine in recent times. Five years ago[1], I heard a report regarding the establishment of the Oriental Herbal Medicine Research Committee in the United Nations. In Tokyo and other areas, discussions on reviving Oriental medicine have been given considerable emphasis. In Korea, people are still receiving plenty of Oriental medical treatments, so discussions on reviving Oriental medicine with the implication of re–establishing it are not relevant. However, further development, elevation and improvement of Oriental medicine is the vital question confronting us. The first thing that is needed when discussing the subject of Oriental medicine, above anything else, is the proper understanding of Oriental medicine itself. Whether one promotes, discards, disagrees with or supports Oriental medicine, without correct understanding of the medicine itself, one should not criticize its validity. To properly understand Oriental medicine, critical comparisons to Western medicine are absolutely necessary.

It is true that bias cannot be avoided in discussing Oriental medicine while looking only from the perspective of Oriental medicine. Also, a biased opinion cannot be avoided in discussing methods outside of Western medicine when coming from a contemporary scientific standpoint. Hence, through comparing and contrasting Oriental and Western Medicine to properly understand Oriental medicine and after clearly recognizing its medical value, society should be educated so that they can have a strong faith in the significance of the existence of Oriental medicine. As the public recognizes its value, public and government support can be acquired. Subsequently, necessary facilities such as research institutes, learning centers, schools, hospitals, etc. will be established. I recognized this point early and devoted every possible effort for seven years so far for the modernization, scientific verification and socialization of Oriental medicine. At this time, I am writing an outline of my humble opinions open to the friendly criticisms and guidance of the readers.

---

1. It should be noted that references to time throughout this book come from the original author's perspective dating back to 1934 or there abouts.

One often hears about the developments of modern medicine or medical technology, but it is an undeniable fact that the moaning of the sick among us is becoming louder and louder. The increase in the so–called modern diseases such as tuberculosis, neurasthenia and all disorders of the digestive system cannot help but put a frown of concern onto our faces.

So–called civilized or modern diseases imply that these diseases have increased in recent times among the people of civilized countries, but upon deeper inspection, it signifies that modern medicine was unable to defend against or eliminate these diseases. Undoubtedly, it is true that complicated living conditions make it easy for people to catch these diseases. The invention of fighter planes was followed with the creation of anti–aircraft guns. When battleships showed their prowess, submarines and torpedo boats were devised. So it is the weakness of modern or Western medicine that it could not alleviate the diseases caused by the stress of modern society even with the power of science.

In a country like the United States, non–pharmaceutical, natural medical schools have considerable influence and try to treat diseases without using drugs from modern hospitals. Recently in Japan, there has been a sudden rise in the use of many kinds of folk medicines. This development illustrates that modern medicine has been unable to satisfy those patients who are receiving these natural treatments.

However, since we have received great benefits from Western medicine, I am not trying to slight or attack Western medicine with these statements. It is solely due to the benefit of modern medicine through the development of serology that there exist many effective preventive measures such as the smallpox vaccine. Due to the development of microbiology, national health institutions are empowered in the prevention of epidemics and many other diseases. As a result of that, a countless number of souls have avoided the misery of epidemics. We must praise the strong points of Western medicine and at the same time supplement the weak points. In my opinion, the method of supplementation can be adopted only from Oriental medicine.

Oriental medicine bases its root in philosophy and Western medicine has built its foundation on natural science. Accordingly, their methods are different and their roles are divided so that the strengths of Oriental medicine are the weaknesses of Western medicine and the superior aspects of Western medicine are inferior in Oriental medicine. The former is holistic and the latter is analytical. The former puts its effort into the observation of living phenomena and the latter puts emphasis on the investigation of the structure of matter. Although Western medicine is superior in defending and eliminating external pathogens that threaten life, Oriental medicine is superior in fundamentally cultivating the internal life force to increase health.

One can compare the duties of Western and Oriental medicine in protecting life or health of the human body to the duties of laws and morals in maintaining peace and order in a society. If both do not support each other, a prosperous society cannot be expected. Having faith in the omnipotence of Western medicine by looking at surgical management or efficacious medicine for curing syphilis, malaria, etc. while disregarding Oriental medicine is a biased faith. Unconditionally protecting Oriental medicine and attacking and deploring Western medicine in cases where chronic illness was easily cured through

Oriental herbal medicine is an equally narrow opinion.

Morality is fundamental and law is temporary. In a similar way, Oriental medicine is a "root–treating medicine"[2] and Western medicine is a "manifestation–treating medicine."[3] Governmental power, for example, is exercised in unavoidable situations for the safety of the public, but morality has a more effective function than law in the daily life of all people.

It is natural for the authorities to adopt Western medicine for prevention of epidemics and forensic medicine, but in actuality, it is Oriental medicine that has contributed more in quantity than all the free medical treatments by the government for the health of each individual. Next, I'm going to state a few concrete examples.

HOLISTICALLY TREATING MEDICINE AND LOCALLY TREATING MEDICINE

Oriental Medicine is a "holistic medical approach" while Western medicine is a "localized (symptomatic) approach." For example, the cause of sinusitis in Western medicine is attributed to an increase in pyogenic bacteria in the sinus cavities (maxillary, ethmoidal, frontal and sphenoidal), which creates pus. Thus, performing surgery in that region has become the method of treatment.

In Oriental medicine, on the other hand, the cause of sinusitis is not found in the nasal region. One's constitution and many physiological abnormalities are holistically observed and synthesized in order to inquire and identify the cause of sinusitis in that person. Even in the treatment, Oriental medicine does not directly perform artificial treatment such as surgery on the diseased region. Rather, physiological abnormalities are holistically and naturally regulated in order to eliminate the disease phenomenon in the nasal region.

Besides the experience of the author in the healing of sinusitis without surgery, researchers have tested the effectiveness of Oriental medical herbs many times and reported successful findings.

Let us now put aside whether that treatment is superior or inferior and investigate the theoretical basis of holistic medical treatment.

It is not incorrect to say that the cause of sinusitis is the pyogenic bacteria acting on the sinus cavity, but thinking one step further, it is true that in any healthy body, pyogenic, pneumonia, diphtheria and influenza bacteria are always present in the nasal and the sinus cavities. Therefore, the cause of sinusitis is not in the pyogenic bacteria but in the reduction of resistance that suppresses and restrains pyogenic bacteria. Sinusitis is called *Bi Yuan* (nose–pool) and *Nao Lou* (brain discharge) if severe. The cause of it can be largely categorized as follows:

1. Sinusitis due to Internal Injury (*Yang* Deficiency sinusitis and *Yin* Deficiency sinusitis).
2. Sinusitis due to External Invasion

---

2. The medicine which treats the root cause of a disease.

3. The medicine which treats symptoms of a disease.

(1) originates from physical constitution and (2) is due to the common cold. Regardless of Internal or External sinusitis, the sinusitis that accompanies an abnormality of the genito–urinary system is called *Taiyang Bi Yuan*[4] and sinusitis that accompanies an abnormality in the digestive system is called *Yangming Bi Yuan*.[5]

The specific Oriental medical treatment for this sinusitis will be presented at some other opportunity. Rather than stating whether holistic treatment or localized treatment is better, either can be better according to the type of a disease. There are times when the former must be used, and times when the latter must be used. Sometimes both treatments must be combined. Thus, viewed from the standpoint of medicine, both are utterly necessary.

As a result of overly venerating localized or analytical medicine, strange events can frequently occur when viewed from the standpoint of holistic medicine. The most appropriate example of this is the #606 (penicillin) injection incident regarding a dentist which was repeatedly reported in the newspaper recently. It became a judicial issue and the judgement which was passed made #606 injections by dentists unlawful. This is a truly humorous thing when viewed from an Oriental medical standpoint. It is like lawfully preventing a dentist, who has been granted the privilege to treat dental disorders, from eliminating the cause of the dental disorder. The reason is that an abnormality frequently occurs in the tooth region due to syphilis, which is easily treated with penicillin. My point is not a discussion about the question of #606 injection privilege, but rather, about the fault of limiting the treatment of the dental disorder to the mouth by isolating dentistry away from treating the cause.

According to the channel theory of Oriental medicine, abnormalities or diseases of the reproductive and urinary system react on the Conception, Governing, Urinary Bladder and Kidney channels.[6] Erosion of the nose, loss of the voice and decaying of the tooth root occur frequently when syphilis invades those regions. Anyone can observe, if they pay close attention, that women develop toothaches and certain abnormalities in the mouth during pregnancy and menstruation. Since the oral region is at the end of the Conception channel, disorders of the reproductive system are clearly reflected in that region and disorders of the tooth root due to syphilis are a common occurrence. Thus, from the holistic viewpoint it seems a major contradiction not to let dentists eliminate the cause of dental disorder. When treating the disease of a human being, who by nature is a holistic organism, such a blunder seems quite obvious as a result of adopting the "locally treating" theory.

NATURALLY TREATING MEDICINE AND ARTIFICIALLY TREATING MEDICINE

One can view Oriental medicine as the "natural medicine" and Western medicine as

---

4. The Taiyang or "Greater Yang" channel is the Urinary Bladder channel and is related to the reproductive system in Oriental medicine. Problems in the genito–urinary system can affect the nasal region. See Chapter 4 on the channels for more details.

5. The Yangming or "Bright/Extreme Yang" channel is the Stomach channel. Any problem in the digestive system can affect the nasal region. See Chapter 4 on the channel for more details.

6. See Chapter 4 on the channels for the details regarding these channels.

the "artificial medicine." In a strict sense, natural treatment cannot be a medicine. Also, a purely artificial treatment cannot exist apart from the natural healing power of a living body. It is classified in such a way only through its main focus. The former guides and promotes natural healing power to eliminate disease through the normal functions of the living body itself and the latter puts effort in artificially adopting emergency measures to eliminate the disease.

Here too, we cannot discuss the superiority or inferiority of Oriental and Western medicine. According to the disease, there are many cases where artificial medicine must be used. Most surgical disorders must be treated by Western medicine. Orthopedic medicine or optometry, which can be viewed as semi–medicine, can easily treat disorders that are quite difficult to treat using Oriental medicine.

However, advocating the superiority of surgery for all diseases just on those grounds is not proper. For example, there are many instances of appendicitis and otitis being cured without surgery using the application of one or two packs of herbs according to the Oriental treatment method. In cases like these, there are some Western medical doctors who say, "Diseases of humans were made to heal naturally, so getting cured with Oriental herbs merely means that the disease was at the level where it could have been healed without surgery." This is a statement that will remain unsettled no matter how much one argues. Even if the disease is at the level where Western doctors feel surgery is absolutely necessary, the disease cured by Oriental herbs cannot be returned to the original state to be tested. It is also impossible to return a person to life who died because of surgery to check to see whether they could have lived without surgery. Here, we can only wait for fair judgement from the public to see which is correct.

Appendicitis, in Oriental medicine, is given medical terms such as Blood Accumulation (*Shang Han* Theory)[7], Blood Hernial disorder (Hernial disorder)[8] and inguinal carbuncle[9] (external medicine). They all have the same meaning, but the treatment methods are not fixed according to the medical terminology.

Another example of Western technique is the application of ice for a febrile disease. Everyone knows that large quantities of heat are consumed when ice is melting and as a general rule, a temperature over 42 degrees Celsius (107.6 degrees Fahrenheit) can be fatal. To prevent this from occurring, cold ice is artificially applied to the head and heart region in order to reduce the heat. This method is not without some benefits, but it has the following disadvantages:

1. Physics already has proven that evaporating–heat requires seven times more calories

---

7. Blood Accumulation occurs as a complication of the Taiyang Syndrome in Shang Han Theory (Theory of febrile diseases caused by Cold). There are symptoms such as lower abdominal mass with pain and distention, aversion to pressure, constipation, fever that gets worse at night, and at times, there is delirium.

8. Hernial disorder describes a diseased condition in which there is protrusion of a part of an organ in the body cavity to the exterior of the body. It is also a collective term for disorders in the external reproductive organs. Furthermore, it can describe a condition that includes severe abdominal pain with difficult urination and constipation. Blood Hernial disorder describes the condition where there is swelling with fixed, excruciating pain in the lower abdomen.

9. Inguinal lymphadenitis (swollen lymph nodes in the inguinal region).

than melting–heat. Therefore, consuming heat through sweating rather than through the ice is the wisest method.

2. The best method for reducing the heat of the human body is by sweating; applying ice actually hinders sweating.

3. To make one area extremely cold when the whole body is warm is not a good idea. Doesn't glass or pottery immediately break when there is discrepancy of temperatures in different parts?

Aside from these points, there are many other disadvantages to the Western approach when assessed through Oriental medicine. So in these situations, I believe that resolutely adopting the "naturally treating medicine" is correct.

An injection is artificial while taking medicine internally is natural. For example, a pancreatic hormone injection is given in diabetes. It is natural for all substances other than air to be assimilated into the body through digestive organs, but injecting a certain substance directly into blood vessels is unnatural. In Western medicine, a hormone preparation must be injected because of the concern for the change in its properties if it is passed through the digestive tract. However, in natural healing medicine, the person's pancreatic endocrine function is promoted instead of borrowing the pancreatic hormone from other animals. "Earth controls Water"[10] indeed demonstrates the opposing relationship between the pancreas (Earth) and Kidney (Water). Thus, this endocrine relationship was already known in the Orient thousands of years ago.

To explain the Oriental medical treatment of diabetes in modern terms, the treatment method chosen is to ingest Oriental herbs through the digestive organs to have a kind of external hormonal function toward the central endocrine nerves of the pancreas to recover pancreatic endocrine function and to totally restore glucose assimilating function.

STRUCTURAL MEDICINE AND PHENOMENAL MEDICINE– IMMOBILE MEDICINE AND MOBILE MEDICINE

Western medicine is "structural medicine" and Oriental medicine is "phenomenal medicine." Western medicine is "immobile (fixed) medicine" and Oriental medicine is "mobile (flexible) medicine." The foundation of the former is in anatomy and the basis of the latter is in the study of syndromes. The former looks for the cause of illness within the changes in the organism's structure and the latter identifies it by the abnormalities in physiological phenomena. Here also, the relative superiority and inferiority between Western and Oriental medicine should not be discussed since aspects of their roles are different. To give a few examples of the diseases that are treated more advantageously with "phenomenal medicine" or "mobile medicine," I would first of all cite mental illness. Mental illness is a subtle reactive phenomenon to a physiological abnormality. Therefore, to look for the cause of illness in the structures of the brain and the spine can only be considered an impossible task. Mental illness, when correctly observed and treated from the standpoint of phenomenal medicine, is an illness that can be cured with one to two packs of herbs at the time of onset.

---

10. In Oriental medicine, the pancreas is seen as a part of the function of the Spleen. The Spleen belongs to the Earth Element. Kidneys belong to the Water Element. For further explanations, please see the section on the Five Element Theory in Chapter 2.

The cause of mental illness is diagnosed through observing symptoms of mental illness such as: (1) type of emotional expression; (2) type of illusion or fantasy; (3) movement; (4) pulse quality; (5) facial color; (6) season of onset; (7) time of progression or decline in the condition of illness; (8) foods enjoyed commonly and (9) abnormal sensation or location on the channel pathway. I will be writing in detail regarding these at another time.

Another example of the disadvantages of "immobile medicine" over "mobile medicine" is the use of calcium injections for lung disease. According to reports on anatomy, areas of a cadaver where traces of the tuberculosis virus were overcome are greater than 80 percent. Since calcium surrounded tuberculosis bacteria in those areas, calcium injections are given to the tuberculosis patient. Observing this through Oriental medicine, there is a big inconsistency because:

1. Even if calcium is needed, it should be taken through the digestive organs with calcium containing foods and assimilated more naturally through other organs. Injecting mineral calcium directly into the bloodstream does not seem beneficial.
2. Tuberculosis bacteria is a *Yang* type of bacteria and in contrast to gonorrhea, which is a *Yin* type of bacteria, it is a germ that is most active when the body temperature is high. This is supported by the fact that pulmonary tuberculosis becomes worse during summer and in the afternoon, dangerous during adolescence and is aggravated during excitement. Since the rise in body temperature by a calcium injection can be proven by the thermometer, it is definitely detrimental to treatment of the disease.[11]

ROOT–TREATING MEDICINE AND MANIFESTATION–TREATING MEDICINE

Oriental medicine is the "root–treating medicine" and Western medicine is the "manifestation–treating medicine." Oriental medicine is superior in the treatment of the root cause of a disease and Western medicine is superior in emergency management.

For example, there is the condition of hyperchlorhydria or excess secretion of stomach acid. Western medicine is superior in neutralizing the already secreted excess amount of stomach acid with something like sodium bicarbonate to prevent harm to the stomach wall, but Oriental medicine is a must in order to regulate physiological abnormality to fundamentally stop the over–secretion of stomach acid.

Hyperchlorhydria in Oriental medicine is called *Tun Suan* Syndrome and its cause is said to be, "Wood overacting on Earth" or "Liver overacting on Spleen." In other words, acid digestive juices of the Liver channel system are said to overcome alkaline digestive juices of the Spleen channel system (which includes the pancreas). The secretion of digestive juices is regulated to prevent excess and deficiency through the external hormonal function of Oriental herbs. Since most kinds of chronic disorders are like that, Root–treating medicine is the superior treatment here.

DEFENSIVE MEDICINE AND HEALTH–CULTIVATING MEDICINE

Western medicine is "defensive medicine" and Oriental medicine is "health–cultivating medicine." In artificially defending against external disturbance through

---

11. Calcium injection for the pulmonary tuberculosis is no longer used in Western medicine.

disinfection, sterilization, serum injection, etc., Oriental medicine cannot compare with Western medicine. In strengthening resistance toward disease by cultivating the internal life force and balancing physiological regulation, Western medicine cannot compare with Oriental medicine. When examining these points, Oriental and Western medicine absolutely must not oppose each other, but must mutually cooperate to give the best possible medical treatment.

INTERNAL MEDICINE AND EXTERNAL MEDICINE

Oriental medicine is "internal medicine" and Western medicine is "external medicine." The Oriental medical doctor even tries to treat the external[12] or structural disorders with internal medicine and the Western doctor tries to treat the internal disorder through surgical treatment (external intervention).

There are many cases where internal treatment is necessary when the cause of external disorder is internal such as with skin disorders and there are cases where surgical treatment is necessary when the internal disease is in the late stage. Therefore, if Oriental and Western medicine communicate and complement each other well, we can avoid leisurely treating external disorders which could be quickly treated with surgery and we can avoid great sacrifices resulting from surgery for internal disorders which could be cured simply with internal medication.

STANDARDIZED MEDICINE AND ADAPTABLE MEDICINE

Western medicine chooses "standardization"[13] and Oriental medicine chooses "adaptation."[14] Western medicine, needless to say, does not ignore the uniqueness of individuals, but it is true that when observing the disease, an isolated discipline called pathology is established to always try to put the disease into the frame of certain universally valid rules of science. It even tries to establish a universal treatment method. Undoubtedly, if that were possible, it would be very fortunate from the standpoint of medical application, but in actuality, it is a difficult problem. For example, in a common cold, there can be among its symptoms, existence or absence of sweat, cough, sputum, nasal congestion, dryness of nose, nasal phlegm, loss of appetite, indigestion, constipation, diarrhea, chills, etc., the combination of which are clinically different syndromes in Oriental medicine. There are many occasions where medicine must not be used as if all common cold syndromes were the same. That is the reason for the development of the *Shang Han* Theory[15] in Oriental medicine. Whether it is a lung disease or neurasthenia, the symptoms and treatment methods are not uniform.

---

12. External disorders can include orthopedic, dermatological or surgical conditions.

13. Standardization here implies that Western medicine has a fixed set of rules which is applied uniformly to everyone without regard for the individual differences.

14. Adaptation here refers to the fact that Oriental medicine is concerned with individual differences and treats the unique presentation of the disease specific to the patient.

15. The Shang Han Theory is the theory on febrile diseases caused by Cold. This theory discusses the diagnosis and the treatment of febrile diseases according to the six channels. They are Taiyang (Greater Yang), Yangming (Extreme Yang), Shaoyang (Lesser Yang), Taiyin (Greater Yin), Shaoyin (Lesser Yin) and Jueyin (Declining Yin) channels. See Chapter 4 on the channels for further details.

To give another example, consider beriberi. The cause is said to be a deficiency of vitamin B–1 according to modern medicine. It is true that the symptoms of beriberi will appear in animals not supplied with vitamin B–1 and there is a deficiency of vitamin B–1 in the body of beriberi patients. Accordingly, ingesting a lot of vitamin B–1 is the method chosen by Western medicine for the treatment of beriberi. However, there are many cases where no matter how much one ingests and injects vitamin B–1, beriberi does not get cured. This is definitely a weakness of the standardized treatment method.

When viewed according to Oriental medicine, even if there is an inseparable relationship between beriberi and vitamin B–1, it is not so much a lack of vitamin B–1 in the diet of the beriberi patient (there is a possibility of that), but rather, a decline in the ability to assimilate B vitamins. The cause of decline in the assimilative function is in a person's physical constitution and abnormalities in weather conditions such as environmental temperature or dampness. This is supported by the fact that beriberi occurs frequently during damp weather and is more severe for the person living in a damp environment; thus, the relationship between weather and beriberi.

A person's constitution determines why person A gets beriberi and person B does not, though they eat the same foods and lead the same lifestyle in the same family. Therefore, the treatment method does not become fixed by a diagnosis of beriberi in Oriental medicine.

When viewed from the standpoint of Western medicine which tries to identify the "principal disease" and the "principal medicine," it is not unreasonable to have thoughts of ambiguity or insufficiency and develop doubt about the possibility of Oriental medicine in the treatment of diseases. Having a guiding principle within the ambiguity is the special characteristic of Oriental medicine. This is not limited to medicine, but is true in all aspects of Oriental culture.

India's poet Tagore has said that Oriental civilization is like the forest and the Western civilization is like the brick house. It is a most fitting comment. No matter how large a brick house is, the number of bricks can be calculated. But when one confronts a large forest, its vastness is indescribable. The types and shapes of plants and trees that exist cannot be known and are all different. However, within its complicated distinctive features, we can still find the uniform rule of nature. Plants that breed in damp ground are located in areas of high humidity, plants of shaded ground in dark, dry areas and plants of sunshine in bright, open areas. Not even a branch or a leaf diverges from this rule. This is the way in which Oriental medicine can make sense of seeming ambiguity and the profound laws within vastness.

Oriental medicine, while disapproving of universally valid treatment methods, includes principles which have universally valid legitimacy. As always, the proof is best judged by the results of treatment effectiveness. So words are not needed as much here. I will only say that medicine may be divided into two types; standardized medicine and adaptable medicine.

MEDICINE USED BY GOVERNMENT AND MEDICINE USED BY COMMON PEOPLE

Western medicine, in contrast to Oriental medicine, is the medicine most appropriate for use by the government. For the prevention of epidemics in a country or for judicially related medical needs such as blood type, finger prints, autopsy, etc., Western medicine is most effective. That is why the support of the government has always been given to Western medicine.[16]

Those who are concerned about Oriental medicine should remember that it is always in a disadvantageous position compared to modern medicine which has formed a trinity with government authority and monetary resources.

Western and Oriental medicine should not oppose each other. It is not a matter of which one is superior. Though the duties undertaken and the direction of contribution may differ, when looking from a wide standpoint as a medicine, there is a feeling that Oriental and Western medicine are like the two wings of a bird. When both fully communicate, complement and cooperate, then it will be possible to give the best in medical treatment.

II. THE SYNTHESIS OF ORIENTAL AND WESTERN MEDICINE

The medicinal properties (pharmacological effect) of Oriental herbs, which have been laughed at up until now, are now being proven with scientific tests. To give a few examples:

A. Human Placenta and P.O.U. Hormone

Human placenta, especially from the first born is said to greatly strengthen the body. Dr. Ishihara of Japan, seeing a complete cure of uterine cancer with herbal treatment, analyzed and researched that herb. He discovered an effective medicine against uterine cancer which he called P.O.U. hormone, contained within the umbilical cord and placenta of the human body.

B. Seaweed and Iodine

In Korea, women who have given birth to a child are given as much seaweed soup as possible. According to herbology, seaweed has a sweet, bland, and slight sour taste and is a mixture of black, green and yellow colors. So with either taste or color, it is an herb that nourishes and regulates the three *Yin* channels of the legs, namely the Kidney, Liver and Spleen channels.[17] In any case, its effectiveness in actuality cannot be disapproved and according to modern medicine, kelp generally contains iodine and seaweed especially is said to have a large iodine content. Since iodine has the following functions, foods that contain iodine are most appropriate for the women who have given birth:

(1) It invigorates metabolism.
(2) It destroys and obliterates diseased cells and germs.

---

16. Even in Korea, Western medicine has the full support by the government.

17. See Five Element chart on page 114.

(3) It neutralizes and excretes toxins in the body.

C. Child's Urine and Male Urine Hormone

Using a child's urine as a medicine in Oriental Medicine has been the subject of much ridicule. Recently, however, Dr. Masao Ito of Japan has researched extracting "an anti–aging substance" from the urine of 17 or 18 year old males.

D. Oyster Shell and Copper

The oyster, more so than any other food, contains large quantities of copper, and copper is said to be absolutely necessary for the production of red blood cells. This demonstrates the theory in herbology that oysters help tonify[18] Blood and beautify the complexion, which is often times a function of healthy blood.

E. Aromatic Fragrance and Disinfecting Properties

"Interior clearing" herbs in Oriental medicine (internally ingested medicine for external diseases such as skin disorders) almost all contain aromatic fragrances and according to modern pharmacology, it has been proven by experiments that fragrant substances have the power of disinfection.

F. Ministerial Fire and Adrenalin

According to Oriental medicine, "Ministerial Fire"[19] implies "Fire within the Kidney" and is said to activate the Monarch Fire. The Monarch Fire is the Heart: Heart is called Fire, since the body temperature is maintained or fluctuates according to its activity. When adrenalin is released from adrenal glands, it strengthens the beat of the heart. This can be seen, indeed, as "Ministerial Fire activating Monarch Fire." There are many examples aside from these and they will be introduced in the following chapters.

III. COMMON CHARACTERISTICS AND DISTINCT CHARACTERISTICS

It is true that the average physical body of an American is bigger than that of the average Korean. However, if you compare certain individual Americans to specific individual Koreans and think that Americans are always bigger physically, it can be misleading.

When thinking from the viewpoint of an organism, amoebas and humans are ruled by common and consistent rules of nature, but taking a step further to conclude that humans and amoebas are completely the same is nonsense. Humans, regardless of the differences in race, class, age, and sexuality, are all included in the common concept called human

---

18. Tonify means to nourish, augment and supplement vital substances in the body, such as Qi (vital energy), Blood and bodily fluids, or to strengthen the functional aspect of various organs such as Heart, Spleen and Kidneys.

19. Ministerial Fire implies the Fire in the Kidney that warms and activates various organs and systems in the body. This Fire contrasts with the Monarch Fire which is in the Heart.

species. However, it is incorrect to consider that persons A, B, C or D all have the same constitutions and personalities, enjoy the same type of foods and can be effectively treated with the same medicine.

Recently, people have been divided into the blood types of A, B, O and AB, so that the body fluids, even saliva and tears, of people with the same blood type show the same reactions. It is said that one cannot possibly find Type B body fluid in a Type A body and it is likely that there are also differentiations even within Type A persons.

PHYSICAL CONSTITUTION AND INDIVIDUAL DIFFERENCES

Ever since human beings appeared on Earth, no two of them have ever been the same. Accordingly, no one has had an exactly identical physical constitution. There is no explanation other than the subtle phenomena of nature that brought about such complicated distinctions in physical constitutions. The great varieties in human constitution come from the combination of what is inherited prenatally from the parents along with postnatal environmental differences and changes due to the living environment. The latter include, for example, the differences in weather and climate, disparities in food due to race, land and social class, and differences in the amount of stimulation of the emotions, etc.

According to the physical constitution, there are people who easily get diseases of the digestive system and people who are prone to develop respiratory organ diseases. Even in diseases of the digestive system, there are *Yin* types and *Yang* types. The diseases of the respiratory system are also divided into *Yin* and *Yang* types. These are the so–called "individual differences" and must be taken into consideration in the treatment of diseases and ingestion of nutrients. It is due to these individual differences that the medicine effective for person A is not effective for person B, even though the medical terminology is the same. This is an important matter, especially since there are many instances in which patients are unaware of their unique constitutional needs and are attracted to exaggerated advertisements. They greedily ingest the medicines sold and indiscriminately test the medicines that are recommended by others. While confused and in a flurry, precious life is gradually melting away.

Clearly classifying physical constitutions and individual differences is the special characteristic of Oriental medicine. Since the distinctive features of the physical constitution and symptoms manifest in each aspect of daily life, by precisely observing them, the treatment methods are established based on individual differences.

Therefore, the "Study of Syndromes"[20] becomes the whole of Oriental medicine. The differences in physical constitution and syndromes appear in likes and dislikes of food, complexion, emotion, pulse quality, changes in the sensations of body surface (channels) and physical frame, time of day or night in which symptoms are aggravated, likes or dislikes of cold or heat and dry or damp of weather. Aside from these general observations, infinite varieties of constitutions and syndromes appear when the differences are observed in detail. Thus, physical constitution must be identified in order to perform the treatment that is appropriate for each individual.

---

20. See Chapter 3, "The Study of Syndromes."

IV. PHYSICAL CONSTITUTION, NUTRIENTS, DIGESTION AND ASSIMILATION

The study of nutrition teaches that certain substances are necessary for the human body to live a healthy life. However, since people who have somewhat sufficient resources in modern society eat without thought, disease often occurs from overnutrition rather than undernutrition. In the life of a human being, there are many points that cannot simply be stipulated with mathematical logic like one plus two equals three, since humans are not containers like a vase or a basin, but are organisms that have digestive functions. Even in a thing like a stove, if the air does not circulate well and combustion is incomplete, no matter how much coal is put into it, most of it becomes smoke. When the digestive power of the human is weak, putting in excessively large amounts of nutrients overstrains the digestive organs.

Even the nutrients, likewise, cannot be thought of apart from the individual constitution, so that the type and quantity of nutrients needed varies according to individual constitutions. The effect of nutrition is manifested for the first time when those nutrients become digested, absorbed and assimilated. For example, even though the nutritional value of fish liver oil is considered high, if one gets indigestion, vomits or has diarrhea after taking it, it does not become a nutrient in any way. The relationship between beriberi and B vitamin that I mentioned earlier, indicates this faulty "assimilation" well.

V. MYSTERIES OF LIFE'S OPERATION

There is nothing in nature that is as exquisite a machine as the human body. It is truly a precision instrument whose mysteries of organic perfection bring only marvel to our minds.

When a person sees food, it is obvious that there is a production of saliva, secretion of gastric acids and gradual preparation for the activity by other digestive organs. Vomiting is rejection of harmful or excessive food and diarrhea is quick elimination of harmful intestinal contents or excess water out of the body.

When eating a certain food for a long time, one is said to get "fed up" so that the food that once tasted delicious gradually becomes disliked because the body is demanding other nutrients. The preference for food differs from person to person because each person demands the foods necessary for him or herself.

It is to attract the opposite sex for the reproductive function that there is a ruddy and genial expression, with a constant smile on the face during adolescence. It is to prevent the approach of the opposite sex and to avoid danger that pregnant women get freckles on the face, look unattractive and have rougher personalities – they easily cry and easily get angry.

During the growth and developmental stages, the thymus gland suppresses the reproductive function to concentrate all energies towards the direction of development. When development is completed, the thymus gland deteriorates, the function of the thyroid gland becomes active and the secretion of the reproductive glands become sufficient.

When there is a disease, the cause of disease is eliminated with high fever, thus the so–called "High fever treatment method" is an excellent natural cure. There are many examples such as cases of gonorrhea that are completely cured due to the fever of malaria or progressive paralysis getting relieved by some other febrile disease. So the Korean saying, "Malaria in elders is a sign of longevity" is not without meaning. There are many cases of emaciated people becoming lustrous after smallpox or typhoid fever.

Ticklishness sensitizes one to external disturbances so that one can quickly take action for escape or to defend oneself. Itching is a demand from the body for treatment stimulation on the skin. The reason for the appearance of hypersensitive lines (Head's belt or channels) is to prompt a change in the normal sensation on the exterior into a sensation which elicits treatment.

When angry, the complexion shows a blue/green color to sink and suppress the activeness of the opponent. When fearful, one manifests the color of a corpse to make the opponent lose thoughts about killing him or approaching near.

Of all disease symptoms that we abhor, there is not one that is not a treatment effort[21] on the part of the body for the protection of life. Here are a few things that I would like to examine.

PERSONAL OPINION ON TONSILLECTOMY

Tonsils are considered useless remnant organs or as a gate for bacterial invasion. The usual practice is to remove them when one goes to the hospital. However, I have doubts about this because even though tonsils are considered a door for bacterial invasion, they are not doors to give entrance to bacterial invasion. It is more proper to consider them as a barrier and an epidemic control center for defending against bacterial invasion. In tonsillitis, bacteria attack with fierce intensity so that fighting them with the usual defensive system of the body is insufficient. The enlargement of tonsils is analogous to the temporary expansion of an epidemic control center or the establishment of a new prisoner's barrack. The accompanying fever should be seen as an effort to eliminate germs which have invaded the body.

The mouth is the easiest location for the invasion by various types of harmful substances together with foods. Since tonsils are located at the most strategic place inside the mouth to keep those organisms from entering the body, they are very unlikely to be remnant organs. Given the perfection of the human body, it is most unlikely that a useless organ would be placed in such a vital spot. Even if there is no obvious harm done by removing tonsils because of the compensation by other organs, it is by no means beneficial to the body and tonsillitis is a disease easily treated with Oriental herbs.

---

21. Symptoms are an indication that the body has already begun to heal itself.

A STUDY ON SALIVA

The opinion of Oriental and Western medicine on saliva is completely different and I would like to examine a theory here.

Observation through bacteriology shows that there is no place dirtier than the human mouth. When we awaken in the morning, we do not know how many hundreds of types of bacteria are in the mouth. The number is said to be around 3 to 4 billion and at night when the mouth is cleaner, at least 300 to 400 hundred million are present, of which at least 70 to 80 million are alive. It is difficult to know how correct this is and it differs according to each person, but in any case, it is true that the number of germs living in the mouth are almost immeasurable. This is why saliva is considered a highly dangerous thing. In herbology, however, saliva is considered to be an antibacterial and detoxifying medicine. For example:

(a) Rubbing saliva on a swollen lymph gland is said to disperse swelling.
(b) Rubbing saliva when bitten by an insect or a snake is said to detoxify poison.
(c) Rubbing saliva on skin disorders is said to heal them.
(d) Saliva dissolves mercury (makes it into powder).

For the above actions, the saliva that is in the mouth before one speaks in the morning is said to be most effective. Let us explore some possible explanations for these actions:

1. It is true that there are many bacteria in the mouth. Are these bacteria useful or harmful to the organism? If they are harmful, then the human body, which is so minutely precise, will secrete antibacterial saliva to prevent their reproduction. Looking at the existence of such a large quantity of germs, what is the reason the body does not kill these germs, but instead cultivates and promotes their reproduction?

(a) "Kill the germs with the germs."

I think that perhaps those germs harmful to the human body are eliminated by the germs in the mouth. There is no way that the body does not use a wise war strategy such as "Control enemy with enemy." Inside the mouth, a considerable number of wounds do not suppurate (generate pus) and heal in a few days. This is presumed to be due to germs in the mouth exterminating suppurative germs. It is for this same reason that the saliva after sleeping, which has the most amount of germs in the mouth, is most effective as a treatment for the enlargement of the lymph gland and skin disorders.

(b) Stomach Heat[22] and bad breath.

In stomach disease, especially when there is Heat in the Stomach, the inside of the mouth ulcerates and bad breath occurs. At this time, germs in the mouth are reproducing in large quantities. This is also not meaningless. An ulceration in the mouth can be seen as the cultivation and placement of a great number of germs in the mouth which are analogous to desperate soldiers for hire. This is done for the purpose of further solidifying

---

22. Stomach Heat is a condition that is caused by spicy foods, alcohol or hot weather.

the defense in the mouth, the first gate, in order to supplement the reduction in the defensive power caused by a stomach disorder.

2. When saliva is spat on mercury and mixed, mercury loses its luster and mobility and turns darker. With this evidence, it is difficult to determine how saliva directly detoxifies mercury toxins, but obviously saliva has a certain chemical action on the mercury.

There are many cases of insects that are harmful to the body such as a centipede immediately dying when spat on. Thus, I like to believe that there is insecticidal power or power of detoxifying insect poison in saliva.

All of the statements above have not been verified through test tubes and microscopes, but are the results of many centuries of observations. Theoretically, they are not altogether without foundation and I look forward to experimental studies by scientists.

VI. ORIENTAL MEDICINE AND THE REGULATION OF ENDOCRINE SECRETION

It is the nerves that regulate the life of an organism and it is the hormones, produced by various endocrine glands, that regulate the functions of the nerves. Many types of hormones exist and there is no need to speak of their profound and complicated relationships, but on the whole, they can be categorized into two types – suppressing and promoting hormones. Nerves are categorized like hormones and the maintenance of a balanced state in the physiological function of the body without excess and deficiency is due to the antagonistic function of the opposing nerves. Accordingly, there are two types of antagonistic functions in hormones to avoid imbalance in the regulation of the nerves. This relationship in Oriental medicine is called the "Harmony of *Yin* and *Yang*."

The suppressing and promoting functions of nerves or hormones are not uniform, but they usually have a suppressing action on one organ while having a promoting action on another organ. This relationship is called the "Generating and Controlling cycle" of the *Zang Fu* organs.[23]

Human disease refers to the abnormal physiological phenomena that occur when there are abnormalities in the regulation of the endocrine system and the control of nerves. In other words, when *Yin–Yang* are in disharmony. As a result, it is enough to correct this imbalance in the endocrine function for a recovery from disease.

Oriental medicine is a medicine that fundamentally and naturally helps recover health by regulating the function of the endocrine glands. Oriental herbs always have a hormonal action on the central nervous system and the endocrine system. The functions of herbs are divided into *Yin* or *Yang* according to the Herb's *Qi*[24] and the organs acted upon are specified according to the "taste."

---

23. See Chapter 2 on the Zang Fu Organs for further details.

24. "Qi" in Oriental medicine has a variety of meanings. In herbology, Qi mainly refers to the temperature of the herbs (warm, cool, cold and hot – the "Four Qi"). See Chapter 6, section 5 on the Qi, Taste and Color Theory.

As for the details regarding this, readers will be able to understand certain points after reading through the book. At any rate, I would like to say that those who intend to research Oriental medicine should concentrate on the study of endocrinology more than anything else.

VII. A REQUEST TO STUDENTS OF MODERN MEDICINE

Everyone recognizes that modern medicine has made rapid progress. However, it is not yet satisfactory. Despite this, there are many modern doctors who adopt arrogant attitudes and sneer at treatment methods outside of modern medicine without ever wanting to find out the facts about them.

Since the duty that we entrust to modern doctors has such an impact on our lives, we cannot avoid giving modern doctors candid advice, even if it is not what they want to hear. Arrogance implies satisfaction, and satisfaction is that which obliterates progressiveness and striving effort. Let us examine just how far modern medicine has really developed.

THE SUBJECT OF MEDICINE

Modern medicine is said to be one of the natural sciences. However, there is no science like medicine that builds a foundation on merely hypotheses and assumptions. The true nature of "life," which is the subject of medicine, is yet unknown and still remains a riddle. Hence, it is an unavoidable fact that Western medicine itself cannot transcend its limitations. As various branches of medical science, the following are listed: histology, anatomy, physiology, biochemistry, biophysics, pathology, pharmacology, hygienics, microbiology, helminthology, psychology, forensic medicine, medical history, etc. Adding these branches and all the other branches does not establish a truthful and complete medical science.

Those studies might become basics or have assisting roles in medicine, but they cannot truly be the medicine itself. The medicine, which has the life of a complex organism as its subject, will become a complete science for the first time after the essence of life has been brought to light.

The following is a list of efficacious treatments and disease management protocols in modern medicine:[25]

(1) Treatment of malaria with quinine.
(2) Extermination of syphilis with salvarsan.
(3) Treatment method based on the extermination of intestinal parasites.
(4) Prevention of smallpox with vaccination.

---

25. These statements were written around 1934 and although protocols have increased in number, so has the number of side effects from these protocols.

(5) Various types of effective surgical management.

Aside from these treatments, there are those that have the effect of prevention or treatment with antitoxins or serum treatment, but have not reached the level of a wonder drug.

Even if the few examples mentioned above can be fully relied upon, their number can be counted with less than ten fingers, so the foundation of modern medicine is insufficient to boast of its greatness with only those examples. As an example, consider malaria. A person with a weak resistance against the bacteria of malaria, one or two episodes may pass with the ingestion of quinine, but relapse occurs. There are many instances where a person has to take a huge amount of quinine in one year. For these people, the "root treatment" will not take place unless Oriental herbal medicines such as *Bu Zhong Yi Qi Tang* (Tonify the Middle and Augment the *Qi* Decoction)[26] are combined with the Western treatment. In the Western treatment of syphilis there are some in whom the "root treatment" does not readily occur and relief remains elusive.

In diseases aside from these, Western treatment performs emergency, temporary and momentary symptomatic treatments to temporarily avoid pain, reduce fatigue and rest the affected part or the whole body. Not only are there just a few examples of modern doctors facing patients with 100 percent confidence, but in the management of weak persons, Western treatment can actually bring about negative results. Thus, it seems preposterous for Western doctors to have thoughts of satisfaction or self–pride.

Therefore, I hope that medical doctors research Oriental medicine with an open mind and avoid relying wholly on Western medical doctrine.

---

26. For more details regarding this formula, see Chapter 7 on prescriptions or appendix II.

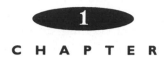

C H A P T E R

YIN AND YANG

*J*n studying Oriental medicine and utilizing its techniques, it is enough to classify *Yin* and *Yang*.[1] Since the distinctions of *Yin–Yang* can be found in the physical constitution, in the conditions of a disease and in the properties of an herb, the disease manifestations can be naturally eliminated by distinguishing the *Yin–Yang* of the physical body, observing the *Yin–Yang* of disease conditions and by matching the *Yin–Yang* of the herbal properties.

I. THE CONCEPT OF YIN AND YANG

There are many people who think that Oriental medicine itself has no scholastic value since the explanations about Oriental medical principles are expressed in non–modern terms such as *Yin–Yang* and Five Elements,[2] and only a few Oriental medical doctors try to make their explanations understandable to the layman. However, its principles and facts should not be rejected just because the methods of explanation are weak or because people do not understand them.

The *Yin–Yang* Theory has roots in Oriental philosophy and the laws of the universe and nature are explained with this *Yin–Yang* Theory. The substances of Five Elements are created according to differences in the mixture of *Yin–Yang* and the seasons change according to the rise and fall of the two Qi of *Yin–Yang*.[3] It is said that *Tai Chi*[4] created

---

1. Polar opposites. Mutually interdependent forces in nature that create and transform all phenomena. They are the positive and negative forces in nature.

2. The Five Elements are Wood, Fire, Earth, Metal and Water. They represent not only the physical substances, but also the energetics of generation, growth, transformation, harvesting and storing. Together with the Yin–Yang Theory, the Five Element Theory forms the basis of Oriental medicine. See Chapter 2 and 3 for more details.

3. Qi is the fundamental force in nature that is the basis of all change. It is manifested in two ways, Yin and Yang. Qi can be roughly translated as "life force," "bio–energy," or "life energy."

4. Tai Chi means "grand ultimate." One interpretation of Tai Chi is that it is a state in which all phenomena are encompassed, but is not yet differentiated. It can be compared to a seed which can later grow to be a tree or it can be compared to a zygote which can later become a human being. Another interpretation is that Tai Chi represents something that is complete or whole. A tree or a human being or the entire universe itself can be Tai Chi. Tai Chi, therefore, is a state which is extremely small and simple yet infinitely large and complex.

Yin–Yang and *Yin–Yang* gave birth to Four Symbolic Forms. The Four Symbolic Forms created the Eight Trigrams and the Eight Trigrams gave birth to the 64 Hexagrams.[5] Thus, the distinct phases in the mixture of *Yin–Yang* spread out to infinity. Here, all things in nature are created.

Five Element Theory (see Chapter 2 on Zang Fu organs) is pluralistic, *Yin–Yang* Theory is dualistic and *Tai Chi* Theory is monistic. This is the beauty of Oriental studies – pluralism being regulated by dualism and dualism unifying into monism. To philosophically comment and completely explain *Yin–Yang* Theory would be too voluminous of a job. So here, only a few comments that are essential in understanding *Yin–Yang* Theory of Oriental medicine are presented.

In simple terms, *Yang* implies movement and *Yin* implies stillness. *Yang* is active and *Yin* is passive. Vigorous activity consumes many calories so that the body temperature increases, while insufficient activity decreases body temperature. That is why heat is *Yang* and cold is *Yin*.

This *Yin–Yang* must be well balanced in order for us to maintain a healthy body in a normal physiological state. When the balance of physiological regulation breaks down, due to the disharmony of *Yin–Yang*, the disease phenomenon is produced. Anything above or below the bounds of the normal physiological state is illness. A body temperature that rises above 39 or 40 degrees Celsius (102.2 or 104 degrees Fahrenheit) or drops below 35 or 34 degrees Celsius (95 or 93.2 degrees Fahrenheit) is considered an illness. A pulse beat above 90 or 100 per minute or below 50 or 40 per minute is considered an illness. In the former, the activity of *Yang* is strong and *Yin* weak. The latter is a manifestation of strong *Yin* and weak *Yang*.

PHYSIOLOGICAL INQUIRY OF YIN–YANG

There are two types of opposing forces in the physiological function of a human. One is the force which promotes the function of organs and the other is the force which suppresses that function. Let's look at the nerve distribution of the heart as an example:

A. The suppressing or parasympathetic nerve of the heart (*Yin* type of nerve) passes through both sides of the vagus nerve and arrives at the heart nerve plexus.[6] Based on experimentation, cutting one side (stronger if both sides are cut) of the vagus nerve and stimulating the tip where the nerve was cut produces the following actions:

1. Reduction in the number of beats and momentary stoppage of the heart beat (*Yin* type chronotropic action).
2. Reduction in the force of contraction (*Yin* type inotropic action).

---

5. This is the beginning of all phenomena in the universe. From Tai Chi, all phenomena are created through this differentiation. The Four Symbolic Forms are Taiyin (Great Yin), Shaoyang (Small Yang), Shaoyin (Small Yin) and Taiyang (Great Yang). From these forms, eight basic trigrams, which are like the archetypes, are created. They are Earth, Mountain, Water, Wind, Thunder, Fire, Lake and Heaven. Through the combinations of the eight trigrams, 64 hexagrams are formed. They represent all phenomena in nature.

6. "The parasympathetic fibers that supply the heart arise from neurons in the medulla oblongata and make up parts of the vagus nerves." "Human Anatomy and Physiology" by John W. Hole, Jr. P. 667

3. Slowing down of conduction (*Yin* type dromotropic action).
4. Reduction of excitation (*Yin* type bathmotropic action).

Excitation of parasympathetic nerve centers of the heart increases when oxygen becomes deficient and carbon dioxide accumulates in the bloodstream (Blood does not move without *Qi*) and increases when blood pressure rises (*Yang* in the extreme produces *Yin*).

B. The central axis of the accelerating nerve of the heart (*Yang* type of nerve) is the sympathetic nerve and its function is the opposite of the suppressing nerve.

If the heart has only the stimulating nerve without the suppressing nerve, the beat of the heart will reach 100 or 1,000 or an infinite frequency per minute. Consequently, the body will all at once "burn" and disappear. On the other hand, if there is only the suppressing nerve without the stimulating nerve, the action of the heart will stop and life will be lost instantly. This is why, for a human to maintain an approximately fixed heart beat, excitation of those two nerves must be well regulated. This is called the Harmony of *Yin–Yang* in Oriental medicine.

When the stimulating nerve is permanently in an excess state of excitation, due to disharmony of *Yin–Yang*, so that the body temperature is higher than in a normal person with strong pulse beat, the condition is called "Deficiency of *Yin* and Dominance of *Yang*," "Deficiency of Water and Exuberance of Fire" or "Deficiency of True *Yin*." When the suppressing nerve is continuously in an excess state of excitation, so that the body temperature is deficient and vitality is weak, that condition is called "Deficiency of *Yang* and Dominance of *Yin*," "Deficiency of Fire in the Gate of Life" or "Deficiency of *Qi*."

It can be presumed that substances which regulate excitation of each nerve to harmonize *Yin–Yang* are hormones (endocrine) and catalysts (stimulating substances other than hormones). Therefore, it is appropriate to define Oriental medicine as "hormone regulating medicine."

The following is a description of the physiological phenomena manifested by *Yin* constitution and *Yang* constitution persons.

■ Exuberance of Yang (Yin Deficiency)
1. high body temperature
2. likes coolness
3. pulse is strong and rapid
4. strong exhalation
5. emotional activity is intense and cannot stay calm physically
6. demands lots of water, especially cold water
7. likes plain, clear and cool food
8. has good digestion and strong appetite
9. has reddish complexion
10. urine is dark, scanty and infrequent
11. easily becomes constipated
12. likes cold season

■ **Exuberance of Yin (Yang Deficiency)**
1. low body temperature
2. likes warmth
3. pulse is weak and slow
4. strong inhalation
5. likes to stay quiet
6. has little thirst and likes warm water
7. likes warm and spicy food
8. has poor digestion and poor appetite
9. has dark complexion
10. urine is clear, copious and frequent
11. tends to get diarrhea or constipation
12. likes warm season

The above description divides a person's constitution into two main types – *Yin* and *Yang*. However, one should not try to fit a living body, which is mysterious and complicated, strictly into the above frame of references. The physical constitution can be studied, from the above descriptions, by carefully observing which description a person's body best matches.

YIN–YANG AND PSYCHOLOGICAL PHENOMENA

The existence of a human must be thought of in terms of synthesizing "Heart" and body or in other words, mind and physical body. Physiological change inevitably occurs with corresponding psychological change and psychological change also occurs with physiological change. The physiological and psychological changes cannot possibly be thought of as separate, not because both are different, but because both are no more than observing the same phenomenon from two directions.

Though stimulation of the human can be classified into mental stimulation and physical stimulation, the result of either type appears identical. Type A emotion implies a Type A physiological state, and a Type B physiological state implies a Type B psychological state. An emotion such as joy is associated with a joyous facial expression and joyful emotion cannot be found with a gloomy facial expression. So facial expression is obviously a physiological manifestation of an emotional change.

When one is excited, breathing becomes hurried and the pulse quickens. A person with breathing and pulse faster than others, in ordinary situations, is always in a psychologically excited state. For example, most patients with lung disease have uncommonly devious dispositions and the degree of deviousness fluctuates according to the extent of the progression of the disease.

The physiological activity of a lung disease patient is intense because they are desperately struggling against, for example, the tuberculosis bacteria. The breathing is hurried, pulse is rapid and body temperature is high. Psychologically, the patient is always in an excited state of rage and hostility. Hence, there are many occasions when the patient burns with feelings of hostility as if he or she is facing the enemy, frequently cursing and making perverse speeches. The patient becomes furious like a blazing inferno and seems ready to wield a knife towards family members or the nurse, who with ceaseless sincerity, put their effort into caring for the patient. These all imply the oneness of physiological phenomena and psychological change.

In the Orient, getting easily angered is said to be "injurious to the Lung" or "Short *Qi* (short temper)." This expression of language comes from observing the relationship between the mind and the body.

When a person is excited due to various reasons, mentally stimulating the person further through speech or physically stimulating the person with alcoholic drinks will result in sudden rise in physiological activity and intensification of emotion.

When insulted by others, there are some people who get angry and some people who become saddened. The same person can even get furious sometimes and get saddened at other times. Since fury is active, it becomes the motive for a fight and since sadness is passive, it makes a person bear resentment. When a person is in good health and has the ability to fight, he or she gets furious. If not, he or she harbors sadness in order to prepare for the decisive battle at a later time. If there is power, sadness can change into a fury at anytime.

When drinking alcohol, there are some who cry in their beer and others who get good feelings with ceaseless laughter. This happens because the reaction to alcohol can become active or passive at different times according to the physiological need.

Having an appetite implies that preparation for digestion has occurred physiologically and the body is demanding intake of food. Having sexual desire implies that the sexual organ has become congested with blood, eager for the sexual act.

The physical constitution and state of health can be assessed by observing and investigating a person's psychological and emotional states because the psychological manifestation does not stray from the laws of *Yin–Yang*.

■ **A Comparison Chart of the Psychological State of Yin–Yang**

YANG	YIN
active	passive
dynamic	static
rage, fury	grudge, resentment
light–heartedness	melancholy, depression
joy, delight (laugh easily)	grief, sadness
courage	cowardices
uncontrolled desire	discretion, prudence

NITROGEN AND OXYGEN IN THE AIR AND YIN–YANG

It is said that *Yang* is the life energy and *Yin* is the death energy. The functions of *Yin–Yang* can be compared to the functions of nitrogen and oxygen in the air towards certain organisms. Oxygen is a gas needed for human breathing and nitrogen is a gas that suffocates animals. From this perspective, oxygen can be viewed as life energy and the nitrogen as death energy.

However, even though oxygen is absolutely needed to maintain our life, if there is only oxygen without any nitrogen, all things will burn and disappear. Thus, there is an occurrence of a strange phenomenon. Nitrogen, which harms our life, being suitably mixed into the air is absolutely necessary for the preservation of our lives. In precisely the same manner, death energy (that force called "*Yin*") tries to take our life away by interfering and stopping activities of all of our internal organs, but is absolutely necessary for maintaining our health.

YIN–YANG AND INQUIRY ACCORDING TO BIOCHEMISTRY AND PHYSICAL CHEMISTRY

Yin–Yang in Oriental medicine is identical to acidity and alkalinity in chemistry. From the viewpoint of the chemical reactions, acidity and alkalinity exist relative to each other. Both have a completely reciprocal nature, but when they combine with each other, they become a neutral substance that has the property of neither side. Between the two, when the power of one is stronger, the property of the stronger side appears.

The life phenomenon of the human body, which is *Yin–Yang* according to life reaction, is always relative. Although the human body is formed through the blending of *Yin* Qi and *Yang Qi*, the human body that is formed by those two *Qi* is neither *Yin* nor *Yang*. It is similar to neutral properties in chemistry. A neutral property is neither acidic nor alkaline. Therefore, *Yin–Yang* is well balanced in a completely healthy body so that neither a *Yang* nor *Yin* pathological phenomenon occurs.

When abnormality in life occurs due to breakdown in the balance of *Yin–Yang*, a disease manifests. This rule agrees with the pathology of modern medicine which teaches that the body fluid of a human must be neutral (slight alkaline) in order to be healthy. If it inclines toward strong alkalinity or acidity, disease occurs.

From the viewpoint of electrophysiology, when a disease occurs in a human body, the negative electrical potential rises in that diseased region. At its opposite pole, positive electrical potential rises. For example, when there is disease in an internal organ, negative electrical potential rises in that organ and its opposite must exist at the body surface, where positive electrical potential rises. (This can be interpreted as "Exterior is *Yang* and Interior is *Yin*"). This region where positive electrical potential rises is namely an acupuncture and moxibustion[7] point according to the Channel Theory of Oriental medicine. The disease is eliminated when the electrical potential is neutrally converted by giving stimulation to that region where positive electrical potential has risen.

---

7. Moxibustion is the application of heat using a substance called "moxa" which is Chinese mugwort. Moxa can be applied directly to the body or indirectly with garlic, ginger, salt, etc. The action of moxibustion regulates the Qi and Blood in the body to bring about healing. It is especially effective in patients with weakness and coldness in the body.

II. YIN–YANG OF SEASONS AND HEALTH OF HUMANS

Even in seasons, there are times when *Yang* is exuberant or *Yin* is exuberant. The season of *Yang* exuberance is from the vernal equinox (approximately March 20th) to the autumnal equinox (approximately September 20th). The season of *Yin* exuberance is from the autumnal equinox to the vernal equinox. *Yang* reaches its peak at the summer solstice (approximately June 20th) and *Yin* reaches its peak at the winter solstice (approximately December 20th).

In the season of *Yang* exuberance, all things are dynamic, active, growing, developing and breeding. All plants sprout anew, flowers blossom and fruits are produced. Even in the animal kingdom, the activity and breeding function becomes vigorous in every aspect, so that hibernating insects go into action and mating becomes prevalent. In the season of *Yin* exuberance, all things are static and inactive. The plants wither and animals hibernate.

Looking at the relationship between season and health, there are diseases that occur with or are aggravated by certain seasons. It is common for younger people to get sick during spring and summer and for diseases of the elderly and weak to get worse during fall and winter. When this idea is classified into principal parts, it expresses itself in the following way:

1. In spring, there are many diseases that develop from fatigue due to the inability to endure the overly exuberant physiological activity: "Spring sickness" or neurasthenia, etc.
2. In the summer, there are many disease that develop due to excessive body heat such as lung disease and hysteria.
3. In autumn, there are many diseases that are caused by the reduction in physiological activity: digestive disorders such as vomiting, diarrhea, cholera, etc.
4. In the winter, there are many diseases that occur due to lack of warmth in the body or getting injured by cold temperature: common cold, cough in the elderly, asthma, kidney disease and other diseases due to declining metabolism.

Dividing this into *Yin* Syndrome and *Yang* Syndrome, *Yin* Syndrome worsens during winter and *Yang* Syndrome worsens during summer. When a person with Excess *Yang* is exposed to the summer season, the *Yang* inside the body and the *Yang* of the air (hot temperature) join force to make *Yang* even more exuberant. Consequently, the degree of disharmony of *Yin–Yang* becomes such that it is difficult to maintain health and eventually transforms into a form of disease. When an Excess *Yin* person is exposed to the winter season, *Yin* inside the body joins forces with the *Yin* of air (cold temperature) to form *Yin* Syndrome disease.

STATISTICS ON MORTALITY AND YIN–YANG THEORY

When a person dies due to a natural cause such as chronic disease or old age, the time of death is generally fixed – during cold season and at night. Looking at the natural death of the elderly, there are many examples of the person's mind becoming confused after sunset. As it comes close to 11 o'clock at night, his mind strays and goes into an unconscious state. Around two o'clock in the morning, the person becomes even more endangered and continues in a state as if life is about to expire at any moment. Then between five to ten o'clock in the morning, life expires. This can easily be understood if individuals reflect on their experience and gather many obituary notices, paying attention to the time when death occured. Even regarding the season people die in, the percentage of deaths is greater during winter. Many obituary notices are received during the winter. If one researches dates when memorial services are held in many households, they are greatest during winter and early spring. Looking at this, one cannot disagree that many people die during the period of *Yin* exuberance. To explain it in *Yin–Yang* terms, *Yang* is life energy and *Yin* is death energy. While *Yin* of the body becomes exuberant and constantly tries to stop physiological activity, external *Yin* is also exuberant. The inside and outside join forces to eventually take away the life of a person.

III. TIME AND CHANGE IN SYMPTOMS

There is a classification of *Yin–Yang* even for a day: day is *Yang* and night is *Yin*. A clear day is *Yang* and a rainy day is *Yin*. Hence in a disease too, some are worse in daytime and others are worse at night according to the physical constitution and symptoms.

■ **Yang Symptoms**
1. The body is more tired after sunrise.
2. The body is comfortable and the mind is refreshed after sunset.
3. The body is comfortable on cloudy days.
4. The person dislikes bright light.
5. The person feels worse around three o'clock in the afternoon.

■ **Yin Symptoms**
1. The mind feels refreshed and the body is comfortable after sunrise.
2. The disease is worse and the person has no energy at sunset.
3. The body is comfortable during clear days.
4. The person likes bright light.
5. The person feels worse around five o'clock in the morning.

This information is highly useful in differentiating the syndromes according to *Yin–Yang* in Oriental medicine.

AFTERNOON FEVER

Body temperature generally goes up to its highest level from two to four o'clock in the afternoon. The timing of fevers in malaria and lung diseases is highly predictable. Aside from those diseases, there are many instances of fever developing in the afternoon. The reason is that two to three o'clock in the afternoon is when the *Yang* is the most extreme during the day. Though the sun is closest at midday, *Yang* is most extreme at two to three o'clock in the afternoon instead of midday. This is because the rise in temperature on the surface of the Earth is not due to direct heat of the sun, but because the surface of the Earth receives the sun's heat and is warmed by its radiating heat. Consequently, the surface of water is cool and there are arctic plants in the highest mountain peaks of the tropics.

Around two to three o'clock in the afternoon when the radiating heat is most strong, the body heat rises to its highest because the *Yang* of the body has its most exuberant activity in the afternoon due to the principle: "When *Yang* meets *Yang*, there is exuberance of *Yang*." So, when the Yang of the body meets the external *Yang*, there is twice the *Yang* inside the body leading to fever. Another way of looking at this is since the disease–causing agents that lie dormant within the body become active at this time, the *Yang* of the body can be seen to act vigorously in desperation. Either way, afternoon fever does not contradict the principle: "When *Yang* meets *Yang*, there is exuberance of *Yang*."

EARLY MORNING DIARRHEA

The time during the day when *Yin* is most extreme is just before sunrise. Since the surface of the Earth does not receive heat from the sun after sunset until sunrise of the next day and because it keeps radiating the heat acquired during the daytime, heat on the surface of the earth gradually weakens and reaches its lowest point at dawn. Thus, *Yin* becomes extreme around five o'clock in the morning which is the worse time for the *Yang* Deficient–*Yin* Exuberant person. At this time, there are people who regularly get diarrhea everyday which is a proof that *Yang* is deficient.

This disease condition is frequent in middle to old age and is common in young people with neurasthenia or digestive problems. A typical patient has a pale face and insufficient *Yang* Qi. The reason for this is that a person with weak physiological activity has insufficient body temperature due to poor blood circulation. Before the sunrise, when the temperature is lowest during the day, even that lower body temperature is difficult to maintain. Thus, diarrhea occurs when the intestine does not absorb water and instead urgently excretes it. The following are reasons why water is excreted when the body temperature becomes low:

1. When there is much water inside the body, maintaining that water at the same temperature as the body temperature consumes even more calories.
2. Water inside the body requires a lot of dynamic calories until it is excreted through breathing, sweat or urination.
3. When water disperses, especially through breathing and sweating, it carries off immeasurably large quantities of evaporative heat.

Therefore, early morning diarrhea is a self–protecting physiological regulation to avoid these phenomena.

IV. YIN–YANG OF THE PHYSICAL CONSTITUTION

The physiological phenomena of a human being can be generally divided into two types. One is based on the innate physical constitution and the other is based on the condition of disease, but the dividing line between them is quite ambiguous. The differentiation of physical constitution from disease differs from person to person and time to time. There will be fluctuations in the boundary of health and disease according to the individual's level of education, the level of culture in a society and especially, on the state of progress in medicine.

Another thing to think about is that a person's disease cannot be considered to be separate from his or her physical constitution, nor the person's physical constitution considered separate from his or her physiological changes. Ultimately, the difference between a so–called physical constitution or a symptom suggests only the difference in their degree and time of occurence.[8]

THE BOUNDARIES OF DISEASE AND HEALTH

The line separating disease and health changes according to person, class and existence or absence of knowledge:

1. One who is not very aware of his or her body does not realize a disease unless he or she is extremely sick.
2. A person who is extremely self–confident about health does not think of slight sickness as a disease.
3. An uneducated person just experiences a fairly tolerable illness without knowing that it is a disease.
4. A person of the working class is pressed by daily living, so he or she has no room to consider sickness as sickness and just bears it.

The threshold of disease for these people goes up to the level where they cannot move and must lie down.

At the other end of the spectrum lies the following:

1. A sensitive person with exaggerated feelings.
2. A person who always complains about his or her weak health due to lack of self–confidence about health and regards oneself as a sick person, always looking for a disease.
3. A person in the educated class who is obsessed with his or her body.
4. A wealthy person of leisure class.

For these people, the threshold of disease greatly decreases. Thus when their nose is slightly itchy, they take cold remedies, cover up and lie down. When they do not have a

---

8. Diseases that are deeply rooted arise from the constitution. Also, diseases that are chronic in nature arise from the constitution.

bowel movement for a day, they make a commotion about getting a headache and having a dull mind, hoping to quickly fix their constipation. Since they overeat and do not exercise, when they have slightly uncomfortable feelings in the stomach, they consider it to be indigestion and pour in anti-acid. When they cannot fall asleep for a few hours in one night, they consider it to be neurasthenia and go to the hospital. So there are no occasions of being healthy.

It is a fact that our life gets shorter every hour since there is a limit to human life. This implies that our health is being robbed every hour. So while our health is being robbed, there must be a corresponding disease phenomenon also at play. Therefore, the boundary of disease and health cannot be set uniformly, but can only be generally divided.

THE YANG ZANG (ORGAN) AND YANG SYNDROME; THE YIN ZANG (ORGAN) AND YIN SYNDROME

"*Yang Zang*" implies a *Yang*–type constitution of a healthy body and a *Yang* Syndrome implies the *Yang*–type symptoms of a disease. "*Yin Zang*" implies a *Yin*–type constitution in a healthy body and a *Yin* Syndrome is a disease that has *Yin*–type symptoms. The term "*Yin Zang*" is not used frequently because a person with a *Yin*–type constitution realizes that he or she is always unhealthy and his or her constitution is incorporated into the *Yin* Syndrome.

DISEASES OF YANG SYNDROME		YANG–TYPE CONSTITUTION
External Cause Yang Pathogen[9] (Acute Disease)	Internal Cause Yin Deficiency (Chronic Disease)	Yang Zang (Organ) (Strong)

DISEASES OF YIN SYNDROME		YIN–TYPE CONSTITUTION
External Cause Yin Pathogen[10] (Acute Disease)	Internal Cause Yang Deficiency (Chronic Disease)	Yin Zang (Organ) (Healthy)

COMPARISON OF PHYSIOLOGICAL PHENOMENA OF YANG ZANG AND YANG SYNDROME

■ **Yang Syndrome**
1. The body temperature is high.
2. The person likes cool things.
3. The pulse beat is rapid.
4. The breathing is short and hurried since exhalation is strong and inhalation is weak.
5. The person is physically and mentally active yet has no stability.

---

9. Yang pathogen implies disease causing agents of a hot nature.
10. Yin pathogen implies disease causing agents that have a cold nature.

6. The person has thirst and demands lots of cold water.
7. The person likes bland and cool food and drinks; eating stimulating foods harms the body.
8. The person has a congested feeling inside.
9. The person has a thick tongue coating, good digestion and good appetite. Still, the sense of taste is not so keen and at times there is no appetite due to fullness inside, even though the food eaten has been digested.
10. The person has a reddish complexion with a look of excitement.
11. The urine is dark and urination is difficult, scanty and infrequent.
12. The person easily gets constipated.
13. The person's body feels uncomfortable during spring–summer seasons and afternoon.
14. The person has no endurance.
15. The person inclines toward emotions of anger and joy.
16. The person is impatient and rash.

■ Yang Zang (Organ)

1. The body temperature is slightly higher than the normal person, but does exceed a certain limit and shows no big change in body temperature due to either physical work or cold weather.
2. The person tends to like cool things, but coldness or hotness does not harm the health in any way.
3. The pulse has strength yet is not rapid, but soft and smooth.
4. The breathing is not hurried, but moderate although exhalation seems to be slightly stronger.
5. The person can be active yet calm, so the person is mentally and physically stable.
6. The person does not have much thirst.
7. Ingesting stimulating foods does not harm the person's body.
8. The person has no congested feeling inside.
9. The person has a normal tongue coating and has a good digestion with tremendous appetite, yet never becomes weak or drowsy even after skipping one or two meals.
10. The person has a reddish complexion yet is emotionally calm and strength seems hidden in the lower abdomen.
11. The urine is copious and infrequent, yet clear and easily excreted.
12. The person has no occasion of having diarrhea and the stool is firm yet soft.
13. The changes in the person's health do not occur according to different seasons.
14. The person is positive and active with perseverance.
15. The person's emotion does not become extreme.
16. The person is calm and brave.

"*Yin Zang*" and *Yang* Deficiency are essentially difficult to distinguish and are almost identical. They are distinguished for convenience by establishing the degree of their difference. In other words, "*Yin Zang*" constitution implies that a certain state of health can be maintained even though vital energy is not exuberant. A *Yang* Deficient person, with a "*Yin Zang*" constitution, has excess activity of *Yin*. Thus if clothing, living place, or food and drink become slightly cold, he or she immediately develops diseases such as the common cold, abdominal pain, diarrhea and vomiting. Aside from those, he or she may have chronic diseases such as incontinence, enuresis, seminal emission, cough, asthma and chronic diarrhea.

One thing to be cautious about here is that even in a *Yin* Syndrome, so long as it is a disease, it too has bodily fever. No matter how weak *Yang* is, as long as we are alive, the body is not completely without *Yang*. Thus bodily fever occurs due to weakened *Yang* in an emergency situation displaying an intense effort to recover health. This heat in Oriental medicine is called "Deficient Heat" or "False Heat."[11] This False Heat can be wrongly treated by mistaking it as true heat. Therefore, the Oriental medical doctors must discern *Yin–Yang*, Excess–Deficiency, and the Trueness–Falseness of syndromes.

V. YIN–YANG OF SYNDROMES

Oriental medicine is said to be the study of treating syndromes. It is the medical science that has the most well developed "Study of Syndromes." The study of syndromes and herbal pharmacology become two wings of Oriental medicine. Prescribing herbs according to syndromes is free and unrestricted. To explain syndromes in detail is limitless and since this can be considered as all of Oriental medicine, I will explain only the fundamentals in the differentiation of syndromes according to *Yin–Yang* by giving a few examples here.

INTERIOR–EXTERIOR AND YIN–YANG

Exterior is *Yang* and Interior is *Yin*. Acute disease is generally an Exterior Syndrome that invades with intensely painful conditions such as chills and fever, headache, joint pain, etc. Since chronic disease is generally an Interior Syndrome, conditions of it are not sudden and recovery is not as easy as an Exterior Syndrome.

The treatment method in Exterior Syndromes is to produce sweat, which is to disperse disease toxins out of the body through the skin and respiratory system by using diaphoretic and antipyretic formulas. The treatment method of Interior Syndromes is to descend, which is to eliminate the cause of illness out of the body through the stool and urine by using diuretic and laxative formulas. Diaphoretics are *Yang*–natured herbs that have pungent and fragrant tastes with an ascending–dispersing nature. Purgatives are *Yin*–natured herbs that have bitter and bland tastes with a descending nature.

The Exterior Syndromes and Interior Syndromes are again divided into *Yin–Yang* so that there are warm–dispersing and cool–dispersing properties in External Syndrome herbs and warming–Middle, clearing–fever and promoting–urination properties in Interior Syndrome herbs.

---

11. A Deficient or False heat/fever occurs when there is a weakness in the body's vital energy (Yin or Yang energy) and is approximately 38 degrees Celsius (100.4 degrees Fahrenheit) or less.

UPPER–LOWER AND YIN–YANG

Fire is hot and water is cold. Heat is *Yang* and cold is *Yin*. Air rises when hot and descends when cold. It is the same for water. Water vaporizes when extremely hot and air liquifies when extremely cold. Air is *Yang* and liquid is *Yin*. Even in a disease, *Yang* Syndrome manifests in the upper region and *Yin* Syndrome manifests in the lower region. Thus, when the region where a disease phenomenon manifests is located above the diaphragm, it is *Yang* and when located below, it is *Yin*. Headache, asthmatic breathing, cough and coughing up blood are *Yang*; beriberi, diarrhea, prolapse of the anus and bed wetting are *Yin*.

When there is a lot of heat, the chest feels uncomfortable, breathing becomes asthmatic, the eyes become red, and the ears ring. When there is a lack of heat, symptoms such as abdominal pain, diarrhea, coldness in the knees, backache, etc. appear in the lower part of the body. When looking at the structure of the physical body, the upper body is developed in men (*Yang*), so that the shoulder region is wider. The lower body is developed in women (*Yin*), so that hip region is larger. A man with narrow shoulders is not considered masculine and a woman with narrow hips can show a greater incidence of infertility.

BREATHING AND YIN–YANG

When the breathing of a person is carefully observed, the intensity of inhalation and exhalation is different. Observing this breathing is one of the easiest and most important things in classifying *Yin–Yang*. The person with high fever (body temperature) has almost no inhalation and only exhales, while the person with deficiency of heat has strong inhalation and weak exhalation. When a person is on the verge of death, he sobs and his jaw rattles and then inhales.

As stated many times above, *Yin* is death energy. Since *Yin* is dominant and *Yang* is deficient at the time of death, there is only inhalation and no exhalation. Looking at the emotions, exhalation is stronger when one feels internally congested due to excitement or anger and the inhalation is much stronger when one is sobbing in grief. Looking at this physiologically, it can be presumed that the inhalation is stronger in a person with a deficiency of body heat (*Yang* Deficiency) because of the greater demand for oxygen. In a person with a lot of heat, the exhalation is stronger to reduce the oxygen supply and at same time to quickly eliminate carbon dioxide from the body. This is done in order to somewhat suppress the body's exuberant combustive action.

NOTE: 1. The average breathing rate is 12 to 14 times per minute.
2. The average intake of oxygen is approximately 2,000 liters per day. The average discharge of carbon dioxide is approximately 450 liters per day.
3. The difference in the duration of inhalation and exhalation in the average adult is six to seven.
4. When excitation on the inhalation suppressing and exhalation stimulating nerve center is great, it is considered to be a *Yang* Syndrome. When the excitation on the exhalation suppressing and inhalation stimulating nerve center is great, it is considered a *Yin* Syndrome.

QI, BLOOD AND YIN–YANG

In Oriental Medicine, the meaning of *Qi* varies greatly so it is difficult to explain in a few words. However, it can be generally considered to be something related to breathing.

"Wind injures Wei, Cold injures *Ying*" (*Zhang Jing Yue)*[12]

Wei means Protective *Qi*, namely it implies that oxygen is furnished through breathing to combust nutrients in order to acquire dynamic energy. *Ying* is Nutritive–Blood that transports and supplies nutrients through blood circulation. Thus, unhealthy air injures the respiratory system, and excessive cold weather interferes with blood circulation.

"Wind is *Yang* and Cold is *Yin*; *Wei* (*Qi*) is *Yang* and *Ying* (Blood) is *Yin*; Wind injures *Yang*, and Cold injures *Yin*. Each follows its type and causes injury." *Classic on Pulse*[13]

This has the same meaning as the above statement.

"In a person with Excess *Qi*, breathing must be coarse and the voice and complexion is in Excess. In a person with Excess Blood, Blood must be stagnated and presents both pain and firmness. In a person with Deficient *Qi*, the voice is weak and there is shortness of breath similar to asthma (difficult breathing). In a person with Deficient Blood, the skin is dry and rough and muscle channels[14] are in spasm." (*Zhang Jing Yue*)

"When there is Cold, *Qi* gathers inward since the *Cou Li* closes and *Qi* cannot move. When there is Heat, sweat pours out because *Cou Li* opens and *Ying–Wei* can move about." *Inner Classic*[15]

Cou Li implies small orifice of the skin. Air pores and sweat glands can be seen as included in *Cou Li*. It would not be entirely wrong to see it as an abstract noun that indicates all of the physiological functions of the skin. The small orifices of the skin contract when cold contacts the body. Since the breathing action, which depends on the skin stops (*Qi* cannot move), the burden on the lungs increases so that they suddenly

---

12. Zhang Jing Yue wrote the famous "Complete Works of Jing Yue" which has 64 volumes in 1624 A.D. His theory was that Yang energy is the basic life force in humans and advocated the "Warm Tonifying" method in his treatments. He said "Yang is difficult to acquire but easily lost – once Yang is lost, it is difficult to recover."

13. The book, "Classic on Pulse" was written around 280 A.D. by Wang Shu He. It comprises of 10 volumes and describes 24 types of pulses. Also, it discusses Zang Fu organs, channels, syndromes, treatment principles, prognosis, etc.

14. There are 12 muscle channels in the body similar to the 12 main channels. They help distribute Qi and Blood of the 12 main channels to the muscles in the body and connect bones and joints, thus helping to maintain the normal range of motion. Unlike the 12 main channels, these muscle channels do not connect with the internal organs.

15. Known also as "Yellow Emperor's Inner Classic," this is the oldest text on the principles of Oriental medicine. It is estimated to be written around 722 B.C. to 221 B.C. It consists of 18 volumes. This classic is divided into two sections: Su Wen (Simple Questions) and Ling Shu (Spiritual Axis). Su Wen mainly discusses the theories of anatomy, physiology, pathology, therapeutics and cultivation of health. Ling Shu mainly discusses the theories of acupuncture and moxibustion.

overwork, resulting in a fever (*Shang Han* fever – common cold, pneumonia, etc.).

There are times when the swelling of the body (edema) occurs due to the Invasion of Cold. This is due to a breakdown in the body's ability to eliminate sweat and since the kidneys have to take up the slack, they become overburdened and nephritis occurs. At this time, warming the body and using a formula with pungent, fragrant, warm, and dispersing properties (*Yang* natured herbs) opens up skin orifices so that sweating occurs and the breathing of the skin recovers its original state. This results in bodily comfort.

Diseases of the respiratory system are diseases that relate to the *Qi* and diseases of the heart and kidneys are diseases that relate to the Blood.

LIGHT–DARKNESS AND YIN–YANG

Liking brightness is *Yang* and liking darkness is *Yin*. When this is compared to the condition of disease, certain patients ask to block off the light by closing the door and they dislike electric lights at night (at the time of an onset of acute lung disease, etc.). Some patients like sunlight shining into the ward and do not want the light turned off at night. The former is considered the *Yang* Syndrome and the latter the *Yin* Syndrome. Why does *Yang* manifest in the *Yin* Syndrome and *Yin* manifest in the *Yang* Syndrome? Since *Yang* is deficient in *Yin* Syndrome, the body requests the support of *Yang* from the outside to physiologically assist the *Yang* on the inside, for the purpose of acquiring the balance of *Yin–Yang*. This results in the desire for brightness (*Yang*) and warmth (*Yang*). It is also for the same reason that the body requests *Yin* in the *Yang* Syndrome.

YIN–YANG SYNDROME IN CONSTIPATION

There are two types of constipation. One occurs due to lack of intestinal movement (constipation from lack of peristalsis) and the other, in contrast to this, occurs due to the excess of intestinal movement (spasmodic constipation). The former is the *Yin* Syndrome and the latter is *Yang* Syndrome. From the viewpoint of physical constitution, I would like to classify them into two types, cold–type constipation (*Yang* Deficiency), and heat–type constipation (*Yin* Deficiency).

In the heat type of constipation, there is an elimination of a large quantity of water through sweating and breathing out of necessity, since there is a lot of heat in the body. To supplement this loss of fluids, the intestines absorb all the available water which makes the stool dry, resulting in constipation. In the cold type constipation, peristalsis of the intestine is slow which slows down the transportation of intestinal contents resulting in constipation. In this condition, the assimilation of water is reduced and absorbed water is eliminated through profuse urination.

Constipation, compared to diarrhea, is a *Yang* Syndrome, but is again divided into *Yin* Accumulation and *Yang* Accumulation. The *Yin* Accumulation is again divided into *Yang* Deficiency constipation and *Yin* Deficiency constipation, so the treatment methods are different. *Yin* Accumulation is a habitual chronic constipation stemming from the physical constitution and *Yang* Accumulation is a constipation that occurs due to acute disease.

I will be writing about the treatment method at another time, but one thing I would like to mention is that purgatives are used too often in recent times. This is something which is usually avoided by both Western and Oriental doctors.

■ Harm of Purgatives

1. They become habit forming so that one cannot have bowel movements unless they are used.
2. Based on the principle of gradually diminishing effect, the dosage of medicine must be gradually increased.
3. There are many occasions where the degree of constipation worsens after ingesting medicine.
4. In the long run, there is no effect after ingesting medicine.
5. Loss of vitality.
6. They unnaturally and forcefully disturb the natural regulation of a person's physiology to cause other side effects.

I believe that without dietary treatment or especially plant type Oriental herbal treatment, a natural "root treatment" will not be possible.

YIN–YANG SYNDROMES OF MENTAL DISEASE

There are many types of mental diseases and in Western medicine, they are classified according to the cause of disease, the age of a sick person, or by the symptoms. They can be classified as dementia (praecox dementia, paralytic dementia, senile dementia, etc.), psychosis, depression, paranoia (fear of being poisoned, delusions of persecution, jealousy, fear of poverty, exaggeration, etc.) or as a mental disease due to heredity, neurosyphilis, arteriosclerosis, alcohol intoxication, etc. Actually, there are times when dementia praecox, which usually occurs around age 20, can develop at age 40 and paralytic dementia, which develops during middle age can develop around age 20. The cause of paralytic dementia is said to be syphilis, but a syphilis germ–killing treatment such as penicillin, mercury or iodine, etc. is not even slightly effective for this. Rather, varieties of albumin therapy, sulphur therapy, fever therapy, etc. are said to have a definite effectiveness. Speaking of symptoms, there is paranoia even in depressive psychosis, dementia and alcohol intoxication, so the above mentioned classifications seem disorderly and ambiguous.

I am classifying this mental illness into *Yin* and *Yang*: psychosis is, for example, *Yang* Syndrome and epilepsy is *Yin* Syndrome and they are again divided into *Yin* and *Yang*.

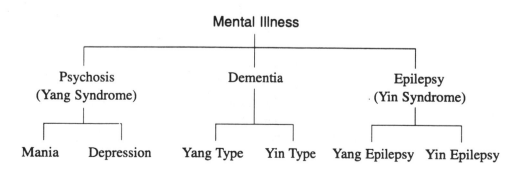

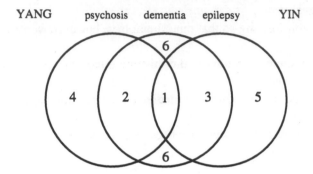

YANG   psychosis   dementia   epilepsy   YIN

Explanation of the above chart (1)
1. Combination of epilepsy, psychosis and dementia.
2. Combination of psychosis and dementia.
3. Combination of epilepsy and dementia.
4. Only psychosis.
5. Only epilepsy (losing consciousness only during epileptic seizures and ordinarily with no deficiency of mental function).
6. Only the mental function is altogether defective without epilepsy or psychosis (dementia praecox usually belongs to this).

A. Epilepsy
■ Yang Syndrome
1. There is fever and rapid pulse during the seizure.
2. The patient shouts.
3. Seizure can easily occur when the patient is excited or is exposed to direct rays of the sun or goes near crowded masses of people or stands in front of fire for a long time.
4. Seizure occurs frequently in daytime.

■ Yin Syndrome
1. The pulse is slow, deep and thready during the seizure.
2. The patient does not shout.
3. Seizure can easily occur when the patient is feeling fear, frightened or goes near water.
4. Instead of the occurrence of seizure, there are times when the patient only loses consciousness and becomes fuzzy or has dizziness.
5. Seizure occurs frequently at nighttime or during sleep.

B. Psychosis
■ Yang Syndrome
1. The patient is talkative, cheerful, fidgety, sings loudly or even acts violently.
2. The patient displays lots of anger and laughter.
3. The patient has paranoia like the following:

"Jealousy paranoia"   – morbid suspicion of wife or husband's chastity
"Exaggeration paranoia" – "I'm a general."

    – "I'm an emperor of heaven."
    – "I'm so–and–so, guardian spirit of the mountain."

4. The patient is afraid of nothing and is extremely bold.

■ **Yin Syndrome**
1. The patient feels depressed and does not move or talk much.
2. The patient usually bears a grudge, feels grief easily, always cries and at times attempts suicide.
3. The patient has the following paranoia:

"Fear paranoia"   – "I'm going to die soon."
                    – "Somebody is trying to kidnap me."
                    – "I am bankrupt and have become a beggar."
"Poison paranoia" – "someone put poison in the food that I ate."

Symptoms can belong to the *Yin* or *Yang* Syndrome according to the expression of the emotion.

As for the treatment method, observe all symptoms in detail and identify which organs have abnormal changes from the viewpoint of the *Zang Fu* organs to make the treatment appropriate for the constitution and symptoms of the individual. One must not carelessly search for miraculous medicine.

VI. YIN AND YANG OF THE ZANG–FU ORGANS

DIFFERENCE IN THE OPINION OF WESTERN AND ORIENTAL MEDICINE ON THE ZANG–FU ORGANS

Before talking about the *Yin–Yang* of organs, one must first understand that the viewpoint on the management of organs by Oriental and Western medicine is different. Here, which one is superior is beside the point. I will give a few examples on the differences:

1.

ZANG ORGANS	
Western Medicine	**Oriental Medicine**
lung	Lung
heart	Heart
spleen, pancreas	Spleen
liver	Liver
kidney (endocrine system)	Kidney (Gate of Life)

2.

FU ORGANS	
Western Medicine	**Oriental Medicine**
stomach	Stomach
small intestine	Small Intestine
large intestine	Large Intestine
gall bladder	Gall Bladder
urinary bladder (pleura)	Urinary Bladder (Triple Burner)

3. Western medicine studies the structure of each organ, connecting relationships between organs and functions of organs through dissection and experiments. Oriental medicine, rather than concentrating on anatomical experiments, classifies physiological phenomena into individual networks and establishes an organ which regulates and represents that system. Thus, the "Heart" in Oriental medicine implies the heart organ of Western medicine and at same time, indicates all functions of the heart and all phenomena caused by the heart. Therefore, the term "Heart" in Oriental medicine has a bit of an abstract meaning. Especially in the case of the "Kidneys," there are even more extensive meanings, so that it can be seen to totally summarize the kidney organ itself, the reproductive system, the urinary system and the endocrine system which regulates vitality.

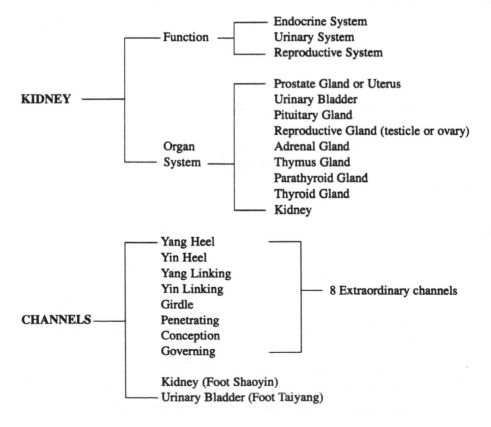

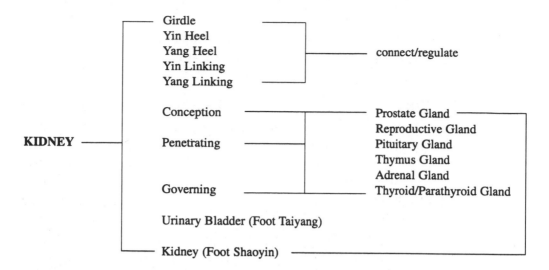

4. The connecting relationships between organs are studied through chemical interrelationship, that is, the relationship between the functions of each organ which are influenced by the hormones, rather than by an anatomical connecting relationship (refer to the Five Element Mutual Production & Control relationship).

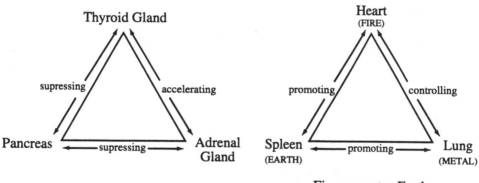

Fire generates Earth
Fire controls Metal
Earth generates Metal

■ **Example 1:**

When the thyroid gland is removed, the metabolism is generally reduced, but the assimilation of carbohydrates speeds up. Yet, the speeding up of carbohydrate assimilation indicates nothing more than the exuberance of the pancreatic function. On the other hand, removing the pancreas increases general metabolism, but the assimilation of carbohydrate is decreased. This relationship corresponds to the principle "Earth controls Water" in Oriental medicine.

The pancreas belongs to the Spleen so it is under element Earth, the adrenal gland and thyroid gland belong to the Kidney so they are under the element Water. The function of Spleen and Kidney suppressing each other is referred to as, "Earth controls Water."

■ **Example 2:**

When the activity of the heart becomes exuberant, breathing is difficult (Fire controls Metal), but digestion is good (Fire generates Earth). However, since the physiological mechanism is truly subtle, the respiratory system, which became fatigued due to the activity of the heart, is indirectly supplemented by the activity of heart (Earth generates Metal). This is the principle of "Mutual Generation and Mutual Control."

This principle is well demonstrated by the fact that a lung disease patient generally has a greater appetite and better digestion than a normal person at the initial stage, but develops fever and cannot endure strain since the heart is always fatigued.

■ **Example 3:** (refer to Chapter 4 on the channels)

ZANG	FU
Lung	Large Intestine
Heart	Small Intestine
Spleen	Stomach
Liver	Gall Bladder
Kidney	Urinary Bladder

Here, spleen and stomach, liver and gall bladder, kidney and urinary bladder can be seen as paired organs without much doubt, but the reason for handling lung and large intestine, heart and small intestine as pairs, is due to the resemblance in the function and connecting relationship of the functions.

Lung & Large Intestine
(a) The lungs eliminate carbon dioxide to the outside of the body and the large intestine eliminates feces.
(b) The lungs disperse water and the large intestine absorbs water.
(c) The lungs breathe air and the large intestine eliminates gas at times.
(d) Constipation occurs when there is heat in the lungs and diarrhea occurs when the activity of the lungs is weak.

Heart & Small Intestine
(a) The heart distributes nutrients to the whole body and the small intestine assimilates nutrients.
(b) The heart sends venous blood to the lungs and the small intestine sends its contents to the large intestine.

These are examples of how Oriental medicine puts greater importance on functional interrelationship rather than anatomical interrelationship.

5. *Zhu Dan Xi*[16] has said: "Liver (Gall Bladder) belongs to the Wood Element and is located on the left side of the body; Lung (Large Intestine) belongs to the Metal Element

and is located on the right side of the body; Spleen (Stomach) belongs to the Earth Element and lodges on the southwest so it is also on the right side." When this is viewed according to anatomy, it is quite unscientific. What is the reason for saying that the liver is located on the left when it is located on right and the lungs and large intestine are located on the right when they are located on both the right and left, and the spleen and stomach are located on the right when they are located on the left? At first, I also questioned Oriental medicine after reading this and had great doubt.

I was only able to resolve this doubt after several years of study and research. What is implied by right or left here is not the position of the organs according to the anatomy, but a location where the physiological response of those organs occurs.

This can be roughly proven by the following facts:

(a) Headache

Habitual headache is generally caused by digestive problems. The painful region is where we put headache liniment[17] and the time of extreme pain is usually two to three hours after a meal. When an equal amount of pressure is put on that region, most will say the right side hurts more. Some will say the right side hurts more as a subjective symptom without putting pressure. This is indeed the migraine headache. Anyone can easily see if they pay some attention that right side migraine is most common.

The headache of a person who is diagnosed as having jaundice or a gall stone is usually more painful on the left side or subjectively complains of a left side migraine.

(b) Shoulder pain – (neuralgia in the shoulder region and adhesive capsulitis of the shoulder)

Most shoulder pains are symptoms that occur when there is habitual constipation or diarrhea, namely dysfunction in the large intestine. Patients usually complain of pain on the right shoulder and wrist.

ZANG IS YIN AND FU IS YANG

Here are examples of differing points that are common in each *Zang* and *Fu* organ:

1. *Zang* organs, as long as there is life, do not rest even for a moment.

The heart, lungs, spleen, liver and kidneys are all like that. Closely resembling a woman's duty in our family life, when viewed from the outside, even her very existence cannot be known, but she does the cooking, sewing, washing and raises the children so that there is not even one day of rest.

The man of the house, even if he goes on a vacation for a day or two or gets sick and becomes bedridden, does not directly affect the daily life of the whole family except for special circumstances. However, if a housewife or maid goes somewhere or becomes bedridden, there is a great difficulty for the whole family, even for the duration of a single day.

---

16. Zhu Dan Xi (1281 – 1358 A.D.) is the founder of the "Tonify Yin" school of thought. He said that all diseases arise from excess heat in the body, so he emphasized treatments that nourish and support the Yin aspect of the body.

17. It is near the acupuncture point STOMACH 8 which is located in the corner of forehead.

Fu organs rest when there is no work and work only when there is a need for labor. The stomach works when food and drink come in and after sending its contents to the small intestine, it rests until food comes in again. It is the same for the small intestine, large intestine, urinary bladder and gall bladder.

2. The existence of the *Fu* organs, more so than the *Zang* organs, can be known more easily from outside or self–consciously.

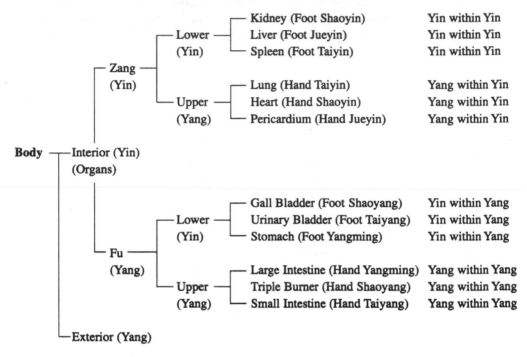

		Lower (Yin)	Kidney (Foot Shaoyin)	Yin within Yin
			Liver (Foot Jueyin)	Yin within Yin
	Zang (Yin)		Spleen (Foot Taiyin)	Yin within Yin
		Upper (Yang)	Lung (Hand Taiyin)	Yang within Yin
			Heart (Hand Shaoyin)	Yang within Yin
Body — Interior (Yin) (Organs)			Pericardium (Hand Jueyin)	Yang within Yin
		Lower (Yin)	Gall Bladder (Foot Shaoyang)	Yin within Yang
			Urinary Bladder (Foot Taiyang)	Yin within Yang
	Fu (Yang)		Stomach (Foot Yangming)	Yin within Yang
		Upper (Yang)	Large Intestine (Hand Yangming)	Yang within Yang
			Triple Burner (Hand Shaoyang)	Yang within Yang
Exterior (Yang)			Small Intestine (Hand Taiyang)	Yang within Yang

3. The reactions of the *Zang* organs appear on the side of the flexors and the reactions of the *Fu* organs appear on the side of the extensors.

Yin–Yang Distribution Chart of the Zang Fu Organs
(See Chapter 4 on the Channels and Collaterals)

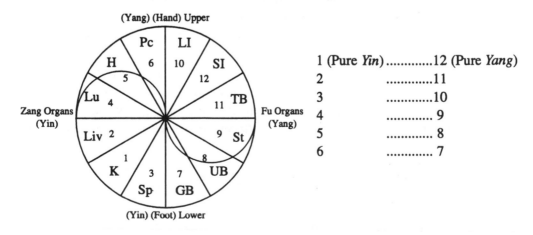

1 (Pure *Yin*) ....12 (Pure *Yang*)
2 11
3 10
4   9
5   8
6   7

Among the Five *Zang* organs, the one whose presence is most difficult to locate is the kidneys and the easiest to know is the heart. The existence of the kidneys cannot be possibly be known without dissection, but the action of the heart can always be observed below the left breast. It pounds on the chest when we get sick or frightened. Therefore, the heart is a *Zang* organ that is "*Yang* within *Yin*" and the kidney is a *Zang* organ that is "*Yin* within *Yin*."

Among the Six *Fu* organs, the one easiest to locate is the small intestine and the one most difficult to locate is the gall bladder. The existence of the gall bladder cannot possibly be known without dissection, but for the small intestine, even a child is able to observe its movement when there is abdominal pain. Therefore, the small intestine is a *Fu* organ that is "*Yang* within *Yang*," and the gall bladder is a *Fu* organ that is "*Yin* within *Yang*."

(a) Small Intestine
The reaction appears on the extension side of the little finger. Its movement can be felt as the winding movement of a snake.

(b) Large Intestine
The reaction appears on the extension side of the second finger. When there is constipation, its existence can be felt as a strong wire–like club standing up in the left lower abdominal region.

(c) Stomach
The reaction appears on the extension side of the second toe. When there is severe indigestion or spasm of the stomach, an uncomfortable sensation can be felt in the abdominal region.

(d) Urinary Bladder
The reaction appears on the extension side of the fifth toe. When one holds urine for a long time, the lower abdominal area feels heavy and painful.

(e) Gall Bladder
The reaction appears on the extension side of the fourth toe. Even when a disease like gall stones occurs, only its symptoms show up and one cannot perceive any change in the right hypochondriac region.

In all of the above, the reaction appears on the extensor (*Yang*) side. This is the common point of *Fu* organs since they are *Yang*.

(f) Heart
The reaction appears on the flexion side of the fifth finger. A heartbeat can be perceived underneath the left breast.

(g) Lungs
The reaction appears on the flexion side of the thumb. Their existence can be known through breathing and expansion–contraction of the thorax. While breathing goes on automatically, the lung is the only organ whose movement can be voluntarily regulated.

(h) Spleen
The reaction appears at the junction between the extensor and flexor of the first toe. There is a disease in children in which the spleen enlarges to the size of a tortoise, but

even in that case, it is difficult to know whether or not it is the spleen.

(i) Liver

The reaction appears on the flexion side of the first toe. The existence of the liver cannot be directly known and only the symptoms show up when there is a disease.

(j) Kidneys

The reaction appears on the sole of foot (flexion side). Their existence cannot be directly known at all and only the symptoms show up, even when one gets a kidney disease.

In the above–mentioned organs, their reactions all appear on the flexor (*Yin*) side.

VII. YIN–YANG OF THE CHANNELS

I will discuss the channels more in detail in the channel chapter, so here, only their classification of *Yin–Yang* will be discussed.

A change inside the human body is inevitably reflected on the outside and the specified reactive regions on the surface of the body that belong to each organ are called channels.

CHANNELS OF SIX FU ORGANS ARE YANG

The Six *Fu* organs refer to the Stomach, Small Intestine, Large Intestine, Gall Bladder, Urinary Bladder and "Triple Burner." The channels of these organs all arrive at the side of the extensors:

Stomach (Foot Yangming channel)	extensor side of second toe
Small Intestine (Hand Taiyang channel)	extensor side of fifth finger
Large Intestine (Hand Yangming channel)	extensor side of second finger
Gall Bladder (Foot Shaoyang channel)	extensor side of fourth toe
Urinary Bladder (Foot Taiyang channel)	extensor side of fifth toe
Triple Burner (Hand Shaoyang channel)	extensor side of fourth finger

Fu organs work only when there is labor and rest when there is no labor.

CHANNELS OF SIX ZANG ORGANS ARE YIN

The Six *Zang* organs refer to the Lung, Heart, Liver, Spleen, Kidney and Mingmen (Gate of Life). The channels of these organs all arrive at the side of the flexors:

Lung (Hand Taiyin channel)	flexor side of thumb
Heart (Hand Shaoyin channel)	flexor side of fifth finger
Spleen (Foot Taiyin channel)	flexor side above big toe
Liver (Foot Jueyin channel)	flexor side of big toe
Kidney (Foot Shaoyin channel)	flexor side of the sole
Gate of Life/ (Hand Jueyin Channel) Pericardium	flexor side of third finger

As long as there is life, *Zang* organs always work without taking a moment for rest.

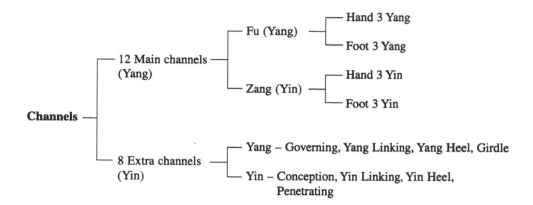

VIII. YIN–YANG OF THE PULSE

I will give a more detailed explanation of pulse in the pulse chapter. Here, I am going to explain quite simply that there is a classification of *Yin–Yang* for the pulse.

CAROTID AND RADIAL PULSE

There are many places on the body where the pulse can be felt:

1. In places where arteries are comparatively large.
2. In places where the distance between the arteries and the surface of body is small.

The places where the pulse can be felt especially clear are the carotid and radial arteries. In Oriental medicine, the carotid pulse is called *Renying* and the radial pulse is called *Qikou*.[18]

The reason why doctors of both Western and Oriental Medicine look for the pulse at the radial artery is because that region is where changes in the pulse can be known most easily.

The diseases of the Five *Zang* and the Six *Fu* organs can be perceived with just the radial pulse in Oriental medicine.

The radial pulse lies on the pathway of the Lung channel and the position can be found by going approximately the width of the first and second finger of one's hand from the transverse crease of the wrist on the thumb side.

This radial pulse is once more divided into three positions, *Cun* (first), *Guan* (second), and *Chi* (third) and becomes six pulse positions by combining the left and right side.

SUPERFICIAL, LARGE, SLIPPERY AND RAPID ARE YANG PULSES

Since the constitutions of humans are not all identical, pulses are truly infinite in

---

18. Renying literally means "Person's Welcome." "Person's Welcome" means that this spot is vital to a person's life. An acupuncture point, STOMACH 9, which is also called Renying, is located here. Qikou literally means "the mouth or gate of Qi." Qikou lies along the path of the Lung channel and the Lungs are in charge of Qi in Oriental medicine.

varieties. Therefore, even though the types of pulses already named according to Oriental medicine are fairly large in number, they are no more than superficial–deep, large–minute, slippery–choppy or rapid–slow pulses when classified generally:

- **Superficial Pulse** – it can be felt by just light contact with the skin surface without pressing with the fingers.
- **Large Pulse** – width of the pulsation is wide.
- **Slippery Pulse** – movement is smooth and soft like a new machine that has been oiled.
- **Rapid Pulse** – pulsation is faster than normal.

Considering the normal pulse rate as 70 beats per minute for an adult, pulses greater than 80 beats per minute must be considered a rapid pulse, even though there are slight differences according to the constitution.

All of the above pulses belong to *Yang*.

DEEP, MINUTE, CHOPPY AND SLOW ARE YIN PULSES

- **Deep Pulse** – it cannot be felt by a light touch and is not felt until heavily pressed.
- **Minute Pulse** – since the width of the pulse is very small and thin, it seems to be almost non–existent.
- **Choppy Pulse** – like a rusty machine, the movement is not soft or smooth and feels rather blocked due to roughness.
- **Slow Pulse** – the pulse rate is less than normal. A pulse under 60 beats per minute can be regarded as a slow pulse.

All of the above pulses belong to *Yin*.

IX. YIN–YANG OF HERBAL PROPERTIES

YIN–YANG OF QI AND TASTE

The fundamental principle of Oriental pharmacology is the "Theory of *Qi* and Taste." Qi is that of classifying the properties of herbs into hot, warm, neutral, cool and cold temperatures. Taste is that of distinguishing pungent, sweet, sour, salty and bitter tastes of the herbs which stimulate the palate. This theory will be discussed later in the pharmacology chapter in detail so here I am going to simply discuss the *Yin–Yang* only.

HOT HERBS ARE YANG AND COLD HERBS ARE YIN

What is meant by hot or cold? For example, things like honey, rice wine or dates warm up the inside and raise the body temperature even when eaten after being kept in ice, while pears or watermelon cool the stomach and can easily result in diarrhea, even when eaten as a warm soup. Accordingly, we can see that honey, rice wine or dates are warm foods and pears or watermelon are cold foods. In the former, the herbal properties are *Yang* and in the latter, the herbal properties are *Yin*.

Pungent taste is *Yang* and bitter taste is *Yin*. Pungent is a taste that is rich and intense, so it implies a stimulating, exciting and aromatic nature. Red pepper, black pepper, mustard seed or garlic all have pungent taste. When these foods are eaten to excess, the face becomes hot immediately and sweating occurs. This clearly shows that they are *Yang*-natured.

Bitter tasting herbs are *Yin*-natured herbs such as lettuce or sophora root. When we eat pungent food, we have to open our mouth and blow out in order to quickly disperse pungent energy upward. When we eat bitter food, we grimace and swallow saliva again and again in order to send it downward.

That is the why "pungent and warm rise and disperse" and "bitter and cold descend downward" are phrases that follow each other and there are no occasions where pungent taste is not included in diaphoretic and stimulating formulas and purgatives and sedative formulas always have a bitter taste.

QI–TASTE THEORY AND WESTERN PHARMACOLOGY

Oriental medical herbs are used as condiments and teas to some degree in Western pharmacology, but they are not generally regarded as medicinal substances, even though a few are classified widely into stomachic (medicine that stimulates and improves appetite and digestion).

COMPLEX OF HERBAL PROPERTIES (see Chapter 7 on pharmacology)

All of the above herbal properties were discussed according to taste and temperature, but in actuality, Oriental herbs do not have just one property. Each has many properties simultaneously, so its complexities are truly beyond description.

Thus, Oriental herbs, which are organic medicinal substances, have the special characteristic of being extremely complicated. Yet that is where the value of Oriental herbs lies and the reason for getting surprisingly beneficial effects.[19]

Nevertheless, Western doctors always try to use only the effective ingredients extracted from the Oriental herbs and there are many who insist that this is the correct method to use herbs. This is not possible in modern times where organic chemistry is in its infancy and can only be seen as a vice of modern science. Analysis should have synthesis as the premise. In modern times, which is a time of analytical science, analysis often has been done for the sake of analyzing so there are many occasions where synthesis is completely ignored.

Let's suppose that ginseng is a very good herb. There are many ingredients in ginseng. So among them, it can be presumed that there is one that helps blood circulation and breathing, one that helps digestive function and one that helps reproductive function.

One cannot possibly discuss the function of ginseng based on an extracted ingredient which is effective for one single organ such as the heart or the stomach. One cannot affirm

---

19. Oriental herbs have effect because of synergistic principles. They influence the body as a whole and are not based on individually isolated constituents. The principle behind the Oriental herbs are the Yin–Yang and the Five Element Theory. See Chapter 6 on pharmacology for further details.

that there are no effective ingredients aside from those and as such, where should the effectiveness be sought and how is the synthesis going to be formed? I know that it will be more appropriate to discuss the holistic effect of ginseng based, preferably, on the *Qi*–Taste Theory.

The effects of ginseng:

- Temperature – slightly warm
- Taste   – slightly bitter
- Taste   – slightly sweet
- Taste   – bland
- Color   – yellow (water ginseng)[20]
- Color   – white (white ginseng)[21]
- Color   – red (red ginseng)[22]

1. Being slightly warm without pungent properties, it does not temporarily raise body temperature due to stimulation, like alcoholic beverages, but invigorates physiological function by assisting Original *Yang*[23] quietly, increasing the body temperature of a person with low body temperature.
2. Bitter taste relieves excitation and fatigue of the Heart and gently and naturally brings down fever due to fatigue because of the slight bitter taste.
3. The sweet taste acts on the digestive system to increase the body's ability to get nutrition from food.
4. The bland taste regulates the function of the Kidney channel, namely the reproductive system.
5. Constituents with yellow color act on the Spleen.
6. Constituents with white color act on the Lung.
7. Constituents with red color act on the Heart.

These diverse constituents become a harmonious whole to act simultaneously on each organ, bringing about a holistic effect by increasing the health totally and intangibly. Since ginseng possesses all these properties not contained in any other herb, there is no better herb than ginseng for the weak person.

To give a few more examples, platycodon and bupleurum are cold herbs that ascend and magnolia and evodia descend even though they are warm. When the lower part of the body is cold as in diarrhea and abdominal pain, it is warmed up with herbs that descend, like magnolia and evodia.[24] When there is heat in the upper part of the body as in eye and throat diseases, it is cooled by using cold herbs that ascend.

---

20. Fresh Ginseng

21. Dried ginseng

22. Cooked ginseng

23. Original Yang is the energy that is stored in the Kidneys and helps to warm up and activate all physiological processes in the body. This is equivalent to the Ministerial Fire or Mingmen (Gate of Life) Fire.

24. For more information on the herbs, see appendix I.

DUAL ASPECTS OF THE EFFECTS OF ORIENTAL HERBAL MEDICINE

In Oriental herbal medicine, a single herb can have dual functions that are contradictory. This is a phenomenon that is only seen in Oriental herbs.

1. The function of ginseng:
   (a) It lowers fever in a person with excess heat and raises body temperature in a person with a deficiency of heat.
   (b) It stops diarrhea in a person with diarrhea and causes bowel movements in a person with constipation.
   (c) It increases urination in a person who finds it difficult to urinate and reduces the frequency of urination in a person who needs to urinate too often.
2. Astragalus reduces sweating in a person who sweats too much and causes sweating in a person who cannot.
3. Zizyphus cures both insomnia and hypersomnia.
4. Apple cures both constipation and diarrhea.
5. Chinese angelica and cnidium can either calm down a restless fetus or induce abortion.

Oriental herbs do not just act in a single direction, but in multiple aspects. They regulate and adjust in order to eliminate both excess and deficiency of physiological function.

X. YIN–YANG OF MOVEMENTS, SHAPES AND NUMBERS

YIN–YANG OF MOVEMENTS

There is a classification of *Yin–Yang* according to movements. Extension is *Yang* and contraction is *Yin*. We open and spread our limbs when hot and curl–up when cold. We open our body during times of elation and curl–up when fearful. This can be seen even in the disease syndromes. The four limbs are generally spread out in *Yang* Syndromes and curled–up in *Yin* Syndromes.

Even in pain of identical magnitude, that which hurts as if being squeezed (spasm and contraction) is cold pain and that which hurts as if burned is heat pain. Naturally, there are exceptions here, but the general rule still holds. Those two types of pain are frequently seen in clinical practice. Hiccup, for example, is a spasm of the diaphragm and is also caused by cold.

YIN–YANG OF SHAPES

There is a classification of *Yin–Yang* according to shapes. A circle is *Yang* and a square is *Yin*. *Yang* is dynamic and *Yin* is static. A circle is not fixed and can always move freely, but since a square is stable, movement is difficult.

1. "Heaven is round, Earth is square" theory[25]

"Heaven is round and Earth is square" theory is interpreted as heaven being circular

---

25. This is an ancient cosmological view held by the philosophers of the Orient.

and Earth being angular. It is disregarded by many as illiterate speech, but in my humble opinion, "Earth" does not literally imply earth per se: Heaven–Earth, Kan–Kun,[26] up–down, dynamic–static, round–square and *Yin–Yang* all have the same meaning.

The words "Heaven is round and Earth is square" mean the same as *Yang* is circular and *Yin* is square and "Heaven is dynamic and Earth is static" is the same as *Yang* is dynamic and *Yin* is static. Above is Heaven and below is Earth. Above is *Yang* and below is *Yin*. Since the surface of the earth is flat, it can remain stable, but the blue heaven looks circular and does not have stability.

The existence of matter is not recognized until it passes through our senses, so seeing the surface of the earth as flat through our observation is not unreasonable in any way. Speaking in the strict sense, the so–called horizon is unscientific and the perception of two vertical lines running parallel is also incorrect.

The circle implies a curved line and the square implies a straight line. "Earth is square" implies that the surface of the earth appears flat and does not imply the appearance of the whole earth. Moreover, let us think about the up–and–down. For the up–and–down of zero degrees longitude and the up–and–down of 180 degrees longitude, the directions will be exactly opposite. Then, is the up–and–down of America correct and the up–and–down of Asia incorrect? No, it is not like that since everything is relative.

In Asia, the up–and–down of Asia is correct and in America, the up–and–down of America is correct. Therefore, Heaven, Earth, Up, Down, East and West are not all fixed and never–changing concepts. However, since they often change relatively according to location, trying to describe fixed existence like the Earth itself in "Heaven is round and Earth is square" is clearly unreasonable.

"Heaven is round and Earth is square" applies even in a human body, so that "Above is round and below is square," that is, "Head is round and foot is square."

Head is *Yang* and foot is *Yin*. Hence, *Yang* Syndromes manifest in the upper body, and *Yin* Syndromes are reflected in the lower body.

2. Curved lines and straight lines, femininity and masculinity

In pictures, masculinity is described as a straight line and femininity is described as a curved line. The horn of a bull is straight and the horn of a female cow is curved. A curved line is *Yang* and a straight line is *Yin*. However, a bull is *Yang* and a cow is *Yin*. Since bulls are *Yang*, they are harmonized by the straight line or *Yin* and since cows are *Yin*, they are harmonized by the curved line or *Yang*. Within the human world, the same principles apply. A man's figure is straight and square while a woman's figure is curved.

Even in a person's age, a woman is harmonized by *Yang* numbers and a man is harmonized by *Yin* numbers.

YIN–YANG OF NUMBERS

1. Odd numbers, even numbers, and circulating decimals

There are *Yin–Yang* characteristics in numbers. Odd numbers (1, 3, 5, 7, 9) are *Yang*

---

26. Two of the trigrams in the I Ching (Book of Change). Kan represents Heaven and Kun represents Earth.

numbers and even numbers (2, 4, 6, 8, 10) are *Yin* numbers. Why are odd numbers *Yang* and even numbers *Yin*? *Yang* is dynamic and *Yin* is static. Dynamic is not fixed and static is fixed. As such, the number that is least fixed is circulating decimals and the factor that is common in the circulating decimals is that a divisor must be an odd number or a number that has an odd number as an exact divisor.

When 1, 2, 4, 5, 7, 8 are divided by 3, all become circulating decimals and when 1, 2, 3, 4, 5, 6, 8, 9 are divided by 7, all become circulating decimals. Eleven, thirteen, seventeen, nineteen and twenty–three are all like that.

1 divided by 3 = 0.333   2 divided by 3 = 0.666   5 divided by 3 = 1.666

2. Round shape and square shape, three (circular constant) and four

In the *I Ching*, it is stated that a circle is three times the diameter and a square is four times the diameter. In modern mathematics, it is said that the circumference is 3.1416 times the diameter and the length of four sides of a square is four times one side. A circle is *Yang* and the circular constant is a *Yang* number. A square is *Yin* and the number of its sides is a *Yin* number.

3. The relationship between age and the sexually active period in men and women

The period of sexual activity in a human is generally fixed with some exception. It is from age 14 to 49 in woman and age 16 to 64 in man. In women, the duration is clear and lasts from the start of the menstruation to menopause. For men, it is not hard to perceive that his attitude toward the opposite sex changes dramatically when he turns age 16.

4. Number seven in women and number eight in men

Women have seven year phases of development and men have eight year phases of development. In woman, two times seven is 14 so the menstruation begins at 14 years of age and seven times seven equals 49. So at 49 years of age, menstruation stops.

Whether or not there is a correlation with this number seven is beside the point. Since the duration of menstruation is proven by the fact, there is no room whatsoever for a different opinion. Therefore, there are scarcely any women who give birth to a child after the age 50. Even when considered as a statistical probability, it is true that the numbers 14 and 49 are multiples of seven.

The difference between chance and natural process is merely in knowing or not knowing the principle. Even when considered a chance phenomenon, if it has universal validity, it is not illogical in any way to infer that certain principles lie dormant within that phenomenon.

Woman is *Yin* (*Shaoyin* or Small *Yin*) and since the number seven (*Shaoyang* or Small *Yang*) is an odd or *Yang* number, *Yin* was harmonized with *Yang*. The *Yang* (*Shaoyang*) of a man was combined with the number eight (*Shaoyin*) which is a *Yin* number.

5. The period of obscure sexual desire and the separation of sexes at age seven

In the book *Elementary Learning*,[27] there is a saying: "Boys and girls should not sit at the same place when they reach age seven." The age of seven was in no way established without a purpose.

When a girl turns age seven, she dimly senses relationship between the opposite sex. Nine years ago, I heard the following explanation during a lecture on sexual problems by Dr. Senzi Yamamoto of Japan.

Dr. Yamamoto said that a woman who never had a sexual experience might merely feel obscure sexual desire, but not a strong physical impulse and not until she has sexual intercourse does she feel the same sexual desire as a man. He also said that the obscure sexual desire occurs when a girl turns to age seven, the proof of which is the activation of shameful feelings.

When I heard this, I thought it was not unreasonable for the ancestors, who held the highest degree of respect for the differences between man and woman, to have said and practiced, "Separation of sexes at age seven."

I do not know if there is such an obscure sexual desire to the level as mentioned by Dr. Yamamoto, but it is true that age seven is a transitional period in development.

According to my observation, one can recognize the following psychological changes when a girl turns seven:

(a) She gets shameful thoughts which cause her to blush.
(b) She pays attention to clothing and on no occasion takes off her clothes or shows parts of her body that are not revealed by a mature woman.
(c) Her sense of beauty gets activated so she gets interested in beautiful clothing, her figure and make–up.
(d) She vaguely understands marriage and the sexual relationship between parents.

These are easily observed by anyone. The following changes can be seen when a boy turns age eight:

(a) He becomes rude and extremely delinquent.
(b) He plays around a lot, easily fights with friends and becomes very detestable since he acts in an undisciplined manner.
(c) Since the notion of despising woman becomes strong, he strongly shows his distaste for all things that are feminine and acts very arrogantly. At this time the characteristics of masculinity become clearly manifested.

6. "Sweet Sixteen"

From the ancient times, there has been a saying "Sweet Sixteen." This is a saying that comes from long experience and is in no way said meaninglessly. It is a saying everyone will acknowledge when they recollect the past and will know well by looking at the adolescents in that age group.

---

27. This is a book on morals for children written by Liu Zi Deng during the Song dynasty (960-1279 A.D.) in China. This book was based on the teachings by Zhu Xi who was a famous scholar of Neo–confucianism.

When a man turns age 16, yearning toward the opposite sex becomes suddenly very strong as if someone provoked it. Since the passion, which burns for the first time at this period, is pure, beautiful and intense, people have been singing much about "Sweet Sixteen." Looking at this, one will not dispute that age 16 is an epoch–making time in the development of a man so what about the man ending sexual activity at the age 64? It is usually difficult to make a definite judgement about this, since the usual custom is to bury sexual activity in darkness in order to keep it in secrecy and elders do not express their emotions well. Even though sexual activity in general is slowed down after the age 56, it is true that there are many elders who have sexual activity until the age of 64. It is a pity that I have not been able to obtain statistical proof.

The following is a quote from *Inner Classic* which speaks about the development of women in cycles of seven years and the development of men in cycles of eight years.

"When a girl is seven years of age, the Kidney *Qi* is exuberant: she begins to change her teeth and her hair grows. At the age of 14, the Dew of Heaven arrives (reproductive organs are matured): the Conception channel opens up and the Penetrating channel is exuberant. The menstruation comes at regular times, thus she can conceive. At the age of 21, the Kidney *Qi* is balanced: the wisdom teeth come in and she becomes fully grown. At the age of 28, her tendons and bones are strong, her hair grows to its peak, and her body is strong. At the age of 35, the *Yangming* (Bright *Yang*) channel weakens, her face begins to darken, and her hair begins to fall out. At the age of 42, the three *Yang* channels are weak in the upper part (of the body): her face becomes dark, and her hair turns white. At the age of 49, the Conception channel becomes deficient, the Penetrating channel deteriorates. Dew of Heaven is exhausted and the menstruation stops. Thus, her body becomes old and she can no longer bear children."

"When a boy is eight years of age, the Kidney *Qi* is full: his hair grows and he begins to change his teeth. At the age of 16, the Kidney *Qi* is abundant: the Dew of Heaven arrives, and the Essence *Qi* (semen) is overflowing. When he has sexual contact with a woman, he can have children. At the age of 24, the *Yang Qi* is balanced: his tendons and bones are strong, the wisdom teeth come in, and his growth is at its zenith. At the age of 32, his tendons and bones are exuberant, and his flesh is full and strong. At the age of 40, the Kidney *Qi* declines, his hair falls out and his teeth decay. At the age of 48, the *Yang Qi* is exhausted in the upper part (of the body): his face becomes dark and the hair on his head and at his temples turns white. At the age of 56, the Liver *Qi* declines, his tendons become inactive, the Dew of Heaven is exhausted, Essence diminishes, the Kidneys weaken and his physical body grows old. At the age of 64, his teeth and hair fall out. The Kidneys control Water and they receive and store the Essence of the Five *Zang* and Six *Fu* organs. Thus, when the Five *Zang* organs are full of energy, they can discharge their essence. Now all Five *Zang* organs are weakened, the tendons and bones are deteriorated and the Dew of Heaven is exhausted so that infertility comes about."

XI. RELATIVITY OF YIN–YANG

Yin and *Yang* are relative. There is neither absolute *Yang* nor absolute *Yin*. For example, even though "phenomenon B" becomes *Yin* compared to "phenomenon A," it can become *Yang* compared to "phenomenon C." The distinctions of all phenomena can be seen due to the differences in the amount of the *Yin* or *Yang* properties they possess.

There is nothing without any *Yin* properties nor is there anything that does not have any *Yang* properties. So the saying, "Within *Yin*, there once again is *Yang* and within *Yang*, there once again is *Yin*" reflects that. We can, like the following example, classify *Yin–Yang* by comparing the characteristics of all matter and when that is once again subdivided without limit, that number will also expand without limit in geometrical progression.

One cannot sufficiently understand *Yin–Yang* Theory without knowing the relativity of *Yin–Yang*, nor understand the fundamentals of Oriental medicine without understanding *Yin–Yang* Theory.

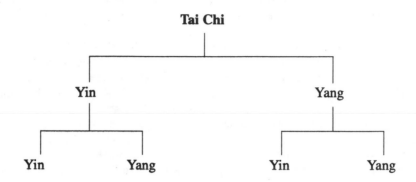

We can see this relationship anywhere.

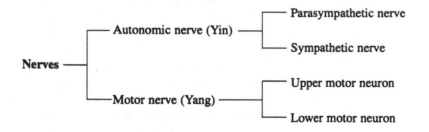

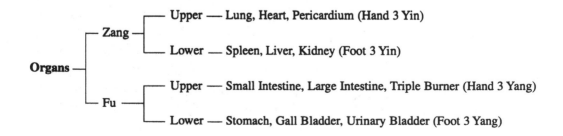

* See Chapter 4 on the channels for stomach being located in lower part and large intestine being located in upper part.

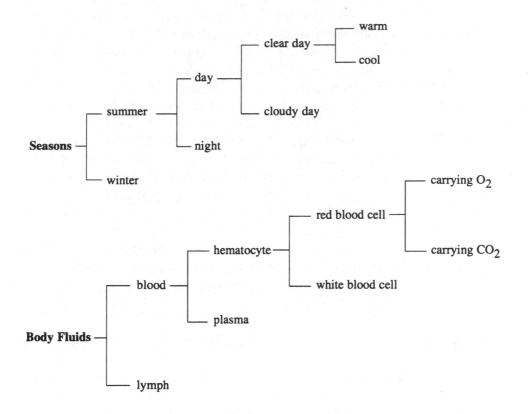

XII. HORMONES AND NERVES

The nerves play a central role in our lives. The brain becomes their source and the spine becomes the main stream, placing branch streams throughout the body to cover the whole surface of the skin as well as organs and bones. The waves of life, similar to electrical current, are sent right down to the individual cells.

One can compare the nervous system of the human body to the telegraphic communication network of a country in a perfect state. It would be suitable to see the system of blood vessels as traffic, transportation and postal network. Those that use this system indirectly to report, petition, demand and request by sending documents or dispatching personnel are the hormones.

Being alive implies that a person carries on the phenomena of life. Carrying on the phenomena of life implies that the metabolic process is carried out without stopping, even for a short time. Life cannot exist without metabolism and metabolism is regulated by nerves, hormones (endocrine) and catalysts (stimulating substances other than endocrine hormones).

WHAT IS A HORMONE?

The tissues of the human body have a variety of mutual relationships. There are two important ways to unify and regulate those relationships. One involves the nerve interconnections and the other through chemical interconnections.

We know that there are interconnections among the nerves because organ (A) can influence organ (B) based on connections by anatomical nerve tissues. For example, when a section of cerebral cortex is stimulated, we can see the contraction of skeletal muscles.

The other important interconnection, which is accomplished by chemical substances, does not borrow the strength of the nervous system. Rather, through the medium of certain body fluids (blood and lymph), these special chemical substances are transported to an isolated area to cause chemical reactions there.

It is not the nerve action, but a chemical action which facilitates the secretion of pancreatic enzymes and bile when the contents of the stomach reach the duodenum. Acidic contents of the stomach act on the mucous membrane of the duodenum forming a substance called secretin which immediately gets absorbed into the blood stream. From there it goes to the pancreas and liver and stimulates the epithelial tissue of those organs to facilitate their secretion. At this time, secretin becomes a messenger to first convey an order to secrete to the pancreas and liver. Thus, the special chemical substances which act on certain tissues or organs are called hormones. Endocrine means internal secretion of a hormone into the bloodstream.

Carbon dioxide, which is the product of the oxidating function of all body tissues, is harmful waste that must be discharged outside of the body. At the same time, it has quite a useful function in regulating breathing. When carbon dioxide stagnates above a certain limit inside the blood, it stimulates the breathing center to make breathing more frequent and deep. Thus, the breathing center responds to the demands of tissues that signal oxygen shortage ("*Yang* can be found within *Yin*" and "Without *Yin*, *Yang* cannot transform"). At this time, carbon dioxide can be considered to act as a hormone in that it is a chemical messenger.

When a woman becomes pregnant, the milk glands enlarge and secrete milk. Up until now, this was regarded as an action of the nerves, but when the nerve connection between the milk glands and reproductive organs is cut or when the milk gland is excised and transplanted near the ear as in experiments with rabbits, the milk glands still enlarge and secrete milk when the rabbit becomes pregnant. This is proof that no nerve connection exists between the milk glands and the reproductive glands. In addition, giving injections of ovary extracts, placenta, endometriotic lining and fetal tissues of the same species of rabbits to rabbits that have not yet become pregnant also enlarges the milk glands and milk is secreted.

There are similar examples in humans, in which one of a pair of siamese twins becomes pregnant and has a normal delivery and the other, although not pregnant, also has notable milk secretion. Since siamese twins are nourished by the same blood, there is no doubt that stimulating substances (namely the hormones) produced by the pregnant woman stimulated the milk glands of the other woman through blood circulation and facilitated the secretion of milk. This is like the following message when compared to our communication network:

> ## To: Milk gland
>
> **A fetus is being created here so please prepare the milk.**
>
> From: Reproductive organ

When such a notice is sent to the blood, it goes around searching for the milk glands and delivers that notice anywhere to the milk gland.

It is difficult to directly prove the existence of hormones because apart from one or two exceptions, their existence has been indirectly proven in a limited way based on clinical pathology, anatomical observation and experiments done on humans or animals. Even though the scope of hormones is not clear–cut and positive proof of the existence of hormones is incomplete, their existence cannot be disproved for the following reasons:

1. Thyroid Gland

(a) When the function of the thyroid gland is lost, the following changes occur: incomplete growth of bone, nutritional impediment of skin, incomplete development of sexual organs, loss of intelligence, decline in metabolism and decrease in body temperature.

(b) When the function of the thyroid gland is accelerated, completely opposite symptoms occur in contrast to when the function is lost: goiter, acceleration of metabolism and increase in body temperature. Also, the patient gets easily excited due to the quickening of mental functions.

2. Sexual Organs

When the testicles or ovaries are removed during childhood, the sexual state of that person's body is changed. Excess development of fatty structures, incomplete development of facial, underarm and pubic hair, childish voice, incomplete development of sexual organs and abnormal bone growth occur in men. Withering of the uterus and amenorrhea occur in women. Personality changes occur in both men and women.

3. Adrenal Glands

Even the chemical structures of adrenalin, secreted by the adrenal glands, have been researched.

Aside from these, there are experimental reports on the endocrine glands such as the parathyroid, thymus, pituitary and the spleen. Their existence can be inferred as stated above and it is not difficult to speculate about the existence of many types of hormones and glands still unknown. Therefore, as research on hormones develops, one will be astonished at the elegant mechanism of the living body.

HORMONES AND ORIENTAL MEDICINE

Oriental medicine is known as – "The Study of Treating the Main Syndromes." I see Oriental medicine as the hormone regulating medicine. There are probably many types of hormones, the functions of which are complicated, but they can be divided into the force that promotes and the force that suppresses. These two forces are *Yin* and *Yang*. When *Yin–Yang* is harmonized, in other words, when physiological regulation by the hormones is maintained, one can indeed stay in a healthy state. In contrast, when abnormality in endocrine secretions occur due to disharmony of *Yin–Yang*, certain pathological changes occur in the body. Observing this pathological change and judging which endocrine system is abnormal is called the "Theory of Excess and Deficiency" (Study of Syndromes). Investigating mutual suppressing (as in the relationship between pancreas and thyroid) and promoting (as in the relationship between thyroid and adrenals) relationships among the endocrine glands is the "Theory of Mutual Generation and Control." Regulating abnormality of endocrine secretions through the use of herbs is the "Theory of *Qi* and Taste" (Study of Herbal Properties and the Study of Prescriptions). I will speak in more detail about Deficiency–Excess in the Syndrome, Mutual Generation–Control in the *Zang Fu* and *Qi*–Taste in the pharmacology sections.

XIII. TRUE YIN AND ORIGINAL YANG

THE ORIGINAL SPIRIT

The so–called True *Yin* and Original *Yang* in Oriental medicine are extremely important and at the same time extremely difficult to understand. In a few words, True *Yin* and Original *Yang* are the forces of life. The invisible power that maintains all physiological regulations and operates proper metabolism through the interaction between nerves and hormones is called the Original Spirit. True *Yin* and Original *Yang* are the two aspects of the Original Spirit.

Original Spirit ⎯ ⎡ True Yin (Original Essence) ⎤ ⎯ Living body
                    ⎣ Original Yang (Original Qi) ⎦

* True Yin is also called Original Yin.

Life = (TRUE YANG / TRUE YIN) = (NERVE / HORMONE)

THE FUNCTION OF TRUE YIN AND ORIGINAL YANG

There are both intangible and tangible *Yin–Yang*. Everything that has been said about *Yin–Yang* thus far can generally be considered as tangible *Yin–Yang*. Through what can the intangible *Yin–Yang*, namely Original *Yang* be known? It can be understood by observing the following physiological actions.

Tangible *Yin–Yang* mutually oppose each other. So the rise–fall and prosperity–decay are in opposition. The Original *Yin* and the Original *Yang* mutually compromise and harmonize solely to maintain life. I offer the following as proof:

1. When there is excess heat in the body, one demands cold things. The foods and drinks requested are also cold. This occurs as a result of the physiological need by the body. On one hand, Original *Yang* creates fever and on the other hand, Original *Yin* regulates the body to stop the heat from reaching an excess level. In other words, it regulates the body to request foods and drinks that can eliminate the cause of heat. When the heat of the body is deficient, we can observe a phenomenon opposite to this.

2. When there is excess heat in the body, inhalation is weak and exhalation is strong. The inhalation becomes weak in order to suppress the combustive action in the body by reducing the supply of oxygen. Exhalation becomes stronger in order to quickly eliminate the carbon dioxide produced by an already exuberant combustive action. At the same time, this reduces fever through a large quantity of vapor diffusion during exhalation. This, too, is the function of True *Yin*.

On the contrary, strong inhalation and weak exhalation is the function of Original *Yang*. Infants all have strong inhalation and weak exhalation. The reason for this is that since infants grow and develop actively, True *Yang* functions as a result. The reason for the strong inhalation and weak exhalation during the period of old age is that since physiological function is weak, the function of True *Yang* is passively strong.

A patient with lung disease generally has strong exhalation and weak inhalation. The reason for this is that he or she has "*Yin* Deficiency with glowing of Fire," according to Oriental medicine.

XIV. THE CAUSE OF DISHARMONY OF YIN–YANG

The cause of *Yin–Yang* disharmony can be directly seen as the cause of a disease. The causes of *Yin–Yang* disharmony are said to result from inherited constitution, post–natal trauma, Invasion by External Pathogen, Internal Injury, overstrain, etc. but they can be seen as the collaboration between internal and external causes. Even though there is an external cause, if the inherent constitution is strong so that there is no internal cause, a disease will not develop. Even if the physical constitution is weak, there will also be no disease if the external cause is avoided. If two people are exposed together to cold weather, one person may catch cold and another will not. When the bacteria of a typhoid fever enters the bodies of two subjects at same time, there will be one who gets the disease and another who will not. This shows that there must be a fulfillment of both internal and external causes in order for a disease to occur. However, it is extremely difficult to determine where the dividing line between internal and external cause is. Therefore, the cause of a disease is divided as in the following for the sake of convenience:

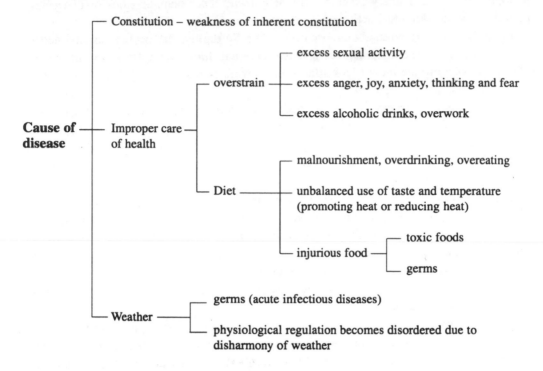

INHERENT CONSTITUTION

The dividing line between inherent constitution and acquired changes is not definite. Contacting germs at the same time, one person gets infected and another does not. Eating the same food, one gets food poisoning and another does not. Under similar stress, one gets sick and another does not. Interpreting in a wide sense, there is not a health–related phenomenon that is not caused by our inherent constitution and yet, the word "inherent" is created by humans, so its boundary can be fixed by humans. In simple terms, "inherent" implies that the cause is unknown. The following are situations that can be considered inherent:

1. Changes in the physical constitution as a result of a certain cause in the mother's womb.
2. Changes in the physical constitution without certain cause after birth.
3. Gradual changes in the physical constitution over a long period of time in minute degrees in which the degree of change is not intense enough to be considered a disease.
4. Changes in the physical constitution during infancy where proper nourishment is missing.

These conditions are all fundamentally based on hereditary factors, but it is also true that environmental factors were added into them. Thus, even an inherently weak person can change his constitution by cultivating his health. Simply stated, even if the condition is inherent, it is definitely not unchangeable.

OVERSTRAIN

Overstrain can be seen as the cause of a multitude of diseases. When a person is mentally or physically fatigued, disease can occur easily because every physiological function is weakened. These include the power of resistance, the power of reparation, the power of compensation and the power of healing. In order for us to maintain health, the following four steps must be followed.

Fatigue develops when one works and when fatigue develops, one rests. By resting, one recovers and when recovered, one works again. Life cannot continue without working and one's health cannot be maintained without rest, so work and rest must always be balanced.

1. The organ that has a direct relationship to work is the heart. Since the heart supplies a dynamic force to all of the systems of the body, being fatigued mentally or physically implies fatigue of the heart and a weak person certainly has a weak heart. Dynamic force is acquired through consumption of calories. Since heat is Fire, the Heart is considered the organ of Fire and the Fire of the Heart is called the Monarch Fire. The heart was compared to the sun by a philosopher/medical doctor in the West. This has the same implication as the Monarch Fire. In Oriental medicine, excess joy is said to injure the Heart. Even though having a joyful emotion is beneficial to health, it becomes an illness in excess. We often hear stories about the old mother who meets her lost son unexpectedly and faints. There are other examples where a poverty stricken person becomes an overnight millionaire through a business success, credit, prize winning, etc. then loses his mental balance.

2. The following statement illustrates the relationship between the organs and the emotions.

"Excess anger injures Liver, excess thinking injures Spleen, excess anxiety injures Lung, excess fear injures Kidney and excess fright injures Gall Bladder." *Inner Classic*

Even emotional activities consume a lot of energy. If one does not get the opportunity to rest and recuperate, the degree of fatigue will gradually intensify due to continued strong emotional activities. In the end, maintaining good health will not be possible. There are many cases of disease occurring as a result of excess anxiety, extreme excitement and strong fear.

3. Excess sexual activity

It has been said since traditional times that fatigue due to sexual activity becomes the cause of lung disease for the most part and this is proven by facts. A large amount of vital energy is dissipated through sexual intercourse. Accordingly, everyone experiences the loss of vitality, especially in the power of resistance.[28] Time is needed in order to replenish

---

28. The weakening of the immune system. In Oriental medicine, excessive sexual activity is one of the causes of a disease. One is said to easily catch cold, especially if he or she goes out in the cold weather immediately after sexual activity.

the vital energy that was used up in sexual intercourse, the duration of which will vary according to the person. Whether it is five days, ten days or one month, if the fatigue constantly accumulates by performing the sexual act again before complete recovery, one will not be able to avoid the ultimate breakdown of health.

4. Excess strain

Continuously exerting excess effort day and night without time for sleep and rest also injures health. When this is accompanied by malnutrition and emotional anxiety, it is even more dangerous.

5. Excessive alcoholic drinks

Drinking excess alcoholic beverages injures health because physiological activity is excessively continued over a long period of time as a result of alcohol stimulation.

6. *Yin* Deficiency and *Yang* Deficiency

As stated above, when the body is fatigued, a *Yang* Deficient constitution occurs if the body reacts passively to the fatigue. A *Yin* Deficient constitution occurs if the body reacts actively. Diseases occur acutely in a person with *Yin* Deficient constitution and chronically in a *Yang* Deficient constitution. The condition resulting from this fatigue can only be attributed to inherent constitution. A person with a *Yin* Deficient tendency should promptly regulate his or her constitution to prevent occurrence of lung disease.

DIET

1. Malnourishment – needless to say, it is not possible to maintain health if one does not ingest plenty of nutrients in his or her diet.
2. Overdrinking, overeating and an irregular eating schedule – not eating at proper times or in proper amounts, will result in a disease.
3. Improper use of heat producing foods or herbs – through ingesting too many stimulating and tasty foods or through taking *Yang* tonics (stimulating aphrodisiacs) excessively to increase sexual energy will incline the body's constitution toward *Yin* Deficiency.
4. Improper use of heat reducing foods or herbs – as a result of being too afraid of becoming *Yin* Deficient and ingesting foods that promote urination and bowel movement in large amounts or overconsumption of formulas with bitter, cold, sinking and settling properties will injure *Yang*. In this way, vital energy becomes depressed and many symptoms of *Yin* Syndrome appear.
5. Toxic substances – ingesting toxic foods or herbs or foods that contain germs will result in a disease.

EXTERNAL PATHOGENS – TOXINS (CAUSE OF ILLNESS)

"Invasion by External Pathogens" is a general term for weather and season related acute disease. A disease that occurs from imbalance in physiological regulation due to sudden change in environmental temperature and humidity is also called "Invasion by External Pathogens." In infectious diseases due to germs, the infectious period is generally fixed, having an intimate relationship with coldness, heat, dryness and dampness of weather. Since the symptoms of the disease occur as an External Syndrome with chills, fever, etc. they are all referred to as "Invasion by External Pathogens."

1. Toxins (germs) – all diseases resulting from germs are considered to be "toxins" in Oriental medicine. In external diseases there may be ulceration, carbuncles, furuncles, cellulitis, etc. In internal infectious disease due to germs, there may be septicemia, plague, malaria, cholera, etc. In combinations of internal and external diseases, there may be smallpox, measles, etc.

2. *Yang* Toxin and *Yin* Toxin – *Yang* Toxin implies a disease causing germ that makes a *Yang* Syndrome occur and *Yin* Toxin implies a disease causing germ that makes *Yin* Syndrome occur. For example, the bacteria of scarlet fever and malaria can be regarded as *Yang* Toxins, whereas the bacteria of cholera can be regarded as *Yin* Toxins.

3. Physiological imbalance – sudden change or abnormal temperature and humidity in the environment disrupts the normal physiological regulation so that many diseases are created: *Shang Han* Syndrome (Injury due to Cold) is the main example of this. The Six Climatic Energies which are Wind, Cold, Summer Heat, Dampness, Dryness and Heat reflect changes in the environment.

4. *Yang* Pathogen and *Yin* Pathogen – invasion by external pathogens of the *Yang* Syndrome is called *Yang* Pathogen and invasion by external pathogens of the *Yin* Syndrome is called *Yin* Pathogen.

DEFICIENCY AND THE PATHOGENIC FACTOR – DISHARMONY OF YIN–YANG AND THE RECUPERATIVE FUNCTION

1. Since Deficiencies are usually chronic, the body itself is weak and cannot be cured in a short time.

2. Since an External Pathogen causes a temporary disease, it can be quickly cured.

3. I want to avoid a lengthy explanation on the relationship between the disharmony of *Yin–Yang* and recovery through these illustrations.

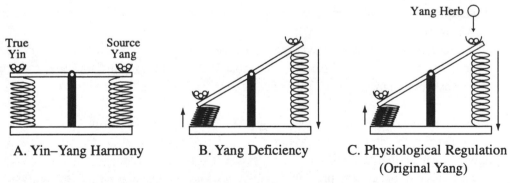

A. Yin–Yang Harmony   B. Yang Deficiency   C. Physiological Regulation
                                                        (Original Yang)

* Illustration (C) is supplementing the deficiency according to physiological demand. *Yin* Deficiency can be thought of as opposite to this.

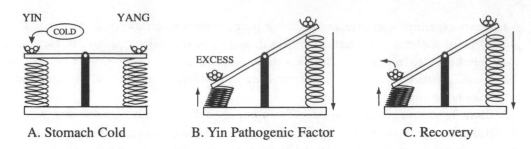

A. Stomach Cold   B. Yin Pathogenic Factor   C. Recovery

* Illustration (C) is eliminating excessive Cold. *Yang* pathogenic factor is opposite to this.

DEFICIENCY–EXCESS OF YIN–YANG AND TONIFICATION–SEDATION

Tonifying the deficiency and sedating the excess is the fundamental principle of treatment. If a deficiency is sedated, then the deficiency will become even more deficient and if the excess is tonified, then the excess will become even more excessive. To give concrete examples:

A. Lung disease is Yin Deficient disease

Lung disease will be cured by supplementing the Deficient *Yin*. Without this, recovery is not possible. To tonify *Yin*, one has to use sweet, cool and calming herbs such as cooked rehmannia, raw rehmannia, peony, ophiopogon, achyranthis, dioscorea, glehnia, etc. Formulas like *Liu Wei Di Huang Tang* (Six Rehmannia Decoction), *Zuo Gui Yin* (Restore the Left Decoction) and *Zi Yin Jiang Huo Tang* (Tonify *Yin* and Sedate Fire Decoction) become the basic formulas to which herbs are added or subtracted and used.[29] If this *Yin* Deficient Syndrome (initial stage of lung disease) is diagnosed as a common cold and mistreated, overstrain will occur. There are two reasons why one can easily mistreat initial stage lung disease as a common cold:

1. Symptoms such as chills, fever, cough, coughing up phlegm, irritability, etc. are similar to a common cold.
2. The patient who is frightened over terms like lung disease and does not want to get that type of diagnosis will insist many times that it is a common cold and will receive treatment for a common cold. This actually nurtures the lung disease.

Diaphoretic (inducing sweat) and anti–pyretic (reducing fever) formulas are used in the treatment of the common cold. Herbs that are frequently used as diaphoretics have pungent, warm, ascending and dispersing properties such as ephedra, cinnamon twig, asarum, aconite, fresh ginger, pinellia, atractylodes, schizonepeta, siler, perilla leaf, etc.

The reason why these herbs are not suitable for lung disease is as follows:

1. Because the herbs with pungent, warm, ascending and dispersing properties are all *Yang* natured herbs, using the above listed herbs first supplements the heat. Supplementing heat to a disease that occurred as a result of excess heat worsens the disease.

---

29. For details regarding these herbs and formulas, see appendix I and II.

2. A *Yin* Deficient person should not be made to sweat. The body's water is insufficient due to excess body temperature. Since sweat is the body's water (namely *Yin*), dispersing *Yin* worsens the Deficiency of *Yin*, which in turn worsens the disease.
3. Since the bacteria of tuberculosis is *Yang*, using *Yang* natured herbs promotes the disease.

For these reasons, it is inappropriate to relieve the heat of lung disease through diaphoretic and anti–pyretic formulas.

B. The Common Cold is referred to as Cold Evil and is namely an Excess Yin Syndrome

The cause of the common cold is "Cold blocking the sweat pores." In other words, the body's skin pores contract excessively due to a sudden contact with Cold Qi, so that breathing and sweating through the skin becomes completely impossible. The body's effort to eliminate abnormality in the metabolism due to that is namely the fever of "*Shang Han*." Even though fever develops, if one looks for its cause he or she will find that the *Yang* is deficient. Among the functions of Yang is its power to re–open contracted skin pores quickly. Therefore, *Yang* natured herbs that are pungent and warm are used to supplement the opening of skin pores. If one misinterprets this as a symptom of lung disease and says that chills, fever, cough, coughing up phlegm, bleeding from the nose and irritability are all symptoms of lung disease or if one becomes worried about a lung disease and uses a *Yin* Tonifying formula to quickly treat the disease, the following will occur:

1. Since sweating does not occur as a result of *Yang* Deficiency, even less sweating will occur by supplementing *Yin*.
2. Skin pores will open by using ascending–dispersing techniques. By astringing–descending, a common cold will get even deeper and become more difficult to cure.

Common colds that are not that simple, and even extremely complicated in actual practice, will be discussed in the prescription chapter.

THE STUDY OF ZANG FU

$\mathcal{T}$he internal organs are classified into *Zang* and *Fu* according to their functions: A *Zang* organ does not rest for even a moment and works as long as a person is alive, whereas a *Fu* organ works from time to time according to the demand.

There are Five *Zang* organs which are the Heart, Lung, Spleen, Liver and Kidney and Six *Fu* organs which are the Small Intestine, Large Intestine, Stomach, Urinary Bladder and Triple Burner. It needs to be understood before discussing *Zang Fu* is that the so–called Heart, Kidney or Gall Bladder in Oriental medicine have a much different meaning than the heart, kidney and gall bladder according to modern anatomy and physiology. Heart according to Oriental medicine has a much wider scope than the heart of Western medicine. When criticized scholastically, the width of this scope is considered too vague. This type of criticism by Western science, which has a limited understanding of the complicated and mysterious functions of living organisms, actually describes a strength of Oriental medicine. It is interesting to note that there have been philosophers in the West who have viewed organs similar to those in Oriental medicine.

I. FUNCTIONS OF ZANG FU ORGAN

Since the theory of *Zang Fu* organs in Oriental medicine is not a study based on dissection, but on physiological phenomena and the syndromes of organisms, it often looks like Oriental medicine ignores the anatomical position of organs. However, this is a result of placing significance on the physiological phenomena rather than a lack of anatomical knowledge. For example, in left–sided hemiplegia, we value the physiological phenomena and consider the disease as being on the left side even though the right hemisphere of the brain is diseased. In the same way, although the stomach is located above and the intestines are located below, according to their reactions, the stomach is called Foot *Yangming*, and is located in the lower position. The large intestine is called Hand *Yangming,* and is located in the upper position (refer to the Channel chapter).

ZANG ORGANS

A. Heart

The organ that represents the "Heart" of the Oriental medicine is the physiological heart and its duty is to circulate the blood throughout the body. The person being alive implies that this heart is active.

The heart distributes nutrients throughout the body and supplies oxygen to maintain body temperature. It offers dynamic force to the operation of life. It transports metabolized products and eliminates them outside the body. It sends blood full of carbon dioxide to the lungs and exchanges it with oxygenated blood. It then sends the constituents that will become urine to the kidneys to be filtered. This is a general duty of the heart when viewed physiologically. In Oriental medicine, however, mental functions of the human also belong to the Heart. When considered superficially, it sounds extremely unscientific. One might ask, "mental functions are carried out by the brain, so what is meant by the heart?" Without connecting mental function to the heart's function, we cannot even begin to imagine. A person with a healthy heart action has a healthy mind and a person with a weak heart has a dull mind. A person with mental instability inevitably shows an abnormality in the activity of the heart. A person who feels fear has a heartbeat particular to fear and accordingly, has a facial color and expression particular to fear. It is the same with anger, joy and all other emotions. Not only that, the region that senses physiological change due to emotional change is the chest, which is the region of the heart. When anticipating joy, the heart throbs. When experiencing intense grief, heartache occurs. When experiencing fear, the heart has a chill of horror. When suffering disappointment in love, we say there is a nail in the heart. These are all due to realizing that the heart is the place where emotional reactions occur. The reason for calling disappointed love a "broken heart" is that one experiences pain, as if the heart is rupturing when disappointed love occurs.

It is neither meaningless nor coincidental that the word indicating heart is identical to the word indicating mental function in both the East and the West. It is not that Oriental medicine does not know the brain. The saying, "The Brain is the Sea of Marrow" implies that the brain is the nerve center and the saying, "The Head is the Storehouse of Spiritual faculties" implies that mental function is connected to the head region.

> "The Heart is a King organ where the spiritual faculties reside ...... Heart is the master of the body, a Monarch organ. There is a physical heart which is shaped like an unopened lotus flower and resides above the liver and below the lungs. There is a spiritual Heart too. Spirit is transformed from *Qi* and Blood and is a Foundation of Life. Prosperity and growth of all matters arise from it." *Introduction to Oriental Medicine*[1]

The reason for considering the Heart as the King organ is because the existence/decline

---

1. This book was written in 1580 A.D. by Li Cun and consists of eight volumes. This book includes charts of the Zang Fu organs, brief biographies of the doctors prior to the Ming dynasty (1368-1644 A.D.), channels, Zang Fu organs, diagnosis, treatment principles and the methods, including acupuncture, moxibustion and herbs. In addition, this book discusses internal and external diseases, gynecology, pediatrics, emergency medicine, unusual diseases, etc.

and strength/weakness of one's body is tied to the Heart, and the Heart presides over emotions such as joy, anger, worry and fear.

B. Lungs

The lungs breathe air. When the venous blood that flows back to the heart is sent to the lungs by a pulmonary artery, the lungs eliminate carbon dioxide from that blood. After the blood becomes fresh by becoming oxygenated, the lungs send the blood to the heart by a pulmonary vein to be circulated throughout the body again. It will be absolutely correct to interpret "Lung governs *Qi*" as breathing air or gas. *Qi* implies life force or Original Energy. In other words, it implies the dynamic force of an organism. Since this dynamic force is acquired through combustion of oxygen, the *Qi* of breath that assimilates oxygen is considered identical with *Qi* of life force.

"Lungs govern circulation of *Ying* and *Wei*, and is an official in charge of mutual transmission." *Introduction to Oriental Medicine*

"Without Blood, *Qi* cannot transform; without *Qi*, Blood cannot circulate." (*Zhang Jing Yue*)

Assimilation of oxygen and elimination of carbon dioxide is carried out by red blood cells, so this is expressed in the statement, "Without Blood, *Qi* cannot transform." When there is no oxygen in the blood, the blood vessels constrict and block the circulation of the blood, resulting in death and stoppage of breathing. There is not even a little blood within the blood vessels when breathing stops. So this is expressed in the statement, "Without *Qi*, Blood cannot circulate" and yet, *Ying* is Blood and *Wei* is *Qi* and the function of the lungs is to facilitate the circulation of *Qi* and Blood and promote the combustive action of the body. This is expressed in the statement, "Lungs control circulation of *Qi* and Blood." Since the lungs have the duty of exchanging carbon dioxide and oxygen, they are referred to as " The official in charge of mutual transmission." There are two types of breathing:

1. External breathing – this implies the lungs discharging the carbon dioxide of venous blood and assimilating oxygen to make arterial blood. External breathing is also done through the skin.
2. Breathing by the tissues (Internal breathing) – this refers to oxygen within arterial blood being assimilated by the tissues which give off carbon dioxide to ultimately create venous blood.

"Lung is a warehouse of skin and body hair." *Inner Classic*
"Lung governs skin and body hair." *Inner Classic*

Even the skin discharges carbon dioxide. The quantity of discharge greatly increases when there is excess sweating and small amounts of oxygen are also assimilated by the skin. Thus, lungs and skin have a common point in their function. Therefore, the skin must be made healthy in order to strengthen the lungs. The reason for the effectiveness of cold water massage, cold wind baths, sun baths, etc. on the lung disease patient, is that the skin is made stronger. When the breathing and sweating by the skin become impossible due to Invasion by the Cold, it is the lungs that are first affected. The lungs are the most developed parts of the skin; this can be clearly observed in the lower animals.

C. Spleen

According to Oriental medicine, the Spleen is said to be in charge of digestion and nutrition. Accordingly, the Spleen is compared to the Earth. Similar to the Earth nurturing all things, the Spleen nourishes the flesh of the whole body. I see the anatomical spleen and pancreas as the organs in charge of the Spleen's function. The Spleen and Stomach become the paired organs as the husband and wife organs and the pancreas secretes digestive juices.

"The Spleen resides in the upper abdomen. It grinds food and grains through which it nourishes the other four *Zang* organs. If the *Qi* of the Spleen is strong, food and grains get ground and digested. Since the Spleen resides in the middle, it transports the essence of food and grain to nourish the flesh and face, making them lustrous. If the Spleen is strong, the buttocks are well developed, but if the energy of the Spleen is cut off, muscles of the buttocks disappear." *Introduction to Oriental Medicine*

1. Physiological Function of the Spleen

The spleen has slow and regular contractions and the following are presumed to be its functions:

(a) Formation of white blood cells – the venous blood of the spleen has a greater white blood cell count than its arterial blood.
(b) It destroys white blood cells.
(c) It destroys red blood cells. Cells that contain many levels of the breakdown of red blood cells can be seen inside the spleen pulp.
(d) It is also said to produce new red blood cells.

The spleen is notably enlarged during times of various kinds of infectious disease. It can be presumed that the duty of the spleen is to make pathogens harmless through the large amounts of cells produced. So–called "tortoise stomach" or "abdominal malaria" in children is the result of a disease that combines the enlargement of the spleen with alternating chills and fever, poor appetite and fatigue of the body and extremities. I do not know to what extent the function of the spleen will be investigated according to physiology in the future, but at the present level of understanding, we cannot say that we know all the functions of the spleen.

2. Function of the pancreas

The pancreas secretes alkaline digestive juices. The secretion of pancreatic juice starts after the ingestion of food and is significantly increased following the transfer of acidic stomach contents into the intestine.

Included among the digestive juices of the pancreas are enzymes that dissolve starch into maltose and maltose into glucose. Thus, a sweet taste is said to belong to the Spleen and a sour taste to the Liver. This is the reason for using barley sprouts in the digestive formulas in Oriental medicine.

Stomach juice and bile are acidic digestive juices and pancreatic juice is alkaline digestive juice. When these are not secreted adequately, indigestion will result. "Wood overacting on Earth," that is, "Excess Liver overacting on Spleen" implies that indigestion has occurred due to secretion of large amounts of acidic digestive juice (Liver) in comparison to alkaline digestive juice (Spleen).

Pancreatic juice is said to be able to transfer from the duodenum to the stomach. It is difficult to affirm whether pancreatic juice or a juice similar to it is secreted there, but alkaline digestive juices all depend on the function of the spleen when viewed according to Oriental medicine.

3. The reasons for attaching the pancreas to the Spleen

(a) The Spleen is in charge of digestion and the pancreas secretes digestive juice.

(b) Sweet taste belongs to the Spleen and the assimilation of carbohydrate, namely sugar, is carried out by the pancreas. Diabetes is related to the pancreas.

(c) "Wood controls Earth"–the functions of the Spleen and Liver are in mutual opposition. This relationship can be found in the acidity of bile and the alkalinity of pancreatic juice.

(d) Earth controls Water – the functions of the Spleen and Kidneys are in mutual opposition. This relationship refers to the "mutual suppressing function" between the adrenal gland (endocrine) and the pancreas (endocrine).

(e) The special point on the Spleen and Kidneys – among the practitioners of Oriental medicine, some say tonifying the Spleen is not better than tonifying the Kidneys and others say tonifying the Kidneys is not better than tonifying the Spleen. In other words, all diseases disappear when the digestion is good and health comes about when the vital energy is flourishing. Setting aside which is correct or incorrect, one cannot disagree that the Spleen and Kidneys are the most important of all the organs for regaining or maintaining health. It is rather natural for the Spleen, which is equally as important as the Kidneys, to have an endocrine gland (the pancreas) that belongs to it, while there are adrenal glands, reproductive glands, prostate gland, etc. that belong to the Kidneys. Viewed according to the channels, the Kidneys and the Spleen have special channels that other organs do not have.

> "There are 12 Main channels which are the three *Yin* and three *Yang* channels of the hand and foot. There are 15 *Luo* (connecting) channels; each of the 12 Main channels has one *Luo* channel. The Spleen has one Great *Luo* channel which together with the *Luo* channels of Conception and Governing channels makes 15." *Difficult Classic*[2]

The Conception and Governing channels belong to the Kidneys.

---

2. This classic is reputed to have been written around 300 B.C. by Bian Que. It consists of 81 chapters and expounds on the difficult information contained in the Inner Classic through question and answer format.

D. Liver

1. Physiological Function of Liver

(a) It produces urea – the liver is the region where urea is produced in large amounts from ammonia. Immediately after a dog dies, artificially injecting blood with added carbon ammonia into its liver and making it flow through a portal vein results in decreased ammonia content and increased urea content in the blood at the time of the flow. Also, by directly connecting the portal vein with the inferior vena cava to artificially remove the liver from the blood circulation, or at the time of various liver disorders, the quantity of urea discharged will decrease and the quantity of ammonia and amino acids discharged in the urine will increase.

The purpose of producing urea from ammonium salt is to transform harmful ammonia, which is the end product of protein metabolism, into harmless chemical compounds. When the liver is removed, certain symptoms that are peculiar to ammonia poisoning occur.

> "Liver controls urination. If there is Deficiency of Blood in the Liver channel, use *Si Wu Tang* (Four Substance Decoction) with gardenia. If there is difficult urination with pain in the urethra, it belongs to Damp–Heat in the Liver, so use *Long Dan Xie Gan Tang* (Gentiana Combination)."[3]

Thus, the statement "Liver controls urination" is in accord with Western medical theory.

(b) It destroys and produces red blood cells.
(c) It secretes bile.
(d) It has a detoxifying function.
(e) It stores nutrients.

2. The Power of Combat and Liver

The Liver is said to be a "general" which implies that it presides over fighting. The Oriental saying of "having a thick Liver" and the western saying of "having a lot of Gall" all imply facts about the relationship between fighting and the Liver. Anger, which is the motive power for fighting belongs to the Liver.

```
                    ┌─ nutrition (preservation of individual)  – Spleen ─┐
Life of human ──────┼─ reproduction (extension of life)        – Kidney ──┼── Foot 3 Yin Channels
                    └─ competition (attainment of goal)         – Liver ──┘
```

3. Liver stores Blood

The blood implies nutritive substance and the liver stores nutrients called glycogen. Blood that has newly absorbed nutrients from the intestine passes through the liver by way of the portal vein and goes on to the heart. Liver oil, highly recommended by Western doctors, is said to be beneficial to the body. Eating the liver of an animal is miraculously

---

3. For the herbs in these formulas, see Chapter 7 on prescriptions or appendix II.

effective for nightblindness due to malnutrition.

E. Kidneys

The physiological kidney is simply the organ that excretes urine, but the Kidney according to Oriental medicine is extremely vast in its scope.

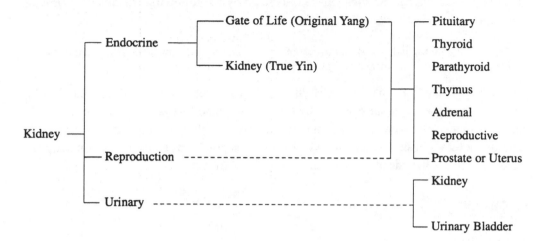

The Kidneys are the source of life force in a broad sense. So–called Original energy, Original power, Vital energy and Vitality, all imply intangible functions of the Kidneys. When the Kidneys are sufficiently understood, it is not an exaggeration to say that one's foundation in Oriental medicine has been established.

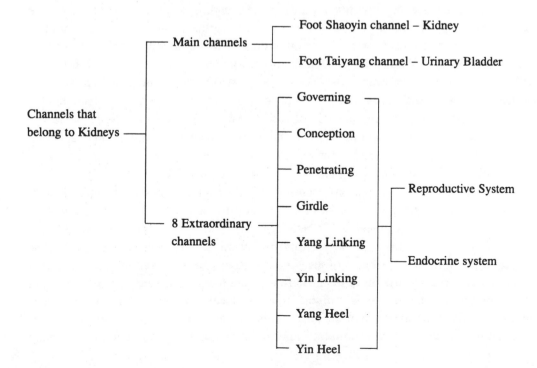

Even though these Eight Extraordinary channels are all made to belong to the Kidneys, it can be inferred that there is an intimate relationship between the Penetrating channel and the Spleen/Stomach and the Girdle channel and the Liver/Gall Bladder. The thyroid gland is at the end of the Penetrating channel and when the thyroid is enlarged, there are cases where the metabolism accelerates unusually so that the appetite becomes several times that of an average person. This is illustrated by the following statement in Oriental medicine:

> "Fire enters Spleen and Stomach; the person eats all the time but constantly feels hungry and drinks all the time but constantly feels thirst."

The Fire is the "Fire within the Kidneys" or "Ministerial Fire." "Ministerial Fire" is presumed to be the hormone secreted by the thyroid gland that promotes *Yang*. When the metabolism increases enormously due to the oversecretion of the thyroid gland, the appetite increases in surprising amounts in order to supply and replenish the raw materials burned up by the increased metabolism.

FU ORGANS

A. Stomach

The stomach is the most important of the digestive organs. When food comes in, the stomach secretes digestive juices and compacts food to make assimilation by the body easier. At the same time, it issues work orders to each of the digestive organs. The official messenger with a command for bile secretion is sent to the liver and the official messenger with a command for pancreatic juice secretion is sent to the pancreas.

The stomach has a most important duty among many organs. It is the organ in charge of nourishment for the whole body. Hence, the stomach must have an intimate communicatory relationship with all the other organs. It is analogous to the Treasury or Ministry of Finance. When each government institution notifies the Treasury of its budget demand, the Treasury considers the demands and establishes the budget. Similarly, the stomach refers to each organ of the body to determine the amount of food intake. Accordingly, appetite and preferences of food speak for the person's state of health. Although stomach abnormalities such as indigestion, nausea/vomiting, poor appetite, excess hunger, etc. are confined to the region of the stomach, their cause must be sought out holistically from the physiological state of the person's whole body.

Many people state that a strong stomach is all a person needs to maintain health. Needless to say, it is a justifiable statement. A healthy person does not have digestive problems, but many sick people do. Whether or not a person has a disease can be based on whether or not there is a digestive problem. Yet tracing back to the cause, a disease usually occurs due to a weakness of the body resulting in a weak stomach, rather than a weak stomach causing the disease. Aside from acute stomach disorders due to harmful foods, treating the chronic stomach disease through "local treatment" of the stomach does not necessarily result in effective treatment. This indicates that the fundamental cause of stomach disease is not in the stomach. This can be demonstrated through the following facts:

1. When a person gets assaulted or receives a physical injury, he or she often has a complete loss of appetite for a short time. Until the moment of encountering that assault or injury, there was no trouble with digestion or anything that could have injured the stomach, but losing the appetite due to physical injury is not as a result of any breakdown in the stomach region. Rather, the loss of appetite results from the body putting all its effort into the recuperation of the fatigue due to external injury. The body gives a message to the stomach that there is no available energy to digest incoming foods, rejecting the ingestion of food beforehand.

2. Eating at the table with a regular appetite and the same taste as usual, but losing the appetite immediately upon hearing about an upsetting event is not a result of a stomach disorder.

3. In so–called "love–sickness," a person is not able to digest even a bowl of soup, but upon meeting the person he or she is longing for, not only does his or her appetite and digestion recover in a day, they thrive over their usual limit. In the same way, vomiting immediately upon discovering a bug in the soup one is enjoying is not the result of an abnormality in the stomach region itself.

The following are quotes regarding the importance attached to the stomach in Oriental medicine:

"When food is well digested, no disease will develop and Five *Zang* organs will be at ease. The Stomach controls the production of *Yang Qi* and is the origin of Six *Fu* organs." *Introduction to Oriental Medicine*

"The Spleen and Stomach are the Sea of Water and Grain, the Gate of Life is the Sea of Essence and Blood, equally, they are the foundation of Five *Zang* and Six *Fu* organs." *(Zhang Jing Yue)*

Pulse diagnosis and Stomach Qi

In pulse diagnosis, there is great importance attached to having Stomach *Qi* and having Stomach *Qi* means there is a harmonious and relaxed feeling in the pulse beat.

Channels and Stomach

Among the channels, the Stomach channel is the only *Yang* channel located on the anterior side of the human body. When examining the intersecting and communicating relationship between the channels, the Stomach channel has an intimate relationship with the Spleen, Lung, Kidney, Penetrating, *Yin* Heel, *Yang* Heel, *Yin* Linking and *Yang* Linking channels. It connects with the Small Intestine, Large Intestine, Pericardium, Triple Burner, Gall Bladder, Urinary Bladder, Heart, Lung, Governing, Conception and Girdle channels. The mammary glands that nourish the infant belong to the Stomach channel and the milk is secreted by hormonal action, which gives us a glance at the complicated mechanism between Stomach and Kidney – between digestive and reproductive organs.

B. Small Intestine

The small intestine absorbs digested nutrients. Since the heart distributes these nutrients, there seems to be an intimate relationship between the heart and small intestine.

"Small intestine connects with stomach above and receives its dregs. It transports and transforms those dregs and sends them to the urinary bladder and large intestine below. Small intestine and Heart correspond with each other." *Introduction to Oriental Medicine*

The reference here, "sends to urinary bladder" sounds unreasonable. "Sends to large intestine" is reasonable according to anatomy, but "sends to urinary bladder" sounds unscientific. By observing the following phenomena, however, we can see that there might be a certain relationship between the small intestine and the urinary bladder:

1. When the Heart is fatigued, the color of the urine always turns dark yellow and becomes difficult to eliminate. Viewed according to the channels, the Heart, Small Intestine, Urinary Bladder and Kidneys are all related as one network.

2. In diarrhea, there are times when using the so–called "Separating water treatment technique" cures it easily. *Si Ling San* (Four Ingredient Powder with Poria), *Wu Ling San* (Five Ingredient Powder with Poria), *Wei Ling Tang* (Calm the Stomach and Poria Decoction), *Xiao Fen Qing Yin* (Minor Separate the Pure Decoction) and *Da Fen Qing Yin* (Major Separate the Pure Decoction) are all anti–diarrhetic medicinal formulas based on diuretics and *Da Fen Qing Yin* (Major Separate the Pure Decoction) is the most frequently used formula for gonorrhea.[4]

"In diarrhea, the cause is frequently in water and grain not separating, so the best treatment method is to promote urination. (*Zhang Jing Yue*)

Here, too, the emphasis was put on the phenomena. An observation was made that among the contents of the small intestine, water is discharged to the urinary bladder and solid matter comes out as feces through the large intestine. The small intestine and urinary bladder are adjacent to each other anatomically. So when water builds up excessively within the content of the small intestine, instead of that water being absorbed by the large intestine and circulated a few times inside the body and passed through the kidneys to come out as urine, it can be presumed to permeate the wall of the small intestine and urinary bladder, going directly from the small intestine to the urinary bladder. In accord with the progression of physiology and anatomy, some day this fact will be proven by experiment.

3. According to the theory on the autointoxication of the stomach and intestine, many changes are said to occur in the constituents of urine according to the condition of the intestine.

C. Large Intestine

The large intestine receives contents of the small intestine and absorbs water from it while the dregs are discharged as feces. It also occasionally discharges gas produced in the intestine.

The large intestine is a paired organ with the lungs. The lungs disperse water and the large intestine absorbs water. The lungs breathe air and the large intestine discharges gas. When there is heat in the Lungs, the stool is dry and when the function of the Lungs is

---

4. See the appendix II on the formulas.

weak, the stool is loose. There is constipation at the initial stage of a lung disease and there is tenesmus[5] at the end stage.

D. Gall Bladder

The gall bladder is attached to the gap in the liver and stores bile, which is the secretion of the liver. It then discharges bile to the small intestine when the contents of the stomach start to come out through the pylorus. Bile, discharged by the liver, contains three percent solid matter. When the intestine is empty, bile does not discharge directly into the intestine, but first goes to the gall bladder and becomes thickened due to the loss of water. It is then mixed with mucus from the gall bladder, which results in the percentage of solid matter increasing to 17 percent.

Jaundice is a disease that develops from a spilling over of the stagnated bile constituents into the blood due to gallstones (cholelithiasis), inflammation of the biliary tract, liver abscess, etc. In a severe case of jaundice, coma or convulsions can occur. This is presumed to be caused by the acidic salt of the gall bladder, which spilled into the bloodstream, invading the central nervous system. When an injection of acidic salt is given to an animal, similar symptoms are said to appear. This is the reason for referring to diseases of the nervous system as "Wind" and as diseases belonging to the Liver in Oriental medicine. Then, has the function of the gall bladder physiologically been sufficiently covered by the above explanation? No. The explanation of the gall bladder's function is still in the boundaries of ambiguity and immaturity. Next, I am going to discuss the gall bladder from the viewpoint of Oriental or philosophical medicine:

1. The Liver is presumed to be an endocrine organ that produces the dynamic force of combat.

Plato, considered to be the father of Western scholastics, classified man's personality into four types. Among the four types, a man with a serene composure and firm character, is also the most appropriate for combat and was called a "Bile Type." In the Orient, statements such as: "having a large Gall Bladder," "power of the Gall Bladder is strong" and "has a thick Liver" all imply that the dynamic force of combat comes from the Gall Bladder. Violent combat comes from strong rage and strong rage changes facial color to blue/green. This blue/green color of rage is considered to originate from the function of the Liver (refer to the section on color in the Chapter 3).

2. The Gall Bladder is a Central Organ among *Zang Fu* organs. Although by classification the Gall Bladder belongs to the *Fu* organs, its character has differing points compared to other *Fu* organs. Thus, I think it should belong to the *Zang* organs. The following is a comparison of the functions of the *Fu* organs:

- Stomach receives external substances.
- Small intestine transmits external substances.
- Large intestine excretes external substances.

---

5. Tenesmus is a condition resulting from spasm of the sphincters of the anus and bladder with pain. There is a constant urge and ineffectual straining effort to empty the bowel or bladder.

- Urinary bladder excretes wastes that are produced in the body together with water.
- Gall bladder processes useful digestive juice secreted by the liver and supplies it to the small intestine.
- Pancreas secretes useful digestive juice by itself.

Thus, there are no big differences between the functions of the gall bladder and pancreas. The gall bladder is also presumed to be an organ that secretes certain types of hormones. A philosopher–medical doctor of the West compared the heart to the Sun and the gall bladder to Mars. Since the Heart is Monarch Fire and the Gall Bladder is Ministerial Fire in Oriental medicine, the viewpoint of the Gall Bladder being identified with the *Zang* organs is in agreement in both the East and West.

(1) Gall Bladder channel viewed in relation to the other channels.
Viewed according to the channels, the back of the body extends, is exterior and *Yang*. The abdomen contracts, is interior and *Yin*. The gall bladder is located on the flank and is neither back nor abdomen, exterior nor interior, *Yin* nor *Yang*, extension nor contraction, but it has one half of both sides. Therefore, the Gall Bladder channel is called "half–exterior and half–interior" or "half *Yin* and half *Yang*." According to the channels, since the Pericardium, Triple Burner, Gall Bladder, and Liver are considered as one system, it can be inferred that the Gall Bladder has an important duty in regulating the functions of all organs.

E. Urinary Bladder

The duty of the urinary bladder is that of discharging urine sent from the kidneys to the outside of the body. In Oriental medicine, too, the duty of the Urinary Bladder is to discharge urine, but when viewed according to the channels, the Urinary Bladder channel occupies almost one half of the whole body. It accompanies the Governing channel and covers the posterior one–half of the body. Among its acupuncture points are the Back–Shu points[6] of the Lung, Heart, Governing channel, diaphragm, Gall Bladder, Liver, Spleen, Stomach, Triple Burner, Kidney, Large Intestine, Small Intestine, Urinary Bladder, etc. and it appears to supervise all *Yang* channels.

F. The Gate of Life, Triple Burner, and Pericardium

1. The Gate of Life and the Endocrine System.
The Gate of Life and the Triple Burner are difficult subjects according to Oriental medicine. One must not go without knowing them, yet knowing them is difficult. The statement, "It has a name but no shape and has no shape but has use" is the best description of this Gate of Life and Triple Burner. They appear only as functions or phenomena, so it is difficult to grasp the nature of these organs. Thus, the explanations and assertions

---

6. The Back–Shu points or Associated points are acupuncture points that are located near the spine along the Urinary Bladder channel. They are associated with all of the Zang Fu organs. Thus, they are used in diagnosing and treating the disorders of the Zang Fu organs.

among Oriental medical scholars regarding the Gate of Life and Triple Burner are diverse.

I see the Gate of Life as a general name for the endocrine system. It is difficult to directly prove the existence of the endocrine system by modern medicine. Their existence is proved or assumed, in a limited way, indirectly with the phenomena and reactions based on clinical observation and experiments performed on humans and animals. This is expressed in the statement, "has no shape but has use."

When the Gate of Life is considered to control and regulate the operations of life by means of hormones, its function can be embodied in the following two ways:

(a) Operation of organs (Triple Burner).
(b) Prevention of breakdown (Pericardium).

For example, when the heart continuously beats and the lungs continuously breathe, the power of those functions is called Triple Burner. When the heart and lungs ceaselessly move, both organs mutually rub so that inflammation and heat are developed. If extreme, they will burn and breakdown. What prevents that is the power of the Pericardium. If machine oil is not put on a rotating machine, that machine will immediately break down. All organs have an apparatus like the oil of a machine that smooth out their movements and prevents breakdown due to friction. The pleura, peritoneum, etc. perform that function and the Pericardium represents this type of apparatus. Similar to machine oil being related to the machine operation, the Pericardium and related apparatus are ruled by the Gate of Life.

When the function of the Gate of Life is expressed physiologically, it is through the functions of both the Triple Burner and the Pericardium. The Triple Burner (Hand *Shaoyang*) and the Pericardium (Hand *Jueyin*) channels manifest functional states of the Gate of Life to the outside of the body and there is no separate Gate of Life channel. With this, one can suppose the relationship and classification of the Gate of Life, Triple Burner and Pericardium.

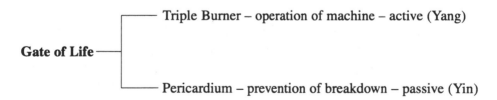

Gate of Life ─── Triple Burner – operation of machine – active (Yang)

Pericardium – prevention of breakdown – passive (Yin)

The force that operates organs is called the Triple Burner. The reason for this is that even though there are numerous organs, our metabolic activity can be usually divided into three stages:

(a) Ingestion (nutrients).
(b) Transportation and Transformation (assimilation).
(c) Elimination (by–products of metabolism).

Our metabolic activity does not go beyond these three stages.

2. Upper Burner and the Transportation/Transformation function.

Transportation and transformation of *Qi* and Blood, or the assimilation of substances, will not be able to be completed without blood circulation by the heart and oxygen supply by the lungs. Heart and lungs are located in the upper part of the body. Since the Upper Burner is above the diaphragm, having a disease in the Upper Burner implies that an abnormality has developed in the heart and lungs.

3. Middle Burner and the assimilation of nutrients.

Assimilation of nutrients is done through the process of digestion. The organs in charge of the digestive process are the stomach, pancreas (Spleen) and gall bladder. All of these organs are located in the central part of the body so the domain of the digestive organs is between the diaphragm and transverse colon. This is the Middle Burner.

4. Lower Burner and elimination.

The organs that are in charge of the elimination of waste are the kidneys, urinary bladder and large intestine. These are all located in the lower part of the body. Changes in the bowel movement and urination indicate that an abnormality has occurred in the Lower Burner.

Like the above, there is division of Upper, Middle and Lower Burners, but there is no definite dividing line between the Middle and the Lower Burner.

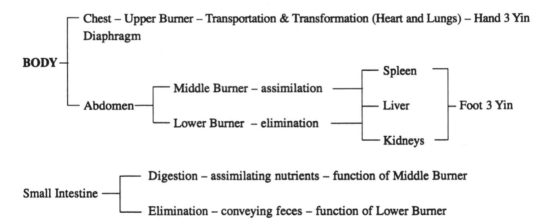

Since the Triple Burner can be envisioned as the location of the organs, I am going to give a traditional explanation.

"There is no explanation in the *Inner Classic* about the meaning of the Gate of Life. Yet, *Qin Yue Ren*[7] said that there exist two Kidneys, but both are not Kidneys; the left one is the Kidney and right one is the Gate of Life. The Gate of Life is a place where the mind resides. Original *Qi* is connected to the Gate of Life, and man stores Essence through it, and woman's uterus is connected to it." (*Zhang Jing Yue*)

---

7. Also known as Bian Que. He was a famous medical doctor in the period of the Warring States (403 – 221 B.C.).

"Gate of Life, located in the right Kidney, is not an ordinary *Zang* organ and Triple Burner is not an ordinary *Fu* organ." *Introduction to Oriental Medicine*

What is meant by right or left here is not the anatomical location, rather it is an explanation about the left and right of the manifestation of the Kidney's functional state. According to pulse diagnosis, the Kidney is examined on the left hand third position and the Gate of Life on the right hand third position. This is illustrated in the following quote.

"Kidney unites with Urinary Bladder. It is located in the left third pulse position and is pure Water. The Gate of Life unites with the Triple Burner, is located in the right third pulse position and is pure Fire." *Inner Classic*

Again, the function is utmost. The left Kidney is called True *Yin* and right Kidney (Gate of Life) is called Original *Yang* (refer to *Yin–Yang* Chapter).

In Oriental medicine, "Jing" or "Essence" is said to be stored in the Kidneys. It is the product of the endocrine system and implies hormones. Marrow implies the central nervous system, brain marrow and cerebrospinal fluid. Tendons imply motor nerves. Problems of physical movement are all diseases of the tendons. Kidneys dominate Jing and the Marrow. The Gate of Life is that which regulates the functions of the endocrine and central nervous system.

II. SCIENTIFIC DATA ON THE FIVE ELEMENT THEORY OF ZANG FU ORGANS

The Five Element Theory, according to Oriental medicine, explains the Five *Zang* organs of a human by associating each with one of the Five Elements. I am not going to explain, with this Five Element Theory, the principle of change in nature from the viewpoint of the *I Ching*, but I will try to explain the relationship between the organs, through Five Element Theory,[8] with simple interpretations that are easily understood.

A VIEW OF THE FIVE ZANG ORGANS BY THE PHILOSOPHERS OF EAST AND WEST

Matching the Five *Zang* organs with the Five Elements is done not only in Oriental medicine, but the philosopher–medical doctors of West also compared organs to celestial bodies. The following is the comparison between the two:

---

8. In ancient Greece, the universe was thought to be made up of four elements, these being Fire, Air, Water and Earth. In ancient China, there was a similar approach to the constituents of the universe, though the number of elements was five, these being Wood, Fire, Earth, Metal and Water.

		East	West
Heart	Heart – physical heart	Monarch Fire	Sun
	Brain – spiritual Heart (residence of mind)	Spirit	Moon
	Gate of Life – Ministerial Fire within Kidney	Ministerial Fire	
	Gall Bladder – Shaoyang Ministerial Fire	Ministerial Fire	Mars
Spleen		Earth	Saturn
Lung		Metal *	Mercury
Kidney		Water *	Venus
Liver		Wood	Jupiter [9]

1. There is a similarity in the Heart being called Fire (Monarch Fire) in the Orient and the heart being compared to the sun in the West.
2. The brain was compared to *Taiyin* (moon) in the West. Mental disease is sometimes called lunacy in English, which comes from the Latin word – luna, meaning "moon." This suggests that brain disease is related to the moon.

In the East, mental functions are seen as the intangible phenomena of the Heart. The following statement explains the relationship between the Heart and the mental function.

> "There is a Heart of spiritual faculties. The Spirit, transformed from *Qi* and Blood, is the foundation of life. All things in nature grow because of the Spirit. There is no color or shape attached to it. Spirit is said to exist but where can it be? Spirit is said to be non–existent, but it exists. It governs all things in nature." *Introduction to Oriental Medicine*

Looking at the statement, "Brain is the Sea of Marrow and the residence of Mind," shows that the relationship between mental function and the brain has not been entirely disregarded. Mental function is considered *Yin* in the East and corresponds to the theory which relates the brain to the Moon in the West. The following chart illustrates the phenomenon of life as interpreted by Oriental medicine.

---

9. In the Orient, Sun represents Yang and Moon represents Yin. The correspondence of planets to the Five Elements in the Orient is as follows: Mars is the planet of Fire, Saturn is the planet of Earth, Mercury is the planet of Water, Venus is the planet of Metal and Jupiter is the planet of Wood.

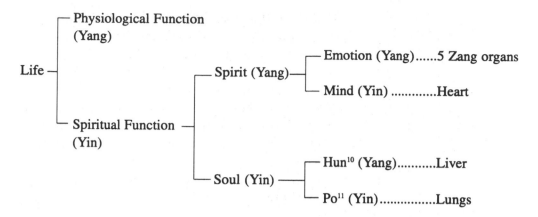

Po denotes an extremely stupefied function of the brain nerves that persists until the last moment of life. The Lungs are said to store *Po* since the stoppage of breath, the dispersion of the *Po* and death occur at the same time.

Looking at the process of going from health to death:

(a) When the body is healthy, emotional activity is proper.

(b) When the body is weak, emotional activity "tilts toward one side."

(c) When the body is extremely weak, the gamut of emotions do not function much and there is only dispassionate mental function.[12]

(d) After the loss of mental function, certain abnormal brain nerve functions such as delirious speech, emotional activity during dreams, etc. can be observed. This is called *Hun*. It is said that, "*Hun* travels and *Po* stays still." So *Hun* is *Yang* and active in comparison to *Po*.

(e) Right before death, there is not even delirious speech; only breath is gathered in the state of coma. At this time, it is said that there is no function by *Hun* and only *Po* remains.

(f) *Po* disappears at the same time the breath stops. At this instant a person dies. The boundary of life and death is fixed here, but in a strict sense, for all tissues of the human body to die, a certain amount of time is needed after the breathing stops.

3. The gall bladder, being compared to Mars in the West, does not differ much from the comparison made in the East. The Gall Bladder is recognized as Fire in the East and is called Ministerial Fire in comparison to the Monarch Fire.

4. Lung (Metal) and Kidney (Water) is changed to Water (lung) and Metal (kidney) in the West. However, since the Metal and Water are in a mutual generating relationship in Five Element Theory, even though they are interchanged, there is no particular difference in the relationship between the kidney and the lung.

---

10. Ethereal soul.

11. Corporeal soul.

12. The person becomes "cold" mentally, without much emotion.

THE GENERATING AND CONTROLLING CYCLES OF THE FIVE ELEMENTS AND THE SUPPRESSING AND PROMOTING RELATIONSHIPS OF THE ORGANS

Five Element Theory is an ideological system that tries to observe and explain all phenomena in the universe through the mutual suppressing and promoting relationships between five symbols which are Water, Fire, Metal, Wood and Earth.

In contrast to the *Yin–Yang* Theory which observes the phenomena of the universe through two opposing symbols, the Five Element Theory deals with the serial relations and circulating nature of the five symbols. All phenomena, such as the movement of the heavenly bodies, weather of the seasons, prosperity and decline of organisms, etc. eternally circulate without beginning or end and can be explained and unified with the mutual generating and controlling cycles of the Five Elements.

Regarding the Five *Zang* organs in the Five Element Theory, rather than explaining why Heart is considered as Fire and Spleen is Earth, I believe that inquiring whether or not the suppressing and promoting relationships between the organs agree with the principles of mutual generating and controlling cycles in Five Element Theory will facilitate the understanding of this theory.

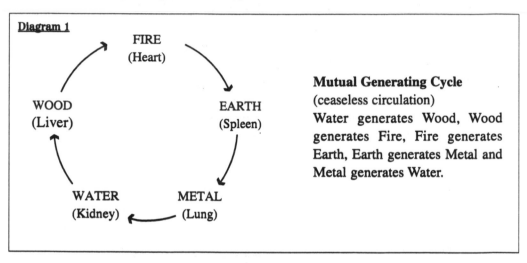

Diagram 1

FIRE (Heart) — WOOD (Liver) — EARTH (Spleen) — WATER (Kidney) — METAL (Lung)

Mutual Generating Cycle
(ceaseless circulation)
Water generates Wood, Wood generates Fire, Fire generates Earth, Earth generates Metal and Metal generates Water.

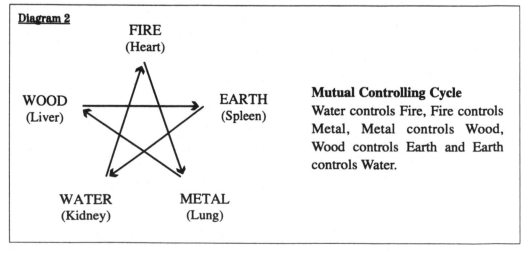

Diagram 2

FIRE (Heart) — WOOD (Liver) — EARTH (Spleen) — WATER (Kidney) — METAL (Lung)

Mutual Controlling Cycle
Water controls Fire, Fire controls Metal, Metal controls Wood, Wood controls Earth and Earth controls Water.

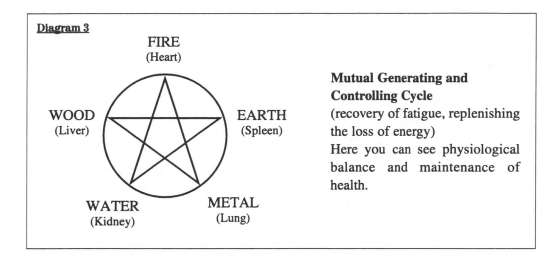

Diagram 3

FIRE
(Heart)

WOOD
(Liver)

EARTH
(Spleen)

WATER
(Kidney)

METAL
(Lung)

Mutual Generating and Controlling Cycle
(recovery of fatigue, replenishing the loss of energy)
Here you can see physiological balance and maintenance of health.

- The curved line is the Mutual Generating Cycle
- The straight line is the Mutual Controlling Cycle

A. Fire generates Earth - The Relationship between Heart and Spleen

Since Fire implies heat, the body temperature increases when the activity of the heart is exuberant. Persons with low body temperature often have digestive disorders and persons with vigorous blood circulation have hearty appetites and sound digestion.

A lung disease patient, in the initial stage, has a stronger appetite and digestive power than the average person. We can often observe in some people that their appetite thrives when they catch a common cold. This implies the empowerment of digestion as a consequence of mild fever – equivalent to Fire generating Earth. Even in common sense, there is a need to supply large amounts of fuel when combustive action is exuberant. Our body is physiologically structured that way.

It would also be possible to describe the relationship between spleen and heart through the destruction and production of red and white blood cells that occur in the spleen.

B. Fire controls Metal - The Relationship between Heart and Lungs

When the activity of the heart becomes exuberant, the lungs become weak due to fatigue. The breathing becomes difficult as a result of extreme fever. Violent exercise such as running also makes breathing difficult. This relationship is referred to in Oriental medicine as "Fire controlling Metal." When large amounts of carbonic acid build up inside the body due to vigorous blood circulation, carbonic acid inside the blood stimulates breathing centers, creating excessive activity by the lungs. Continuing for a long time, this weakens the lungs, thus creating lung disease. Deficiency of *Yin* with Exuberance of Fire signals the initial stage of lung disease in Oriental medicine.

Although the Exuberance of Fire can be attributed to the heart's activity becoming accelerated in order to resist the invasion of tuberculosis bacteria, tuberculosis bacteria can invade our body at any time. The reason it does not become the cause of disease is that the lungs are strong and the bacteria cannot invade. Lung disease can develop easily when the mind and body are maintained in a highly excited state (exuberant activity of heart), by excessive sexual activities, anxiety or other reasons over a long time, so it is valid to see Exuberance of Fire as the cause of lung disease.

Once a disease develops, a fever occurs as a result of the bacteria. However, since the fever is not totally caused by the bacteria, acquiring tranquility of the mind and body to eliminate the cause of intense activity of heart is the prerequisite in the treatment of lung disease.

C. Earth generates Metal - The Relationship between Spleen and Lungs

I have not been able to discover the material that physiologically and pathologically proves the generating relationship between the Spleen and Lungs yet, but in the beginning stage of a lung disease, when the patient is not extremely weak, the digestion is better than the average person. This can be seen as a physiological phenomena which supplements the weakening of the lungs – Earth generating Metal.

The physiological mechanism is truly subtle. On one hand, it works and gets fatigued and on the other hand it recovers. On one hand, it consumes and on the other it supplements. This is the fundamental principle of the Mutual Generating and Controlling cycle (refer to third diagram).

Though Fire controls Metal, it generates Earth which generates Metal. In another words, the lungs are fatigued when the activity of the heart becomes exuberant, but the heart indirectly supports the Spleen which supplements the lungs, making sure that there is no long term damage.

D. Earth controls Water - The Relationship between Spleen and Kidneys

The following relationship can be seen between spleen and kidneys:

1. The thyroid gland and adrenal gland have a mutually suppressing relationship toward the pancreas (Spleen). That is, when the thyroid gland is removed, general metabolism is decreased, but the assimilation of carbohydrate is greatly increased. This increase in the assimilation of carbohydrate indicates the exuberance of pancreatic function. In contrast, when the spleen is taken out, general metabolism increases but the assimilation of carbohydrate is decreased.

2. When the spleen of an organism is removed, the quantity of mineral elimination is increased. It is said in *Li Shi Zhen*'s *Materia Medica*,[13] "All plants and herbs dislike metal containers – especially the Kidney tonics. If the herbs are kept in metal containers, they will instead weaken the Liver and the Kidneys." With this statement, experiments of Western medicine and theories of Oriental medicine coincide. Herbs that tonify the Kidneys dislike metal. Not surprisingly, a large amount of minerals are eliminated from the body upon removal of the spleen, supporting the Oriental viewpoint that metal

---

13. Li Shi Zhen (1518 – 1593 A.D.) is one of the most famous of all doctors in Oriental medical history. "The Compendium of Materia Medica" was compiled by Li Shi Zhen in 1578 A.D. It consists of 52 volumes and took him nearly 30 years to complete. There are 1,892 types of herbs and over 10,000 prescriptions in this compendium. This compendium has been translated into various languages including Korean, Japanese, English, French and German.

suppresses the Liver and Kidneys. The reason for this is that minerals, consumed by the Spleen in order to suppress the Liver and Kidneys to which it has a mutual controlling relationship, are in surplus due to the removal of the spleen.

E. Metal generates Water - The Relationship between Lungs and Kidneys

Since the Earth Element controls the Water Element, the Earth Element generates the Metal Element which in turn generates the Water Element in order to supplement the Water Element. I have not yet found out whether certain nerve or chemical relationships exist between the lungs and kidneys, but in a common sense, the lungs disperse water and kidneys eliminate water. When the Lungs are fatigued, urine is dark and scanty with difficult elimination and when the Lungs are healthy, urine is clear and easily eliminated. The condition of the urine reflects the state of the kidneys. Conversely, when there is a kidney disease, diseases that relate to the lungs such as pulmonary edema, dyspnea or phlegmatic asthma occur.

F. Metal controls Wood - The Relationship between Lungs and Liver

1. The beta and acetic acids, which occur at the height of acidosis, are oxidized and change into carbon and water in a healthy person. The small amount of acetin, which avoided oxidation, is said to be eliminated through the urine. However, when these substances accumulate in the blood in large amounts due to insufficient oxidation, liver disease and acidosis result. Since oxidation occurs due to the supply of oxygen and oxygen is supplied by the lungs, this relationship can be seen as Metal controlling Wood. Even if this cause–effect relationship is seen in an opposite way, there will be no change in the mutual relationship between the two organs.

2. Anger is an emotion that belongs to the Liver, so one gets easily angered when the Lungs are weak. When anger continues for a long time, the Lungs get injured. Getting angry is said to injure the Lungs. In a physiognomy book from the West, I observed that a person with a small chest has an impatient temperament like a fox and does well in short distance running.

3. Autumn is the season of the Exuberance of Metal. Since Metal controls Wood, the activity of the Liver (Wood) becomes suppressed. Thus, the emotion of resentment, which is a passive emotion of the Liver, acts strongly to make one feel depressed.

G. Water generates Wood - The Relationship between Kidneys and Liver

1. In the last stage of jaundice, degenerative changes in the epithelial tissue of the kidneys, liver abscess, gall stones, inflammations of the biliary tract, etc. demonstrate the relationship of Mutual Generation. Due to the inability to mutually generate, when trouble develops in one region, another region is directly influenced.

2. There is a so–called *"Zi Xian"* syndrome which resembles uremia. A convulsion occurs during pregnancy or childbirth and according to anatomical examination of people who died of *Zi Xian*, there are many times when bleeding from the liver or a blood clot is confirmed.[14]

H. Water controls Fire - The Relationship between Kidneys and Heart

The heart is related to Fire since the body temperature increases when the action of the heart is exuberant. There is a certain force in the body which suppresses the heart's action so that it does not become excessively exuberant. This force is called Water. The function of Water is presumed to be based on a certain type of hormone which stimulates the nerve center that suppresses the heart. The endocrine gland which secretes this hormone is seen to belong to the Kidneys.

In actuality, everyone has had experiences of developing body fever when the reproductive system gets fatigued due to continuous sexual activity. This is called, "Deficiency of *Yin* with Activation of Fire" or "Exhaustion of Water and Exuberance of Fire " in Oriental medicine. It implies that since the power of Water which suppresses Fire is weakened, Fire becomes exuberant. Here, the Kidneys are not the Kidneys in the Western scientific sense, but the Kidneys of Oriental medicine which store True *Yin*.

In Oriental medicine, the Ministerial Fire is said to generate Monarch Fire. The Ministerial Fire is the Fire within the Kidneys. It refers to the function of the sex hormones of the reproductive glands. Adrenalin exciting the sympathetic nerve to increase blood pressure and heart beat is the Ministerial Fire generating the Monarch Fire.

I. Wood generates Fire - The Relationship between Liver and Heart

The portal vein, which arises from the capillary vessels of the abdominal cavity organs, subsequently divides into capillary vessels in the liver, which then drain into the hepatic vein. With this fact alone, it is not hard to presume that the liver has a special relationship towards blood circulation. This coincides with how Oriental medicine views the Liver as an organ that relates to the blood. In Oriental medicine, the Liver is called "The Sea of Blood" and it is said to "store the Blood."

Now, I am going to give a few examples of the functions of the liver:

1. The liver stores nutrients (glycogen).
2. Bile, a secretion of liver, is a liquid that has a strong bitter taste. Bitter taste settles down the excitation of the heart (refer to Chapter 3, section 1). The heart cannot take a break at all and can only regulate its work condition by settling, recovering and supplementing its excitation and fatigue. It is the liver which presides over this duty. In jaundice, when the constituents of bile flow into the blood in large quantity, we can see the slowing of the pulse. This is due to the liver operating excessively to reduce the work of the heart. Chemically, it can be assumed that acidic salt of the bile has acted on the heart and the vagus nerve.
3. The liver is an organ which detoxifies toxins in the blood.
4. Since acid dissolves calcium, in the event that calcium deposits build up on the wall of the blood vessels and harden, we can suppose that the acid dissolves and eliminates the deposits. This greatly reduces the burden on the heart.

---

14. The author here is relating pregnancy and "Zi Xian," its disorder, to the Water Element; and Liver/blood clot to the Wood Element. Refer to footnote 6 on page 123.

The above four functions all have roles in supporting the heart. "Wood generates Fire" can be sufficiently understood with those examples.

In Oriental medicine, the Heart is Monarch Fire and the Gall Bladder is Ministerial Fire. The Gall Bladder, similar to the Minister having the duty of assisting the Heart, is said to eliminate dangerous and injurious things as they come in order to prevent them from invading the Heart.

J. Wood controls Earth - The Relationship between Liver and Spleen

1. Bile (Liver) and pancreatic juice (Spleen) are in opposition to each other. Bile is acidic and the pancreatic juice is alkaline. In Oriental medicine, acid digestive juices all belong to the Liver and the alkaline digestive juices all belong to the Spleen. The cause of excessive acid in the stomach is said to be "Wood overcontrolling Earth" or "Liver overcontrolling Spleen."

2. There is a theory which presumes that cirrhosis of the liver is the result of poisoning by abnormally fermented products of food created from chronic catarrh (inflammation of mucous membrane) of the stomach. I do not know how much truth there is in this theory, but we can assume that there is a certain relationship between liver and stomach from this.

3. There is even a theory that states when an abnormality in the endocrine function of the pancreas occurs from large amounts of acid contained in the blood, diabetes occurs due to over abundance of sugar within the blood.

Sour is a taste that belongs to the Liver and sweet is a taste that belong to the Spleen so acidosis in diabetes is due to the opposing relationship of the Liver and Spleen. This is similar to soldiers of an opposing country forming a balance of power.

THE STUDY OF SYNDROMES

*O*riental medicine in its totality is the "Study of Syndromes."[1] Hence, there is no need to discuss the study of syndromes here, but in order to facilitate learning for the beginners of Oriental medicine and enable them to use it as a reference when faced with clinical syndromes, I have created this "Syndrome" chapter by generally gathering information that is not contained in the "Study of Pulses" and the "Study of Channels."

I. TASTES
(refer to Chapter 6 on Herbal Pharmacology)

According to Oriental medicine, taste is very important. The foundations of the study of herbal properties are taste and *Qi* (temperature)[2] and taste holds an important position even in the "Study of Syndrome." A person's physical constitution and syndrome can be examined and identified by observing changes in the sense of taste and taste preferences.

Just as everyone's face is different, the tastes for foods are also different because the physical constitution of every individual is different. A person who likes spicy foods, a person who likes sweets, a person who eats salty foods, a person who eats bland foods or a person who enjoys eating bitter and sour foods are all different. Even among the persons who like spicy foods, the selections are all different: red pepper, black pepper, garlic, mustard, etc. So by no means can one force person B to have the same taste as person A. The following proverbs talk about this fact:

---

1. The word "syndrome" in Oriental medicine not only includes signs and symptoms, but also includes the location, nature and cause of a disease. In addition, it implies the dynamic relationship between the "pathogenic" or disease causing factor and the body's "Zheng Qi." The "Zheng Qi" or "Upright Qi" refers to the three factors which are the body's normal physiological process, resistance against the disease and the ability to recover from the disease once you fall under the disease.

2. In Oriental medicine, the term "Qi" not only refers to the vital energy in the body and in nature, but also to the reaction of an herb (including temperature) and sense of taste of an herb. See Chapter 6 on the pharmacology for further details.

"A sour pear tastes different to different people."

"There can be no saying about the interest and taste of a person."

The taste influencing the body can be generally observed from two points of view; one is through sensory nerves and the other is through chemical action.

A. Gustatory Nerve

The way we perceive taste is through the sensations of the gustatory nerve which is distributed on the tongue. The areas of perception are determined according to the types of taste: pungent taste in the anterior tip, sweet taste in the middle and bitter taste in the posterior region.[3]

One cannot particularly perceive sweet taste by putting a candy deep inside the mouth and pressing with the tongue: it does not taste much different than putting in a steamed rice–cake.

When spicy foods are eaten in excess, one feels a burning sensation on the tongue (especially anterior tip) and a hot feeling in the body which makes one sweat. This is proof that there is a specific organ and tissues which are influenced by a specific sense of taste.

To give an example of the pungent taste, it has the following actions:

1. Deepens breathing.
2. Stimulates sympathetic innervation to the heart to produce heat.
3. Promotes sweating.
4. Opens the mouth, nose and sweat pores of the whole body.

B. Chemical Action

I think that the above stated physiological changes due to taste are not simply due to the action of the sensory nerves, but more so by chemical action. The chemical action can be divided into two stages:

1. It can be assumed that due to the stimulation of taste, a certain type of chemical is produced (hormone) in the tongue tissue which is then absorbed into the blood and stimulates a specific organ, producing specific physiological changes. The above mentioned chemical action is supported by the fact that when pungent or sweet tasting foods are ingested, a unique kind of mucus peculiar to each taste is produced on the surface of the tongue.
2. It can be presumed that after food is digested and absorbed, while the blood is circulating, it has the role of a hormone that acts on a specific organ according to the individually unique components of taste.

THE TONGUE, THE SENSE OF TASTE AND THE FIVE ZANG ORGANS

There is no organ in the body that is unimportant, but few organs have as many important and complicated duties as the tongue. Here is an outline of its functions:

---

3. As is evident by the taste locations on the tongue, Oriental and Western theories do not always match up. However within each system, there is an equal amount of logic.

1. Our feelings are expressed through words. The tongue is intimately related to the sexual organs since it is located at the end of the Conception channel. In animals, both nose and tongue have an important role during the time of sexual intercourse. In humans too, one cannot say that there is no action of the tongue during the arousal of passion or during sexual intercourse. The nose is the end of the Governing channel so it corresponds to the male sexual organ and the mouth is the end of the Conception channel so it corresponds to the female sexual organ. Additionally, the tongue can be seen to correspond to the clitoris (refer to Chapter 4 on the channels).

2. Tongue has an important function in digestion and in nutrition.

(a) It mixes food during chewing.

(b) It pushes food downward when swallowing.

(c) It examines and selects food through the sense of taste, reports items of food received to the central nervous system and notifies each organ.

The mouth is the gate that imports all goods and since the tongue is the supervising office that handles all goods, it seems as though the messenger on an official trip from each organ resides on the tongue. For example, when a certain organ demands a sweet substance, it orders the ingestion of sweet tasting foods to its dispatched official; accordingly, a delicious taste is then perceived when sweet foods are ingested. Ingesting all of the demanded quantities will make one lose the desire toward that food. This is the reason why the taste and demand for foods are different according to each person and taste changes according to age and physiological state even in the same person.

After passing through the digestive organs and going to the heart, food is distributed to each organ. Hence, the conditions of the digestive organs and the heart appear on the tongue. Furthermore, the condition of each organ appears on the tongue. The saying, "The tongue is the mirror of the Heart" implies that the heart presides over the health of the whole body since it is a monarch organ and the tongue is an organ that manifests the state of health of the whole body.

SELF–PERCEIVED TASTE IN THE MOUTH AND THE STATE OF HEALTH

I have already mentioned that according to the state of his or her health, a person will desire foods with a specific taste and will find these specific foods delicious. Even when there is no food in the mouth, it is possible to have a taste in the mouth according to the state of health. All of these are acts of the "messenger" residing on the tongue on an official trip from each organ. The following are a few examples of frequently experienced tastes in the mouth:

1. Bitter taste – anyone can usually experience this when they are extremely tired or when they worry too much.
2. Pungent taste – sometimes, the inside of the mouth burns and feels hot.
3. Sweet taste
4. Sour taste – sour and astringent
5. Salty taste

6. Bland taste
7. Fishy taste
8. Rotten taste
9. Burning fragrant taste – similar to fried sesame seeds

The above tastes in the mouth have actually all been complained of by many ill people – they are not randomly enumerated. Tastes other than bitter were generally heard from married women. There are probably a lot of people who, according to their physical constitution, have never experienced these "tastes in the mouth," but if one pays attention to the people around him or her, these complaints can be frequently heard. This phenomenon is not only confirmed by the sense of taste in the mouth, but also by the fact that phlegm has distinctive tastes.

TASTE AND ITS GOVERNING ORGAN

A. Bitter Taste and the Heart

In Oriental medicine, it is said: "Bitter taste goes to the Heart" and "Bitter taste first goes to the Heart and is able to drain and dry." There is no taste which does not go to the heart, but "Bitter taste goes to the Heart" implies that bitter tasting substances have the specific characteristics of a hormone that acts on the heart. The following facts prove this:

1. Regardless of Western or Oriental medicine, purgatives generally have a bitter taste. Bitter taste settles excitation and reduces fever. When we eat spicy food, we open our mouths in order to disperse upward, but when we eat bitter food, we incessantly keep swallowing the saliva.
2. Bitter taste acts on the heart and its parasympathetic nerves, lessening the workload to make the heart settle down and recover. The slowing down of the pulse that appears in jaundice, when large amounts of bitter tasting bile flow into the blood, is a disease phenomenon resulting from an over–reduction in the workload.
3. When the heart is fatigued, a bitter taste can be perceived.
4. A person with exuberant activity of the heart has an easy time eating bitter lettuce or other bitter tasting vegetables, but a person with deficient body heat will immediately get nauseous if he eats even one piece of bitter lettuce.
5. Beer, more so than any other alcoholic drink, has a cool and refreshing taste and one recovers faster from it after being drunk. The reason is that beer is quite bitter. When a constitutionally cold person drinks a lot of beer, he or she gets diarrhea and anybody who drinks beer frequently eliminates large amounts of urine. Accordingly, beer is an alcoholic drink of the summer; a type of cool and refreshing drink. Recovery is quick because even though the heart is stimulated by alcohol, the stimulation is settled down by the bitter tasting substance.

B. Pungent Taste and the Lungs

We can infer from the following examples that pungent foods act on the lungs.

1. When pungent foods are eaten, one breathes deeply, opens the mouth, lifts the tip of the tongue and breathes out.
2. A person with slow breathing usually likes pungent foods.
3. In diaphoretic formulas[4] for common colds and cough, pungent and warm herbs are generally used.
4. For cough in a lung disease,[5] pungent and warm herbs are avoided. Thus, there is a tendency in these patients to dislike pungent foods and to like bland and sour foods.

C. Sweet Taste and the Spleen

The Spleen is the organ in charge of digestion and nutrition. Unrefined sugar has a high nutritional value. Most patients of "Consumptive Disease"[6] request sugar.

Since pancreatic juices dissolve starch into maltose and maltose into glucose, we can infer that sugar or sweet tasting substances are related to the Spleen. Diabetes is seen as an excess of sugar in the blood that results from changes in carbohydrate metabolism due to pathological changes in the Spleen. Sweet taste tonifies, harmonizes and relaxes. The statement "Sweet taste enters the Spleen, and harmonizes and relaxes" reflects this. Looking at a child's face after giving him or her sugar, one can see that his or her expression is very harmonious and relaxed. It is the same for adults: when they ingest sugar, it softens the mouth to make them enjoy the taste and their facial muscles relax and give them a fulfilled expression.

D. Sour Taste and the Liver

Acids in the body all belong to the Liver. For example:

1. Bile is an acid digestive fluid.
2. Acidosis is a phenomenon resulting from pathological changes in the liver, proving the relationship between acids and the Liver.

Pregnant women, due to psychological changes, become highly sensitive, emotionally intense and demand a large quantity of sour tasting foods. Irascibility is an emotion related to the Liver and the preference for sour tasting foods comes from the Liver. Thus, it is an absolute fact that pregnant women require especially powerful activity of the Liver. What is the reason for this? It is difficult to show precise data on this fact, but I will give a few examples as they come to my mind. The following is only a hypothesis, so it will need to be substantiated by further experiments.

    (a) The Liver and the Gall Bladder are the organs that produce dynamic force for combat. Since a fetus is in the mother's body, it can be observed that the activity of both the Liver and the Gall Bladder are vigorous in order to protect it well. Being highly emotional during pregnancy is further proof of the involvement of the Liver in

---

4. The herbal formulas that increase perspiration. Also known as sudorific formulas.

5. The lung diseases mentioned in this book generally refer to pulmonary tuberculosis.

6. This disease is equivalent to diabetes in Western medicine.

pregnancy.

(b) The Liver stores Blood – the Liver has a mutual generating relationship with the Heart and is called the "Sea of Blood." It is in charge of the *Qi* in men and in charge of the "Blood Level"[7] in women, i.e. menstruation and fetal nutrition. In general, young women like sour tasting foods more than young men and this is more extreme in pregnant women. This fact is observed during pregnancy when the activity of the Liver is very high because there is a demand for large amounts of sour tasting foods.

(c) The liver destroys and produces red blood cells.

(d) The liver has a detoxifying action and it can be presumed that its action becomes more vigorous to prevent toxins from invading the fetus.

(e) It can be assumed that the liver sends large amounts of acid into the blood to make the pancreas release large amounts of sugar into the blood to indirectly nourish the fetus.

(f) It can be assumed that the liver invigorates the metabolism of substances, aside from carbohydrates, by restraining the pancreas. The functions of the kidneys (Kidneys control the bones) are accelerated to invigorate calcium metabolism, which is responsible for the production of bones in the fetus.

(g) Sour taste is regarded to have the power to stop loss of energy due to its astringent nature.

E. Salty Taste and the Kidneys

The relationship between salty taste and the Kidneys can be observed through a few examples:

1. Salt in the body, other than being eliminated in small amounts through sweating, is eliminated in greater part through urination.

2. It is said in Oriental medicine that "Salty taste enters the Kidneys and softens what is hard." Salt softens and dissolves many types of substances. Fresh vegetables droop when salt is sprinkled on them so it can be presumed that salt has a similar action toward blood corpuscles and all cells inside the body.

Drinking solutions of salt when coughing or vomiting blood can calm those symptoms down and drinking solutions of salt at the onset of an epileptic seizure can safely relieve it. This shows that salt weakens vigorous blood circulation and that it has the power to soften muscle contractions and spasms. It is "Water controls Fire," namely the function of the Kidneys, that restrains the circulating force of the blood. Relaxing spasms of the muscles is "The Liver controls the tendons" and "Water generates Wood," so it is certain that the functions of salt also belong to the Kidneys.[8]

3. People who crave large quantities of salt in their food are generally not energetic,

---

7. The body's physiological function can be divided into two levels: Qi level and Blood level. The Qi level is the route in which the Lungs, Spleen and Kidneys (the organs which are intimately related to the Qi) function. The Blood level is the route in which the Heart (controls Blood), Liver (stores Blood) and Kidneys (help produce the Blood indirectly) function.

8. For the explanation on the Five Element correspondence with the Zang Fu organs, see the section on the Five Elements in Chapter 2 (Zang Fu organs).

have a dull sexual life and possess a passive physical constitution. It is true that salty substances suppress the life force. The power that suppresses the life force is *Yin* and *Yin* is Water. Since Water belongs to the Kidneys, the conclusion is that the function of salty substances is governed by the Kidneys.

4. When large amounts of salt are ingested, there will be a simultaneous craving for large amounts of water. The craving for water comes from the Kidneys. In Western folk medicine, rubbing oil (organic) mixed with salt is said to have miraculous effects on burns and putting salt on a charcoal fire when rice is burning takes away the burnt smell. These can explain "Water controls Fire" and the relationship between the Water Element and salt.

5. I have seen a woman, who for many months after childbirth, did not eat even one spoonful of salt and ate pure rice only. This is presumed to be the physiological rejection of salt until the loss of large quantities of blood during childbirth is replenished. This is illustrated in the following statement in Oriental medicine: "Salty taste enters the Blood and when the Blood acquires salt, it congeals and thirst occurs."[9] So the rejection of salt was an effort by the body to avoid congealing of the blood and to assist the activities of the life force.

6. Edema is caused by a kidney disease. In this disease, one can see an excessive retention of water and salt in the body, as in hydremia and hypernatremia for example.[10]

F. Bland Taste and the Kidney

Bland taste has no distinctive taste, but is different from tastelessness. The reason is that there is a difference in taste between various bland substances. Poria, an Oriental herb, has a bland taste and tomatoes have a bland taste with a tinge of sweetness; so, pure and clear tastes are generally called bland tastes. The function of bland tastes, according to Oriental medicine is said to be "Benefits orifice,[11] permeates and drains" and is said to facilitate all types of elimination. The bland taste is also a taste related to the Kidneys. Poria is an herb that promotes urination and eliminates Phlegm. Watermelon is also an excellent diuretic to clear heat. Tomatoes hold an important position in Western dietary therapy and are said to be effective for consumptive diseases and especially, bone diseases – bones belong to the Kidneys in Oriental medicine. It is certain that tomatoes, like their taste, are a medicine that belong to the Kidney system.

II. COLORS

People's complexions are different because their physical constitutions are different. Even for the same person, the complexion constantly changes according to the fluctuation of the emotions and the difference in the state of health. The complexion turns bluish when

---

9. Yellow Emperor's Inner Classic.

10. Hydremia refers to an excess amount of watery fluid in the blood and hypernatremia refers to an excess amount of salt in the blood.

11. The orifice here refers to the urethra.

extremely angry, reddish when happy, blackish when fearful, whitish when worrying and yellowish when overthinking. The proverbs that say, "The face is turning like black ink" and "The face is becoming black and blue" imply sudden emotional changes such as fear, shock or rage. The face of a teenager coming out after being interrogated for charges of theft is whitish and the face of a student coming out of an examination hall is yellowish. Also, a person who thinks too much usually has digestive problems and a person with digestive problems has a yellowish complexion. A person who laughs a lot has vigorous activity of the Heart and a reddish complexion and a person who worries a lot sighs constantly and has a whitish complexion. Accordingly, the conditions of the internal organs can be observed with the colors that show on the surface of the body. These colors are not just manifested on the face, but there are also differences in the pigment of feces, urine, menstrual blood, vaginal discharge, tongue coating, lips, eyes, phlegm, etc.

COLOR AND ITS RELATED ORGAN

Red is related to the Heart, white to the Lungs, yellow to the Spleen, blue/green to the Liver and black to the Kidneys.

ORGAN	Heart	Lung	Spleen	Liver	Kidney
COLOR	red	white	yellow	blue/green	black

A. Red and the Heart

Red is the color of the Fire Element, so red light is a light that is related to the Heart. A face turns reddish when the activity of the Heart is exuberant, thus joyful emotion, fever or even drinking alcoholic beverages turns the face reddish. All of them definitely arise from the exuberant activity of the Heart. However, the health of the Heart should not be inferred from the appearance of the color red. There are both healthy and unhealthy shades of red. Red is the color with the longest wavelength so it is a *Yang* color. In bull fighting, shaking a red object in front of the bull's eyes makes him even more fierce. In cardiac edema, the face color becomes reddish purple or brownish.

B. White and the Lungs

White is a color related to the Lungs. A person who worries a lot constantly sighs and has a whitish complexion. Also, a person with constitutionally weak Lungs generally has a whitish complexion. This person can maintain his or her health as long as he or she does not get a reddish glow. However, if he or she does get a reddish glow, like the color of a peach blossom, it is an indication that a lung disease is in progress. A person who has a white complexion with luster is magnanimous with profound thoughts, so there are many who have the character of a big time politician – the so–called noble type – with this complexion.

C. Yellow and the Spleen

Yellow is the color of the Earth Element, so the Spleen and the Stomach are like the Earth. The Spleen produces Blood and the Stomach ingests nutrients in order to produce the flesh, similar to the Earth nurturing all things in nature. A person with strong digestive organs has a yellowish complexion with luster and a person with a disease of the digestive organs has a sallow complexion and is emaciated, fatigued or has a diseased color that is hard to describe with words.

D. Blue and the Liver

A red color is due to the congestion of arterial blood. As the result of strong heart activity, a large amount of arterial blood flows too quickly and the duration in which the blood is in contact with the tissues is too short. Accordingly, a fresh red color shows up because there are large quantities of oxygen within the blood since a small amount of oxygen is transferred to the tissues. A blue color occurs as a result of the stagnation of venous blood in the tissues (or dark purplish or blackish color). The stagnation of venous blood is a phenomenon that appears when the activity of the heart is weak. The organ that regulates the activity of the Heart is the Liver (refer to Chapter 2, section 2). Perhaps the liver secretes a blue colored substance.

Blue is a color with a short wavelength so it settles and calms. One gets excited when looking at the color red, but settles down when looking at the color blue. Having transcendental or sentimental feelings without particular reasons when looking at blue/green mountains or going into the forest is largely due to receiving the influence of that color. It is said that shaking a blue cloth in front of fierce cattle and in front of a horse calms them down.

What is the necessity of the Liver to manifest the color blue? It can be explained by the following reasons. The color blue is a light that settles and calms, thus impeding activities. Recall that the Liver is an organ in charge of combat and a motive for combat is anger. As such, the emotion of anger belongs to the Liver and in times of anger the color blue appears. The color blue has two functions that are needed in combat. One is to internally curtail the activity of the Heart. In other words, it saves and accumulates energy then lets it out forcefully all at once in order to fight fiercely. Another is to show the color blue externally toward an opponent to settle and suppress his activity and at the same time to give him feelings of fear. This is why a person who normally has a bluish complexion becomes highly sensitive, angers easily and often has indigestion. This indigestion arises from the opposing relationship between Liver and Spleen, that is Wood and Earth.

E. Black and the Kidneys

Black is the color of Water and Yin–Coldness.[12] Also, nighttime is dark. The complexion becomes dark when one is cold and also when one is feeling great fear. A person who normally has a black complexion, like a frightened person, is very weak sexually and has little courage. A healthy person with a black complexion is said in a proverb to have "Iron black color," so he is extremely strong sexually and has boundless energy. The color of the skin changes as a sign of pregnancy and there is a black color like freckles and blotches on the forehead, on the bridge of the nose, around the eyes, around the mouth,

---

12. The Kidneys are the most Yin among all the organs and Yin indicates coldness compared to Yang. Here, think of the deepest part of the ocean where it is dark.

etc. In the center line of the abdominal wall, namely the "Conception channel,"[13] a colored pigment settles in which is black and a dark brown color settles in the external genital region and vagina.

In general, the black color can be seen in Basedow's disease, which is seen as the result of hyperthyroidism or in acromegaly (a disease with the enlargement of nose, mandible, ends of extremities and the whole body), which is seen as the result of the hyperfunction of the frontal lobe of the pituitary gland. The relationship of black to the Kidneys can be recognized if a certain amount of attention is paid. Edema due to a kidney disease can be distinguished by the complexion being a dark white color, as opposed to a reddish purple color of edema due to heart disease. The color white belongs to the Lungs and dark color belongs to the Kidneys, so the Lungs and Kidneys are: "Metal and Water Zang organs of mutual generation."

HEALTHY COLOR AND UNHEALTHY COLOR (TECHNIQUES OF OBSERVING COLOR)

It is extremely difficult to explain this healthy and unhealthy color in words. There is no other way than to train the power of observation by paying attention to the color of the complexion of as many people as possible. It is the same as the teller of a bank being able to easily discern counterfeit notes but not being able to explain their method of discovery to anyone else. There will be no other words than merely, "somehow it feels different." The colors of the complexions of people are difficult to explain, but there is something on which to judge whether it is healthy or unhealthy by observation. This judgement of health and sickness on the basis of color has great importance in Oriental medicine: "Observing the shape and watching the color"[14] reflects this. In reality, "Observing the shape and watching the color" is not only necessary in Oriental medicine, but also in Western medicine and in observing the emotions of other people in our daily lives. It is hard to avoid getting blamed for being ambiguous regarding this observation of color, but I am going to state a few essential points.

METHOD OF OBSERVING COLOR

A. Presence of Qi; Absence of Qi; Presence of Spirit; Absence of Spirit

When observing the complexion of a person, one must be careful about the existence or absence of *Qi* and Spirit. In everyday conversation, terms such as "Color of *Qi* looks bad" or "Color of the Spirit is good" are frequently used. "*Qi*" and "Spirit" are abstract expressions of the movement of life which we can sense. When they are further differentiated, *Qi* is an abstract expression of the emotion and Spirit is an abstract expression of the life force or the state of health. The "color of *Qi* not being so good" means that there

---

13. One of the Eight Extraordinary Channels. It is also called the Ren channel. It runs from the perineum to the lower lip. See Chapter 4 on the channels for more detail.

14. Observing the shape implies examining the person's facial and bodily features. Watching the color implies the examining the different colors of the complexion.

is emotional trouble and the "color of Spirit not being so good" implies that it looks as though there is a disease.

Complexion, regardless of the type of its color, must have vitality. As long as there is vitality, the color of Spirit will be good even if one is emaciated and as long as there is no vitality, the color of Spirit will be bad even if one is plump. A person has a particular complexion according to individual characteristics and that complexion changes according to living conditions. A farmer who constantly gets sunlight has dark skin and a scholar who constantly studies indoors has fair skin. However, receiving the same degree of sunlight still results in all different complexions and studying indoors in the same degree also results in different complexions; these are all due to individual characteristics. The skin is a healthy color especially when there is vitality. When there is vitality in a reddish complexion, the Heart is strong and when there is no vitality, the Heart has become fatigued by excessive activity.

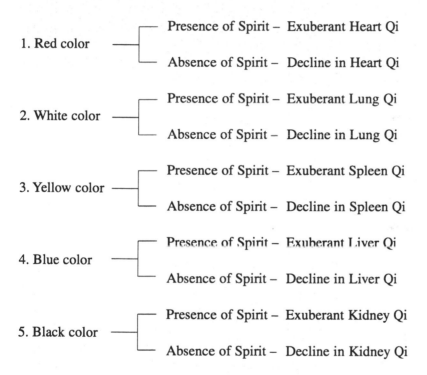

1. Red color
— Presence of Spirit – Exuberant Heart Qi
— Absence of Spirit – Decline in Heart Qi

2. White color
— Presence of Spirit – Exuberant Lung Qi
— Absence of Spirit – Decline in Lung Qi

3. Yellow color
— Presence of Spirit – Exuberant Spleen Qi
— Absence of Spirit – Decline in Spleen Qi

4. Blue color
— Presence of Spirit – Exuberant Liver Qi
— Absence of Spirit – Decline in Liver Qi

5. Black color
— Presence of Spirit – Exuberant Kidney Qi
— Absence of Spirit – Decline in Kidney Qi

B. Mutual Generating and Controlling Cycles in Complex Colors

The color of a person's complexion does not simply appear in one color among the five colors, but the five colors appear in small amounts, thus a so–called red or blue implies the strongest color among them. Accordingly, to observe color in practice is extraordinarily complicated, but it is generally enough to diagnose health or illness entirely through the presence or absence of vitality. Yet there are times when only one type of color shows up strongly or at times two, three, four or five types of colors appear strongly, all individually following the channels. When all five colors appear together, it is a sign that the time of death is drawing near. A color of an autumn leaf showing up on the complexion of a sick person is said to be inauspicious because an autumn leaf has red, yellow, blue, white and black colors.

When many colors are combined, observation under the following standards will generally be very helpful:

1. The colors of Zang organs in a mutual generating relationship are good. For example, a combination of yellow and white (Earth generates Metal), white and black (Metal generates Water), black and blue (Water generates Wood), blue and red (Wood generates Fire), and red and yellow (Fire generates Earth) reflect no problems in general.

2. When the colors of Zang organs in the mutual controlling relationship are combined, it is generally unhealthy. For example:

   (a) Red and White (Fire controls Metal)
   Since this is a color of peach–blossoms, it is the most brilliant color, but it is an extremely bad color when observed from the point of view of health and longevity. This color shows up mostly among patients under 30 years old with a lung disease. The following statements illustrate why this color is unhealthy: "A young man with brilliance, easily acquiring wealth and fame, is a sign of early withering," "A young man with a blossomed flower complexion dies young" and "Men of talent and beauty all die young."

   (b) White and Blue (Metal controls Wood)
   This means having a bluish pale complexion. It is a color commonly seen in older women who were widowed at a young age. This is the complexion of a person weakened by a long time of continued strong resentment (Liver) and grief (Lung). *Yin*–type lung disease patients generally possess this complexion.

   (c) Blue and Yellow (Wood controls Earth)
   A green color results when these two colors are combined; jaundice seems to belong here. Other than the green color in the pigment of bile, I have not been able to find examples to clearly explain this color, but I believe that this complexion will be found if many patients are observed.

   (d) Yellow and Black (Earth controls Water)
   This color can be seen frequently in chronic diseases of the stomach, especially in gastric atony.

   (e) Black and Red (Water controls Fire)
   This complexion has a black color with a red flush, so it seems to look slightly excited: A patient with a lung disease who had a strong constitution prior to the disease generally has such a complexion.

At this point, I would like to caution my readers that these examples must not be over interpreted and presumed as facts. Just because a lung disease patient has the color of (e) above, one must not come to a hasty conclusion that a person having this color has a lung disease. A person with a weak body, searching through the pages of a pathology and symptomatology book, can easily believe that they are suffering from each disease in the book. One should not look at the mirror while reading this and say, "black and red color, blue and yellow color – oh no! I have this disease."

There are mirrors which have a yellow, blue or white tinge, so there are no correct mirrors. Colors look different depending on their relationship to surrounding light rays. There are also some people who have a slight defect in the optic nerves and there also exists a relationship between visual perception and the emotional activity of the moment. There is no need to foolishly be afraid just because something looks a certain way at a quick glance. Therefore, since there is a concern that the main point will be missed in ascertaining the constitution and disease with the observation of color only, the signs and symptoms of *Yin–Yang* should be observed through other methods including: pulse diagnosis, channels, observation of color, food preferences, Deficiency–Excess, Exterior–Interior, Above–Below,[15] etc.

EMOTION AND COMPLEXION

The phenomena of the biological world are truly mysterious and subtle. There is an effort made by all organisms to live longer at any cost and to survive by whatever means necessary. That effort is more subconscious than conscious, mostly instinctive and spontaneous.

Beautiful flowers blossom and secrete honey in the springtime in order to attract bees and butterflies for the spreading of their pollens. The same goes for all fruits, when they ripen, they distinctly show their presence to attract animals for the spreading of their seeds.

People laugh a lot during puberty, especially 17 and 18 year old virgin girls in particular cannot hold back their laughter – this is the same as flowers blossoming in the springtime. In the animal kingdom, there are even more such phenomena. A blue frog changes its color to blue, brown or orange according to its surroundings. An octopus or cuttle fish releases black ink to hide itself when in danger. A weasel or a skunk releases foul gas to stop the pursuit of an enemy when frightened. These phenomena are not conscious, but they are spontaneous. They originate from the will of mother nature. Frequently used terms in recent times like "adaptability," "instinct" and "natural healing power," all imply following nature's will. Since humans are the most developed among all organisms, it is not necessary to say much about how humans have the most superior methods in the protection of their lives. One method is a change in skin complexion or color.

A. Red and Joy; others

A red color appearing on the face can be classified roughly into four types: A flush of joy, embarrassment, passion or fever.

1. A flush of joy not only expresses one's good will, but stimulates another person's feeling of joy, which causes that person to act for the benefit of oneself.
2. A flush of embarrassment expresses good will and other types of emotions at the same time.

---

15. Above and below here refer to the location of the disease. Above implies upper parts of the body such face, neck, and chest and below implies lower parts of the body such as abdomen, waist and legs.

(a) The flush of embarrassment that shows good will and worry is a facial expression that young people get frequently due to either innocence or an insignificant fault; thus, it is asking for forgiveness by signalling a feeling of docility to the other person.

(b) The flush of embarrassment that expresses good will and resentment generally occurs when there is an error by an older person or a person in a position of authority and the error was pointed out by his junior or subordinate; it expresses good will on the part of the person found to be in error by asking for forgiveness of that mistake, but at the same it gives a type of intimidating expression like "how impertinent of you to speak those words in front of me."

(c) The flush of embarrassment that shows good will and fear is the expression of a person when he or she cannot avoid admitting having made a major mistake. The expressions "face turning red" and "so sorry, I don't know what to do," belong to (b) and (c).

3. A sexual flush in a person shows good will to another person and at the same time gives feelings of beauty and incites them to facilitate a spontaneous act.

4. A flush of fever results from a physiological activity. However, we cannot know for sure if the pigment, which appears in the flush of fever, causes a certain type of beneficial chemical reaction in our bodies when exposed to the surrounding light. Other changes in the color of the complexion due to disease all occur for similarly logical reasons.

B. White and Anxiety

White is a color that is pure and innocent, so it dissolves the doubts of others and draws the sympathy of others to avoid present or future difficulties; thus the color of worry is white.

C. Yellow and Rumination

Yellow is a color of rumination, but its necessity has not been found.

D. Blue and Anger

Blue is a calming color, so showing the color blue when someone is extremely angry can calm that person's emotions and at the same time, suppress and restrain any activity.

E. Black and Fear

Black is the color of a corpse, so it shows non–resistance and at the same time, makes an opponent unwilling to get near because of its unsightliness and scariness.

OBSERVATION OF COLORS BESIDES THE COMPLEXION

There are many other ways to observe color besides the complexion. They are all considered in the diagnosis. Changes similar to the color changes of the complexion can be seen in the color of the pupils, lips, phlegm, tongue coat, menstrual blood, vaginal discharge, urine, etc. Especially in children, attention must be paid to feces in order to judge their physical constitutions. Looking at the worsening degrees of diarrhea in an infant, it changes as follows: yellow with slight blue/green (Wood controls Earth), blue/green with slight white (Metal controls Wood) and pure white (exactly like milk).

III. EMOTIONS

ORGAN	Heart	Lung	Spleen	Liver	Kidney
EMOTION	joy	anxiety	rumination	anger	fear

JOY BELONGS TO THE HEART

Although there is no emotional activity which is not related to the Heart, the emotion of joy belongs especially to the Heart. What this implies is that other emotions act greatly on other organs, but it is only the emotion of joy that acts directly on the Heart.

A. Joy and Laughter

When a person is joyful, blood circulation increases greatly, the face reddens and he or she is not bothered by cold. The Element Fire and the color red belong to the Heart, so the emotion of joy, which accompanies that, belongs to the Heart.

Laughter is an expression of joy and a person with vigorous blood circulation laughs a lot. When a person feels slightly drunk after drinking alcoholic beverages, he or she laughs without reason and has endless bouts of laughter.

B. Young Girls and Laughter

The time in one's life when there is the most laughter is throughout adolescence. During that period, girls in particular, laugh a lot. In Korea, there is a saying that goes, "A girl before marriage laughs even at horse feces rolling on the ground" and in Japan, "A 17 year old virgin laughs even at a dog's feces." These illustrate that adolescent girls laugh a lot. It is a fact that when 17 or 18 year old girls gather, they laugh a lot – when their eyes meet, they laugh.

The physiological reason for this laughter is that during adolescence, the activity of the Heart is vigorous in order to grow and develop, regardless of gender. Especially in women, menstruation begins and in preparation for fetal development, a much higher activity of the Heart is required. Accordingly, it is not that there is much to laugh at during this period, but rather they cannot stand not to laugh. When seen as a natural phenomenon, it is merely a way to entice the opposite sex in order bring about conception, like the flowers blossoming in the springtime to attract bees. Therefore, virgin girls during this period, regardless of another person's appearance or personality, never have any reasons to give bad feelings towards others, especially to the opposite sex.

C. Mental Illness and Laughter

Mental patients have many types of behavior. Among them, one who frequently laughs, dances and boasts of his or her high position and fortunate circumstances can generally be regarded as having a mental disorder resulting from a disturbance in the Heart.

D. Excess Joy injures the Heart

When an overly happy event occurs unexpectedly, there can be a disorder of the mind and when extreme, life can be lost. However, this is an extremely rare example.

ANXIETY BELONGS TO THE LUNGS

A. Everyone automatically sighs when they are anxious. The proverb, "He sighed as though ground crumbled" implies that a person is extremely anxious.

B. If a person worries greatly, his or her face turns pale. White color and sighs both belong to the Lungs and so it is certain that the emotion of anxiety also belongs to the Lungs.

C. A person with weak Lungs worries without reason.

D. The saying, "Cucumber flower blossomed on the face" is used to describe a patient with a lung disease or a person who is very anxious.

RUMINATION BELONGS TO THE SPLEEN

A. When a person ruminates, the digestive power diminishes and the face turns sallow. A person who thinks a great deal generally has indigestion and a sallow face.

B. Lovesickness – the "disease" responsible for a major reduction in appetite without any health abnormality is "the love yearning disease." There are many examples of people losing their appetite for several months and recovering digestive ability to a level above average upon meeting their lover.

ANGER BELONGS TO THE LIVER

A. When a person gets angry, his or her face turns to a blue color. The blue color of the face is due to the slowing down of the activity of the Heart. I have already stated many times that it is the function of the Liver which slows down the heart beat.

B. When a person is angry, the outer corners of his or her eyes contract. Recall that the outer corners of the eyes are the ends of the Gall Bladder channel.

C. When a person is angry, there is sometimes an immediate hypochondriac pain, which is in the region of the Liver and Gall Bladder channels.

FEAR BELONGS TO THE KIDNEYS

A. When fear is present, the face turns black. Black is a color related to the Kidneys.

B. When fear is present, the bodily movements and functions of all organs become non–resistant and passive. This is the effect of *Yin* and *Yin* belongs to the Kidneys.

C. When faced with an extremely dangerous situation, one cannot use the waist freely. The waist is governed by the Kidneys.

D. When feeling extremely fearful, one excretes urine and feces. The functions of both sphincters belong to the Kidneys. There are many examples aside from these, but I believe that one can get a general understanding of the relationship between the "Five emotions" and the "Five organs" with these examples only.

EXCESS AND DEFICIENCY OF THE ZANG ORGANS AND THE DUAL ASPECTS OF EMOTION

Although an emotion belongs to a certain *Zang* organ, it can vary according to the Excess or Deficiency of that organ. Thus, when the Heart is strong, there are a lot of joyful feelings and when the Heart is weak, there are a lot of sad feelings. The same goes for all other emotions. A person with an Excess Liver gets angry easily and a person with a Deficient Liver has much resentment. A person with Excess Kidneys is courageous and a person with weak Kidneys is cowardly. A person with strong Lungs does not have quick emotions and is magnanimous. So a person who prudently handles work, a noble person with little worldly desires, a patriot and a person with abundant altruistic feelings generally belong to this category. A person with weak Lungs worries and is anxious over trivial things without reason. A person with a strong Spleen is filled with great administrative abilities and ambition and generally has strong selfish feelings. A person with a weak Spleen fantasizes and daydreams a lot.

ORGAN	Heart	Lung	Spleen	Liver	Kidney
Excess emotion	joy	prudence	greed	anger	courage
Deficient emotion	sadness	anxiety	fantasy	resentment	cowardice

In actuality, each individual exhibits many personalities and emotions at one time. When observing them, a person must analyze which ones are strong or weak. Just as unlimited colors can be created with three primary colors, unlimited distinctions in personalities and emotions can be seen with just five primary emotions.

EMOTIONS AND DIAGNOSIS

A. Relationships between Emotions and the Physical Body

Emotions are an external manifestation of physiological changes. No matter how much stimulation is given to get someone angry, if the physiological changes required to arouse anger do not occur, the manifestation of anger does not occur. An emotional change is nothing more than a physiological change and a physiological change is nothing more than an emotional change. Therefore, observing the state of the physical body through emotional changes can only be a wise method. This is the reason for putting an emphasis on emotions in the diagnosis of health.

B. Mental Illness and Emotional Expression

No matter what the disease is, there is no disease in which emotional change does not occur as a symptom. The most notable among them is mental illness. Mental illness primarily shows changes in emotions as the most important symptom, so let us now inquire into it:

1. The classification of various kinds of paranoia according to the *Zang* organs is as follows:

   (a) **"Fear paranoia"** – Kidney and Liver (deficiency)
   This is a mental derangement with frequent delirious speech such as, "A ghost is coming after me" or "Someone keeps on hitting me" and is generally related to the Kidney and the Liver.

   (b) **"Poisoning paranoia"** – Lung and Spleen (deficiency)
   This is a mental derangement where a person says "Someone put poison in my food" or "There is poison in this water" and then will put his finger in his mouth to throw up; it is generally related to the Lung and the Spleen.

   (c) **Delusions of persecution** – Liver and Lung (deficiency)
   A mental derangement involving delusions with anxiety and resentment such as, "Someone took all of my fortune" or "We became poor like this because of someone" is generally related to the Liver and the Lung.

   (d) **"Pessimistic paranoia"** – Heart, Spleen and Lung (deficiency)
   Poverty paranoia is a type of pessimistic paranoia where a patient fantasizes only about pessimistic things such as, "Our family is becoming poor" or "From now on, I am going to be poor" or "All my family and all the people in the world are praying that I go poor so I can no longer live," etc.

   (e) **"Jealousy paranoia"** – Liver and Kidney (excess)
   This is a paranoia that most frequently involves a morbid suspicion about one's wife's chastity where the patient says, "My wife is committing adultery" and assaults her or even commits murder in the most extreme situation; this is a mental disease generally related to Excess Liver.

   (f) **"Combat paranoia"** – Liver and Kidney (excess)
   This is a megalomania in which there is a strong inclination to fight like: "I am going to teach him a lesson" or "I am going to kill him one day" or "I am going to attack that country to take revenge for our country," etc.

   (g) **Megalomania** – Heart, Spleen, and Kidney (excess)
   "Arrogant paranoia" such as, "I am the most famous general in the world" or "I am a King" or "I am the daughter of God of Heaven" or "I am the Immortal of this mountain," etc. belong to the Kidney. "Happiness paranoia" such as, "I became a millionaire" or "I am the happiest person in the world," etc. generally belong to the Heart. Attacks of "Venturous paranoia" such as, "I am becoming rich now" or "There is going to be a big fortune if I buy these products now," etc. and making insensibly large scale transactions which result in a big loss, can generally be seen to belong to the Spleen. This megalomania is a symptom common among mental patients of the *Yang* type. Aside from these, there are countless types of megalomania.

2. Emotional expression and behavior of mental patients:

   (a) A mental patient who has behaviors such as cheerfulness, verbosity, restlessness, loud singing and dancing, etc. is due to an Excess of the Heart. This mental disorder is frequently seen at the time of a first marriage (mania due to lust), first pregnancy (mania due to pregnancy) and first childbirth (mania due to childbirth).

(b) Melancholic symptoms such as weeping, suicide attempts, etc. are generally due to Deficiency of the Lung and the Spleen. Lamenting frequently is a Lung Deficiency. A person who constantly thinks, "I have to see that person" and continuously says the name of the lover or a person who does not stop saying, "That teacher was really kind to me" or "My mother loved me dearly," has a problem in the Spleen.

(c) Committing acts of violence, shouting or wailing are signs of a mental illness related to the Liver.

(d) Frequently protecting one's body, talking about being scared and asking for a body guard because of foolish fear comes from Kidney Deficiency.

I have had much success in treating mental patients in clinical practice, by observing the mental illnesses using the categories stated above.

IV. TISSUES
(THE FIVE CONTROLS AND FIVE ZANG ORGANS)

ORGAN	Heart	Lung	Spleen	Liver	Kidney
TISSUE	blood	skin	muscle	tendon	bone

THE HEART CONTROLS THE BLOOD

There is no particular need to explain anything about the Heart controlling the Blood.

THE LUNGS CONTROL THE SKIN

The function of the skin has some common points with the function of the lungs:

1. The lungs disperse water as does the skin through sweating.
2. The lungs take in oxygen and discharge carbon dioxide through breathing. The skin also takes in small amounts of oxygen and discharges carbon dioxide.
3. When cold invades and comes in contact with the skin, its influence directly goes to the lungs.
4. A person with a resilient and tough skin does not easily get pulmonary tuberculosis. A person with a soft, weak and elegant skin can easily get pulmonary tuberculosis.
5. A person with a disease of the lungs has a soft skin (adolescent) or a dry–rough skin (elders).

THE SPLEEN CONTROLS MUSCLES

1. The Spleen manufactures blood and the Stomach takes in nutrients to mutually create muscles. Muscles relate to nutrition and tendons relate to movement.

2. A person with a strong Spleen is obese.

THE LIVER CONTROLS TENDONS

1. Tendons relate to movement and movement depends on commands from the motor nerves, so the breakdown of the nervous system relates to the Liver. The reason is that the liver has a detoxifying function and when the function of the liver is incomplete, toxins in the blood invade the central or peripheral nervous system so that abnormalities in the extension and contraction of the muscles occur.
2. The so–called "Wind" in Oriental medicine is a disease of the nervous system. "Wind" is said to belong to the Liver, so its cause is in the Liver. Since its pathological manifestations occur in the tendons, the Liver is said to control the tendons.

THE KIDNEYS CONTROL THE BONES

1. When the function of the thyroid gland is lost, changes such as incomplete development of bones and sexual organs occur.
2. When the parathyroid gland is taken out, abnormalities in calcium metabolism occur, hindering the accumulation of calcium in the teeth and bones. This results in spontaneous fractures or delayed healing of fractures.
3. When the thymus gland is taken out or its function is lost, it leads to marked pathological changes in the bones and sexual organs. The bones, especially long bones, become shortened due to incomplete development and they bend or break easily due to hindered calcium deposits. There is also a hindrance in the generation of sperm.
4. When the pituitary gland of a young animal is taken out, its body becomes dwarfed due to abnormalities in bone development. There is incomplete development of the sexual glands with symptoms such as interruption of the formation of sperm and egg cells. In addition, polyuria occurs.
5. When the sexual glands are taken out, incomplete development of the beard, mustache, underarm hair, pubic hair, sexual organs and bones can be seen. In women, the uterus atrophies and menstruation stops.

With these examples, the fact that there is an intimate relationship between the Kidneys and the bones becomes clear.

V. SEASONS

(THE FIVE EXUBERANCES AND FIVE ZANG ORGANS)

ORGAN	Terrestrial Branches[16]	Lunar Calendar Month (Oriental)	Solar Calendar Month (Western)
LIVER	Yin, Mao	January, February	February, March
HEART	Si, Wu	April, May	May, June
SPLEEN	Chen, Wei, Shu, Chou	March, June, September, December	April, July, October, January
LUNG	Shen, You	July, August	August, September
KIDNEY	Hai, Zi	October, November	November, December

THE SEASONS AND THE ORGANS

Different organs become especially active depending on the seasons; this is what is meant by "Exuberance." Oriental terms of explanation such as, "Season of Water Exuberance" or "Season of Fire Exuberance" or "Month of the Tiger" or "Month of the Rat" do not parallel modern terms. Setting this problem aside, if Darwin's theory of evolution, which is approved by modern science as correct, then this "Theory of Five Exuberance" will be difficult to disprove. The more an organism evolves, the more its tissues and physiological structures grow in complication and subtlety. The reason for developing in that manner is to adapt to its environment and to better maintain life. Since there are changes in the weather according to the seasons, there should be physiological changes to adapt to warmth, coolness, coldness and heat of the weather. Accordingly, the organs responsible for these changes are specifically designated.

Even in plants, seeds sprout and flowers blossom in the spring, leaves are plentiful in the summer, fruits ripen and harvesting occurs in the autumn and energy goes to the roots in the winter. Thus, man too does not escape the rules of the biological world; that is the reason why each organ has a vigorous activity in accordance with its corresponding season.

THE SEASON OF EXUBERANCE OF THE LIVER

This is the "Season of Wood Exuberance" and is the season centered around the spring equinox. This means that the activity of the Liver is exuberant in the months of January

---

16. Terrestrial Branches are ancient devices to denote time. The order of these branches are as follows:

Yin = the month of the tiger (January)
Mao = the month of the rabbit (February)
Chen = the month of the dragon (March)
Si = the month of the snake (April)
Wu = the month of the horse (May)
Wei = the month of the sheep (June)

She = the month of the monkey (July)
You = the month of the chicken (August)
Shu = the month of the dog (September)
Hai = the month of the boar (October)
Zi = the month of the rat (November)
Chou = the month of the cow (December)

and February of the lunar calendar; this can be deduced by synthesizing the following facts.

1. "The Liver stores Blood" – The Liver stores nutrients and with a period of growth and development in nature ahead, it is the duty of the Liver to prepare for the exuberant activity of the Heart. We can infer "Liver stores Blood" through the fact that fish liver oil is often recommended by Western doctors, due to its benefits to the body.
2. As mentioned earlier, a pregnant woman has great activity of the Liver and in the springtime, the whole of nature is in a similar state. This universality cannot be ignored and accordingly, the activity of the Liver becoming exuberant can be inferred.
3. In the springtime, mental illnesses, especially manic–depressive psychosis, are frequent. The diseases of the nervous system belong to the Liver and a person who has a tendency to have an especially exuberant Liver activity, with the demand for additional activity of the Liver on top of that, creates an excessive burden on the Liver. The excitation of the Liver extends over the limit and the person finally has fits of mental derangement.
4. Growth and development, too, are a type of effort and a fight; fighting belongs to Liver.

THE SEASON OF EXUBERANCE OF THE HEART

This is namely the "Season of Fire Exuberance" and is the season centered around the summer solstice. At that period, *Yang* flourishes so that the temperature is at its highest and the growth of all organisms is at a peak of prosperity. The activity of the Heart in a person is at the most exuberant stage at this time.

1. A person with a heat type constitution will develop a disease or an existing disease will worsen at this time. Lung diseases will frequently develop at this time. Thus, it is the time when coughing up blood and nosebleeds are the most frequent.
2. The so–called "Summer febrile disease" implies that such disease is influenced by the seasons of spring and summer. The "Spring Fever" is similar to the "Summer febrile disease." Its cause is due to an excess burden on the Heart and the Liver.
3. There are frequent occurrences of mental illnesses that are related to the Heart and the digestive organs at this time.

THE SEASON OF EXUBERANCE OF THE SPLEEN

This season is not fixed, but follows each of the other seasons while in transition to the next. It is in March, June, September and December, according to the lunar calendar. In terms of the Spleen's exuberance, the month it is most evident in is June (July in solar calendar). Late summer is called the "Season of exuberance of the Spleen" because June follows the "Season of Fire Exuberance" and "Fire generates Earth." Everyone knows that there are many digestive problems during this time.

THE SEASON OF EXUBERANCE OF THE LUNGS

Autumn is the "Season of Metal Exuberance." In the summer, there is a lot of sweating and the skin pores are open, but when the weather gradually gets cooler, the burden on the lungs becomes greater because sweating and breathing by the skin become weak.

1. In autumn, cough in the elderly begins. The cough and asthma of older people are usually fine during the spring and the summer, but they start each year when autumn comes around.
2. Respiratory diseases of the *Yin* Syndrome (*Yang* Deficiency; Invasion by External Pathogen; cough) occur frequently at this time.
3. The Large Intestine is the paired organ of the Lung and also belongs to Metal Element. Disorders of large intestine, especially diarrhea, occur frequently at this time.

THE SEASON OF EXUBERANCE OF THE KIDNEYS

The Kidneys belong to the Water Element; Water is *Yin* and Cold. During the winter solstice, there is a flourishing of the *Yin* and harshness of cold weather. Since the "Season of Fire Exuberance" is centered around the summer solstice and the "Season of Water Exuberance" is centered around the winter solstice, they are in mutual opposition.

1. Kidney diseases occur frequently at this time.
2. Incontinence is frequent during the winter season.
3. Diseases due to *Yang* Deficiency are most frequent at this time.

   (a) Throughout the year, the death rate is higher during this season. The reason for this is that *Yin* is death energy and it receives additional support from external *Yin*.
   (b) Early morning diarrhea is frequent in the winter.
   (c) Cough and asthma among the elderly occur in the winter.
   (d) Injury due to Cold occurs in the winter.

VI. THE FIVE TEMPERATURES, THE FIVE DIRECTIONS, THE FIVE OPENINGS, THE FIVE SOUNDS, THE FIVE SMELLS AND THE FIVE FLUID

There are many more duties and expressions of the *Zang* organs than the ones previously mentioned such as the Five Temperatures, the Five Directions, the Five Openings, the Five Sounds, the Five Smells and the Five Fluids. However, since I have not been able to collect much data regarding these, I will only present a chart and explain only a few of them.

5 Zang Organs	Heart	Lung	Spleen	Liver	Kidney (Gate of Life)
5 Fu Organs	Small Intestine	Large Intestine	Stomach	Gall Bladder (Triple Burner)	Urinary Bladder
Elements	Fire	Metal	Earth	Wood	Water
Tastes	bitter	pungent	sweet	sour	salty
Colors	red	white	yellow	blue/green	black
Emotions	joy	anxiety	rumination	anger	fear
Tissues	blood	skin	muscle	tendon	bone
Seasons	summer	autumn	late summer	spring	winter
Temperatures	heat	dryness	dampness	wind	cold
Directions	south	west	center	east	north
Openings	tongue	nose	mouth	eye	ear
Sounds	laughing	crying	singing	shouting	moaning
Smells	burning	fishy	fragrant	goatish	rotten
Fluids	sweat	snivel (mucus)	slobber (saliva)	tear	spittle (saliva)

Fever

Fever occurs as a result of physiological effort. Fever can be divided into two types: Deficient Fever and Excess Fever.[17] Deficient Fever is a fever that occurs when there is a

---

17. Deficient Fever is a fever due to a weakness in the body's vital energy and is approximately 38 degrees Celsius (100.4 degrees Fahrenheit) or less. Excess fever occurs when a certain pathogen such as bacteria or virus invades the body from the outside and the body puts up a fight to eliminate them. It is approximately 39 degrees Celsius (102.2 degrees Fahrenheit) or higher. See Chapter 7 on the prescription for further details.

weakness in the body's physiological function and the body tries to make up for its weakness by excessively increasing its physiological activity. Excess fever is a fever that occurs when the body actively seeks to eliminate a life threatening pathogen inside the body.

Deficient fever is eliminated by promoting physiological functions – this is called "Tonification." In Excess fever, heat dissipates when the cause of the illness is eliminated – this is called "Sedation."

Deficiency, Excess, Tonification and Sedation are absolutely necessary, but are also difficult to understand in Oriental medical treatment because the relationship between Deficiency and Excess is extremely complicated and subtle.

The so–called "Excess within Deficiency" and "Deficiency within Excess" are combinations of functional weaknesses and the invasion of pathogenic factors, so the skill of a doctor is needed to judge their degree and to discern their relationship.

Cold

Cold has many meanings, but terms like "Intolerance to Cold" or "Detesting Cold" imply the occurrence of cold feelings when the body comes in contact with external cold at a time when the body's temperature is lowered due to the weakness of its physiological activity. This is called "Deficient Cold" or "*Yang* Deficiency with Cold Excess." In such a condition, the cold sensation is quickly eliminated when the body is made warmer and the person is healed when warm tonics are used.

There is also another pathology called "Aversion to Cold" or "chills" which is important in Oriental medicine. In "chills," a person develops a cold sensation physiologically within the body without getting any physical influence from the outside. When there are chills, regardless of how much one lies under a thick blanket in a warm room to warm up his or her body, the cold sensation does not disappear until a certain amount of time has passed.

The distinctive characteristic of chills is that its end result is a fever. There are no chills that do not foretell a coming fever. Sweating is needed to clear up chills. The above stated chills are "pathological chills" and in order to understand this well, we need to inquire into the "psychological chills."

Here are a few examples of contracting chills through a psychological change:

1. One feels chills when fantasizing about an attack by a beast or a thief while taking a walk late at night.
2. One feels chills when listening to a story describing a red hand popping out of nowhere or corpses walking around.
3. There are cases where naive students feel chills when approaching an examination hall for a test.
4. A naive young man feels chills when meeting the person he is attracted to for the first time.

The common cause of chills here is tension in the body and mind. When feeling fear and danger or facing the most important problems in one's life, preparation to give one's best fight and effort at a moment of emergency manifests as feelings of chills. Physiologically, this can be explained as an effort by the body to contract the skin pores to prevent the dynamic force within the body from dispersing to the outside and to accumulate that dynamic force so that it can be put into motion all at once in a focused burst. Furthermore, shivering is created in a severe condition to generate heat or dynamic force within the muscles.

Pathological chills also originate from the same cause. Chills and fever occur in lung diseases, malaria, common colds and cholera. In these diseases, when the invading germs are fiercely active or cause such a strong degree of auto–intoxication that life is threatened, there is no doubt that chills are the preparation by the body to give a desperate fight in an effort to eliminate those germs.

In Oriental medicine, there is a statement, "Simultaneous chills and fever develop from *Yang* and chills without fever develop from *Yin*." "Simultaneous chills and fever" is *Yang* because it is active and "chills without fever" or "Intolerance to Cold" is *Yin* because it is passive. Chills must be treated by "promoting the sweat and releasing the Heat" and "Intolerance to Cold" must be treated by "warming the Middle and supporting the Heat." These types of "chills" and "Intolerance to Cold" differ entirely along the dimensions of *Yin–Yang*, Deficiency–Excess, External–Internal and Tonifying–Sedating.

Sweat

Sweating has two duties in protecting health: one is the regulation of body temperature and the other is the elimination of toxins.

1. It is easy to figure out, by the abundance of sweating during the summer and the lack of it during the winter, that the regulation of body temperature is managed through sweating. Explained in terms of physics, one calorie of heat is needed to raise the temperature of one gram of water one degree higher; to transform it into one gram of vapor, a large quantity of heat (actually 570 calories) is consumed. Therefore, dispersing heat through sweating has seven times the effect of dispersing heat through ice and 570 times the effect of dispersing it through cold water.

2. The elimination of toxic substances is a problem in medicine. This can also be divided into two types:

   (a) Elimination of disease toxins – almost none of the acute infectious diseases get treated without dependence on sweating. The so–called "Injury due to Cold" in Oriental medicine is a general term for diseases that can be treated by sweating. If there is an excess sweating after the occurrence of chills and fever, a person may feel buoyant due to the elimination of toxins.

   (b) Elimination of waste matter – this is excess sweating without a cause such as a fever or disease toxins. It is called "Deficient sweating" and is caused by *Qi* Deficiency. Being *Qi* deficient implies that the function of the Lungs is not exuberant. The person without exuberant activity of the Lungs does not have vigorous activity of the Heart either. Since blood circulation is slow, waste substances within the tissues are not transported quickly enough and they stagnate.

Thus, the direct elimination of waste matter to the outside of the body through sweating is what is called "Deficient sweating." Deficient sweating can easily be cured by promoting physiological function, but when there is an "Excess within the Deficiency," tonification and sedation must be combined.

Deficient sweating has many causes and in order to eliminate the cause, careful observation must be made to differentiate whether it is due to *Qi* Deficiency, *Yin* Deficiency, toxins or a combination thereof.

Dryness

When the air is excessively dry, the respiratory organs are affected first. When there is an overstrain by the Lungs, the body becomes dry.

Dampness

Living in an excessively damp place weakens the digestive function and dampness generally combines with cold to hinder the metabolism. A disease like beriberi is caused by Dampness. An obese person frequently has a "Damp Syndrome."[18] Obesity relates to the Spleen because, "The Spleen controls the flesh."

Tongue

Since the tongue is "The mirror of the Heart," the conditions of the Heart appear on the tongue. When the body is fatigued, a tongue coating occurs. There are white, yellow, blue/green and black coatings, as well as raised red papillaes according to the related organs.

Nose

The condition of the Lungs appears on the nose because breathing is done through the nasal cavities. There is nasal congestion or nasal discharge when one catches a common cold. Breathing done by flaring the nostrils is the terminal stage symptom of lung disease. Since the nose is the end of the Governing channel,[19] abnormalities of sexual organs appear in the nasal region. Abnormalities of the digestive system also appear in the nasal region because the Stomach channel passes through this area. Nose loss due to syphilis and sinusitis are diseases related to the sexual organs. Dryness of the nasal cavity due to indigestion is related to the stomach and the intestines.

Mouth

Since food is ingested through the mouth, the mouth is one of the important organs of

---

18. A person with Damp Syndrome will have heavy sensations in the head, body and extremities, fatigue, poor appetite and digestion, fullness in the chest and epigastric region, abdominal distention, loose stool, scanty urination, etc.

19. The Governing channel is one of the Eight Extraordinary Channels. It is also called the Du channel. It arises from the perineum like the Conception channel, but runs backwards, travelling up the spine and going overhead until it ends at the inside of the upper lips. For more details, see the Chapter 4 on the channels.

digestion. According to the channels, the Stomach, Large Intestine and Spleen channels are all distributed in the mouth region. The mouth has a relationship to the sexual organs because it is the end of the Conception channel. It is the region where the condition of the uterus in females is especially well reflected.

Eyes

The emotion of anger most clearly appears in the eyes. Anger is an emotion related to the Liver. Eye strain is most easily relieved when one looks at the color blue: blue is the color that belongs to the Liver. In jaundice, the eyes get coloration first: jaundice is a disease related to the liver. Since the end of all the channels is concentrated in the eyes, the condition of each organ appears in the eyes. Diseases of the circulatory system are especially evident.

Ears

Since the strength and weakness of hearing is related to the exuberance or decline of the vital energy, the ears are said to belong to the Kidneys. Deafness after a severe illness or in older people is due to the decline in vital energy and the condition of the Kidneys can be observed through the size, firmness and elasticity of the ears. It is for this reason that no one with small ears has longevity from the viewpoint of physiognomy. As for the channels, the Gall Bladder, Triple Burner and Small Intestine channels are all distributed in the ears.

Burnt Smell

When one is fatigued and has a fever, sometimes there is a burnt smell in the nose. Fatigue and fever are directly related to the Heart and accordingly, burnt smell is related to the Heart.

Fishy Smell

There are times when a patient with a lung disease consciously perceives a fishy smell from the throat.

Rotten Smell

Rotten smells can be consciously perceived in certain types of sinusitis. When root canals are rotten, it can be smelled by others or by oneself. These are all physiological abnormalities related to the sexual organs and accordingly belong to the Kidneys.

Fragrant Smell

Fragrant smell is a minty or a savory smell and there are times when a patient becomes aware of such smells. However, there are no data to confirm that this smell belongs to the Spleen.

Goatish Smell – (Unpleasant smell of fat or urine)

There are times when one becomes aware of a goatish smell, but I have not experienced it as being related to the Liver.

Snivel (Mucus)

During the common cold, there is a runny nose which is related to the Lungs.

Slobber (Saliva)

When one feels hungry, there is salivation. Physiologically, saliva is a type of digestive fluid. Some infants salivate excessively and even some adults salivate easily. An intimate relationship exists between saliva and the Spleen, namely the digestive organs. One can even think of the correlation between saliva and the Spleen by making a connection between the enlargement of the spleen during infancy (when many types of germs are conquered and resistance and immunity are developed against them), and the power of sterilization of saliva according to Oriental medicine.

Tears

Tears come out of the eyes and I have already stated above that the eyes belong to the Liver. This is why we can speak of a correlation between the Liver and tears. One scholar has published the results of research which shows that tears have the power of sterilization. Since the duty of the Liver is that of defense, such as detoxifying and sterilizing, this also becomes one of the reasons. Tears imply resentment and resentment is the passive emotion of anger. Therefore, resentment is also an emotion related to the Liver and so tears also belong to the Liver. Crying without reason – as in hysteria in women – is a symptom of Liver Deficiency. Women crying easily during pregnancy is a symptom also related to the Liver because there is an excess burden on the Liver during pregnancy. The reason for this is because a fetus is in the body and defenses must be even stronger. This responsibility lies with the Liver. Also, it is the duty of Liver to supply stored nutrients to nourish the fetus.

Spittle (Saliva)

Phlegm comes out of the lungs, but its cause is in the Kidneys. Excessive phlegm in the cough of older people is entirely caused by the weakening of vital energy. The source of vital energy is the Kidneys. The saying, "When there is weakening of the Fire within the Kidneys, Water overflows and Phlegm is created" implies that older people with *Yang* Deficiency have excessive phlegm. In a lung disease the cause is "*Yin* Deficiency within the Kidneys creating a shortage of Water and exuberance of the Fire" so the cause of phlegm in a lung disease patient is also related to the Kidneys. "Phlegm" in Oriental medicine is a general term for substances within the body that should not be there. The cause for "Phlegm pain" or "Phlegm-Fire" lies within the dysfunction of metabolism and it is the duty of the Gate of Life, namely the Kidneys, to control and regulate the metabolism.

Oriental medicine, as stated above, is the "Study of Syndromes" in its totality, so the topics lacking in this section should be referred to in the chapters on *Yin–Yang*, *Zang Fu*, Channels and the Pulse.

VII. PHYSIOLOGICAL CLASSIFICATION OF BODILY SYSTEMS AND THE CLASSIFICATION OF THEIR SUPERVISING ZANG FU ORGAN ACCORDING TO THE STUDY OF SYNDROMES

The body of an organism is the gathering of multiple systems which perform varieties of actions or functions. The systems that form the body are classified physiologically and their supervising *Zang Fu* organs according to Oriental medicine are as follows:

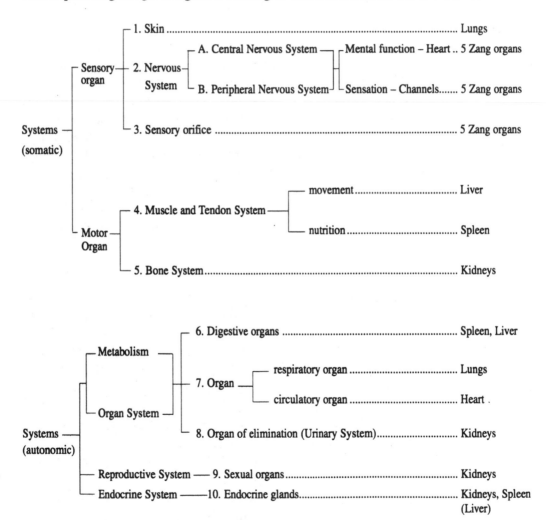

THE STUDY OF CHANNELS

SECTION I • MAIN CHANNELS

I. WHAT IS A CHANNEL?

"Channels" have an extremely important role in Oriental medicine. Discussing Oriental medicine without knowing the channels is the same as trying to understand the state of affairs in a certain country without completely knowing the geography of that country. To know the conditions of Korea well, one must study its mountains, plains, rivers, coastlines, etc. It would also be proper to understand its urban areas, harbors, traffic network, military installations, industry, the "Heart" of people, customs, etc. based on Korea's geographical conditions. The same goes for observing a changing state of affairs: in order to know about good and bad harvests in Chunla province,[1] for example, one would only need to look at the volume of produce transported and exported from various cities around there such as Kunsan, Mokpo, and Daejun[2] – without going around to each house and asking for the harvested volume.

One can know that the weather of Korea is hot by seeing the increased number of passengers – especially first class passengers – departing Seoul and going to Wonsan city.[3] One can also infer that Myungsashipli, Sambang, and Sukwang Temple[4] will be crowded with summer tourists and entertainment seekers without going there.

In a similar manner, our state of health can be known without looking at diseased organs through surgery or by taking X–rays. We can know what type of change has occured in a certain organ by the physiological reactions which appear on the exterior of our body. Consider the fact that changes in our emotion are inevitably expressed on our face. No one will deny that a person's emotional state can be sufficiently observed by

---

1. Located in the southwestern part of Korea.

2. These are cities in Northern Chunla province, Southern Chunla province and Choongchung province (southwestern part of Korea), respectively.

3. A famous harbor city in Hamkyung province (Northeastern part of Korea).

4. Myungsashipli is a famous beach known for its beautiful sands in Wonsan city. Sambang is a famous mineral spring resort near Wonsan city. Sukwang Temple is a famous Buddhist temple near Wonsan city.

looking at that person's complexion and at the tension of the facial muscles. In the *Yin–Yang* chapter, it was stated that psychological and physiological changes are the same thing, so it would not be hard to presume that physiological changes, like psychological changes, must appear on the exterior of our body. Here are a few examples:

1. When there is a problem in the large intestine, blood becomes stagnant on the back of the hand between the thumb and the index finger and the point there (LI–4)[5] becomes extremely sensitive. This is easily seen in anyone who has severe constipation, severe diarrhea or is flatulent upon pressing that region lightly with the finger. Conversely, when LI–4 is very sensitive, one can judge that an abnormality has occured in the large intestine even though a disease of the large intestine is not yet showing up as a subjective symptom.

2. When syphilis is so severe that it appears externally, the areas of outbreak are limited and are related to certain channels:

   (a) Nose region – end of Governing (*Du*) channel, which is the *Yang* channel of the sexual organs.
   (b) Throat, mandible, eye region – end of Conception (*Ren*) channel, which is the *Yin* channel of the sexual organs.
   (c) External side of the Achilles tendon (below the external malleolus) – end of the Urinary Bladder channel.
   (d) Internal side of the achilles tendon (below the internal malleolus) – end of the Kidney channel.

   Aside from these, when there is eczema or enlargement of the lymph nodes, the areas where they appear do not deviate from the Governing, Conception, Urinary Bladder, Kidney and Heart channels. Syphilis is a disease of the circulatory system and so it is reflected on the Heart channel.

3. During menstruation, pregnancy and after delivery, women frequently have changes along the Governing, Urinary Bladder, Conception and Kidney channels as follows:

   (a) Pregnant women develop freckles and liver spots on the forehead, the bridge of the nose (Governing channel), around the eyes and the mouth (Conception channel), and at times, there is an occurrence of discoloration (a black line) on the center line of the abdomen (Conception channel).
   (b) Beriberi of pregnant women – reflected along the Urinary Bladder and Kidney channel.
   (c) At times, women cannot walk at all for a certain period during pregnancy or after delivery – this is involvement of the Kidney and Urinary Bladder channels along the legs.

---

5. LI–4 is the fourth acupuncture point of the Large Intestine channel. It is a Source point, which means that it can be used to diagnose and correct an imbalance in the large intestine.

(d) *Zi Xuan* Syndrome[6] (an upward pressure and oppressed feeling of the solar plexus in pregnant women) – Conception channel.

(e) Tooth pain may occur due to pregnancy – Conception channel.

(f) Boils may appear around the mouth during menstruation or pregnancy – Conception channel.

(g) Eyesight can be lost during pregnancy – Conception channel.

(h) The nasal cavity may ulcerate or become dry during menstruation or pregnancy – Governing channel.

(i) At times, the part of the eyebrows that is near the glabella stands up during menstruation or pregnancy as it does when one shivers from cold – Governing and Urinary Bladder channels.

(j) At times, the color of the lips, especially the lower lip, changes during menstruation or pregnancy to a pale or bluish color – Conception and Governing channels.

(k) Low back pain may occur – Urinary Bladder and Governing channels.

There are numerous examples besides these, so if one pays close attention, one will realize that not even a single pimple appears at any place or any time without having a relationship to the inner body.

---

6. Zi Xuan literally means "hanging fetus" syndrome. This syndrome occurs during the fourth to fifth month of pregnancy. The symptoms include fetal movement, distention and fullness in the chest and oppressive sensation in the epigastric region. The cause of this syndrome is the rebelling of the "Fetal Qi" due to the Liver Qi stagnation or Phlegm stagnation.

II. CHANNELS AND HEAD'S BELT

There is an equivalent to the channels of Oriental medicine in Western medicine – it is called Head's Belt. The names and methods of classification are different, but as far as the fundamentals are concerned, they are in agreement. Both agree that changes of sensation on the body's surface occur because of changes occuring in the internal organs. A detailed explanation of Head's Belt will not be given here. As a brief introduction, Head's Belt is classified according to the areas of sensory nerve distribution.

NERVE DISTRIBUTION:

1. Cervical vertebra (marked by C)
2. Thoracic vertebra (marked by T)
3. Lumbar vertebra (marked by L)
4. Sacral vertebra (marked by S)

Heart Aorta		C3 – C4	T1 – T8 (left side)
Lung		C3 – C4	T1 – T9
Stomach ⌐ Cardia		C4	T6 – T7
Stomach ⌐ Pylorus		T3 – T9	
Small Intestine		T9 – T12	
Large Intestine		T9 – T12	
Rectum		S3 – S4	
Liver		C3 – C4	T7 – T9 (right side)
Gall Bladder		T7 – T9	
Pancreas		T8 – T10 (left side)	
Kidney		T10 – T12	
Urinary Bladder		T11 – L2	S3 – S4
Sexual organ		T10 – T11	S1 – S4

III. PATHWAYS OF THE CHANNELS AND THE AFFILIATED ORGANS

LUG CHANNEL
(belongs to the Lung, collateral⁷ to the Large Intestine channel)

This channel starts approximately four cun (one cun is the width of one's own thumb at the interphalangeal joint) above the umbilicus, passes underneath the clavicle, follows the radial side of the thumb and ends at the exterior corner of the thumb. Its internal branch goes to the radial side of the index finger and connects with the Large Intestine channel. A person with weak lungs makes a fist differently. Almost all of the lung disease patients that I have seen put their thumb inside the fist or they make a fist with the tip of the thumb showing between the second and third finger.

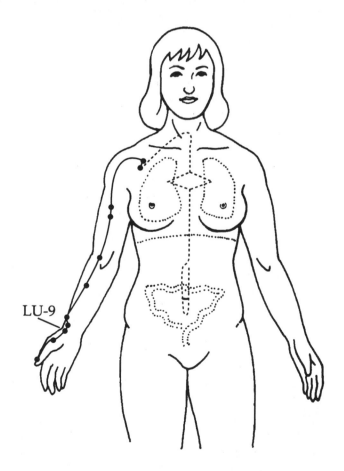

LU-9

---

7. A collateral is a secondary channel that connects two associated primary channels, in this case, Lung and Large Intestine.

LARGE INTESTINE CHANNEL
(belongs to the Large Intestine, collateral to the Lung channel)

This channel starts at the end of the radial side of the index finger and passes through the web between the thumb and the index finger. It then follows the radial side of the thumb, goes over the shoulder and crosses the superior aspect of the clavicle. Next, it climbs up the neck and goes around the mouth to reach the nose region. The internal branch goes to the large intestine from the superior aspect of the clavicle. This channel connects with the Stomach channel at the nose region.

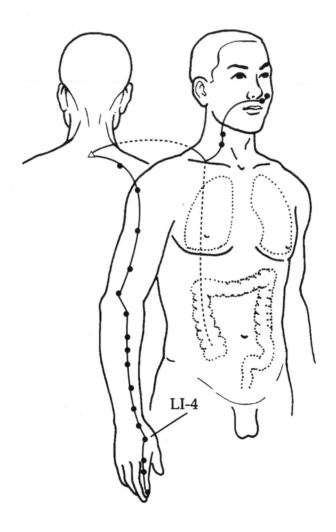

LI-4

STOMACH CHANNEL
(belongs to the Stomach, collateral to the Spleen channel)

This channel starts on the lateral side of the nose then goes up to the eye and comes downward to the side of the mouth. It goes to the angle of the mandible, passes through the nipple and passes down the front of the thigh. It then passes by the patella, follows downward on the anterior and lateral side of tibia, passes by the deepest point on the front of the ankle, and arrives at the lateral side of the second toe. There are many internal branches; from the corner of the forehead, a branch goes to the middle of the hairline of the forehead and another branch goes from the center of the clavicle to the Stomach then down to a point near the inguinal groove (ST–30). There is also one branch from a point below the knee (ST–36) that travels to the lateral side of the third toe.

When there is a problem in the stomach, the top of the sternum feels so sensitive that one cannot put any pressure on it. Also, the place where one puts headache liniment[8] is usually painful and skin problems like pimples (red and hard) develop around the mouth. When the illness is severe as in "Sudden Turmoil,"[9] sometimes all four limbs go into convulsions due to spasms along the Stomach and Large Intestine channels.

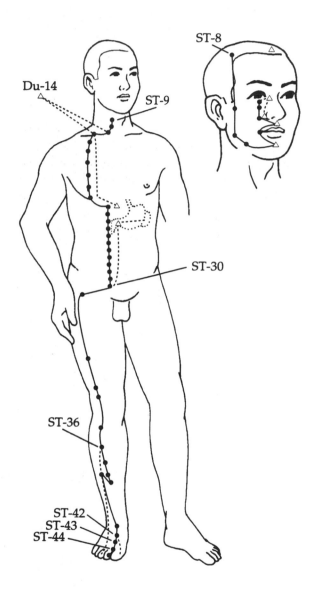

---

8. Headache liniment is put on both corners of the forehead where acupuncture point ST–8 is located.

9. "Sudden Turmoil" traditionally includes any disorder that has simultaneous vomiting and diarrhea as the main symptoms. This syndrome can include epidemic diseases such as cholera or acute gastrointestinal diseases.

SPLEEN CHANNEL
(belongs to the Spleen, collateral to the Stomach channel)

This channel starts from the top of the big toe, passes by the depression in front of the medial malleolus and the medial aspect of tibia, and goes up to the thigh. After crossing the Stomach channel, it goes up the line between the frontal and lateral sides of the abdomen and chest and connects with the Heart channel. An internal branch goes to the tongue.

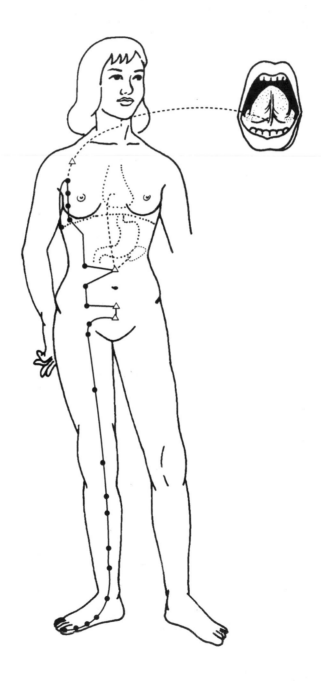

HEART CHANNEL
(belongs to the Heart, collateral to the Small Intestine channel)

This channel starts from the Heart and crosses the thorax towards the axilla and connects with the Spleen channel. Following the ulnar side of the arm, it ends at the tip of the little finger. A branch goes up to the face and by following the muscle that contracts when we laugh, it reaches the eye region.

The cheeks are the regions where facial muscles contract when we laugh, where pimples and smallpox marks frequently occur, where one puts on make–up, and where the cyanosis of patients with a lung disease occurs. The reason for this coincidence is because the cheeks are the regions that reflect the condition of the Heart. A person who has weak blood circulation due to weakness of the heart generally has a cold little finger compared to the other fingers. Besides these, any disease directly related to blood circulation is generally preceded by a change in this channel. In accordance with the progression of the disease, it gradually invades other channels. We can see many examples of this phenomenon. For example, in a disease like leprosy, a few years to several decades before the disease can be suspected with the naked eye, there will be a change in sensations and/or in the tissues along the Heart channel.

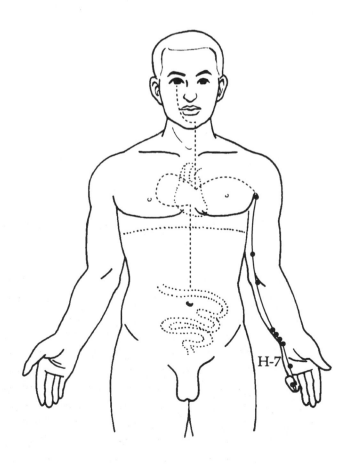

SMALL INTESTINE CHANNEL
(belongs to the Small Intestine and collateral to the Heart channel)

This channel starts at the tip of extensor side of the little finger, follows the ulnar aspect of the forearm and upper arm to the shoulder region, and connects with the Urinary Bladder channel near the spine. A branch goes over the shoulder and divides into two: one going upward to the face, and another going down to the abdominal region.

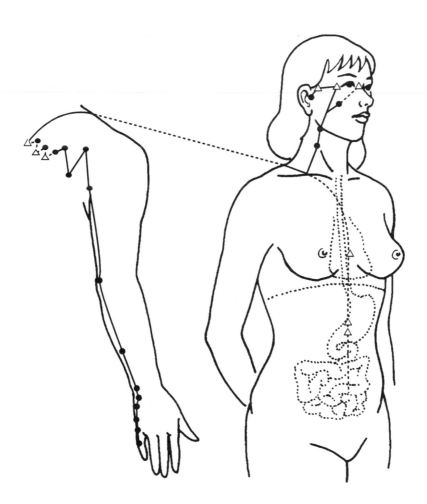

URINARY BLADDER CHANNEL
(belongs to the Urinary Bladder, collateral to the Kidney channel)

This channel starts at the inner canthus, ascends to the top of the head and then descends to either side of the cervical spine. It then separates into two lines on either side of the spine and covers the back. At the lower back region, the inner line goes along the tailbone and the outer line wraps around the buttocks. The two lines gather at the leg, pass through the lower leg and go around the external malleolus, reaching the end of the lateral side of the little toe. The Urinary Bladder channel has the largest domain of the 12 channels. It covers almost one–half of the body's surface. This is the reason why there are the so many *Taiyang* (i.e., Bladder channel) symptoms during the common cold.

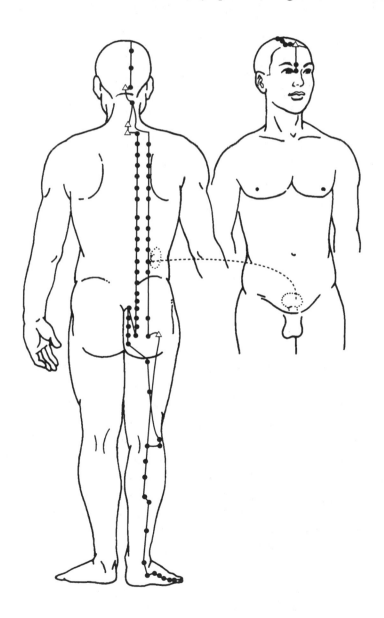

KIDNEY CHANNEL
(belongs to the Kidneys, collateral to the Urinary Bladder channel)

This channel starts at the inferior aspect of the little toe, passes through the center of the sole, goes around the back of internal malleolus, comes up through the inside of the leg and ascends from the side of the genital region to the clavicle.

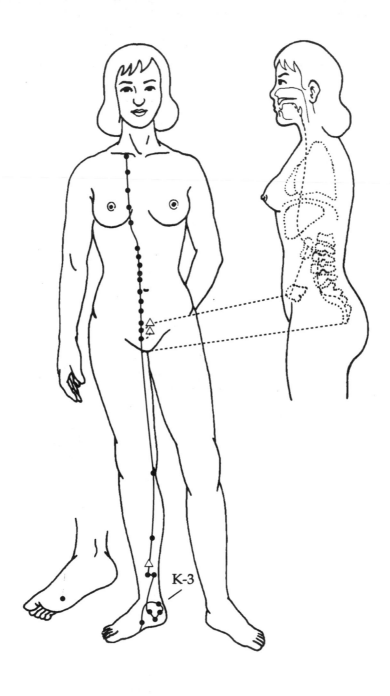

K-3

PERICARDIUM CHANNEL
(belongs to the Pericardium, collateral to the Triple Burner channel)

This channel connects to the Kidney channel in the thoracic region, passes through the center of the anterior aspect of the shoulder, and following the center of the arm, it passes through the center of the palm to reach the tip of the middle finger. It is the strength of the pericardium which keeps the lungs and the heart from breaking down because of the constant friction caused by their ceaseless activities.

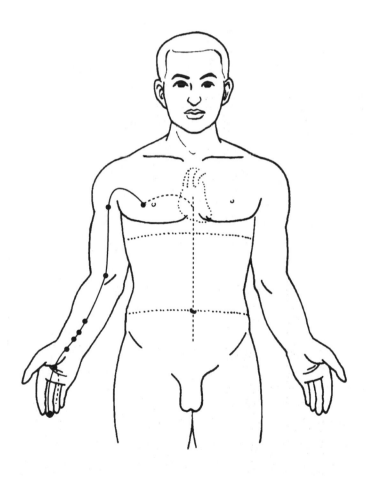

TRIPLE BURNER CHANNEL
(belongs to the Triple Burner, collateral to the Pericardium channel)

Because the Triple Burner does not have a specifically designated organ, it is hard to understand and difficult to explain. Inferring from the *Yin–Yang* relationship it has with the pericardium, which prevents the breakdown of the heart due to its constant friction, it can be generalized that among the functions of the pleura, diaphragm, peritoneum, mesentery and uterine sheath, the *Yin* functions belong to the Pericardium and the *Yang* functions belong to the Triple Burner. This channel starts at the tip of the ulnar side of the fourth finger, goes up through the center of the arm to the shoulder, and goes around the back of the ear to reach the outer canthus. A branch goes over the shoulder and goes down to the thoracic region.

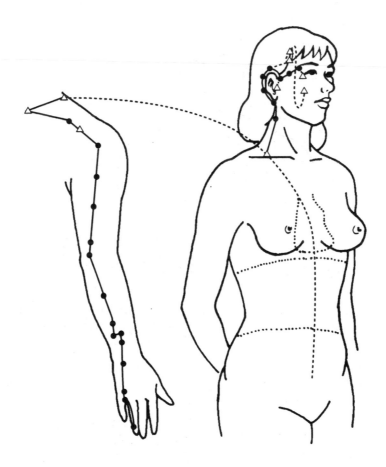

GALL BLADDER CHANNEL
(belongs to the Gall Bladder, collateral to the Liver channel)

This channel starts at the outer canthus, passes the side of head and following the angle of the head, goes around the back of the ear, then down to the shoulder. From the axilla, it goes down the center of the lateral aspect of the body, passes in front of the external malleolus of the foot, and goes to the lateral end of the fourth toe.

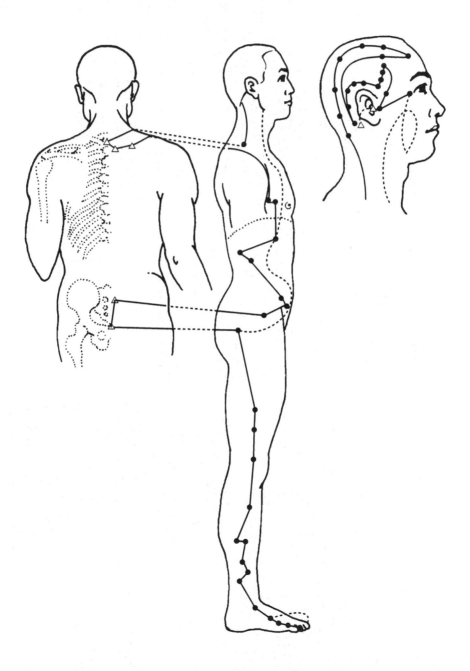

LIVER CHANNEL
(belongs to the Liver, collateral to the Gall Bladder channel)

This channel starts from the lateral side of the big toe, passes by the internal malleolus, and goes up the center of the medial aspect of the leg. Then it takes a very winding course through the abdomen and the thoracic region, goes up to the head region and penetrates the eye region.

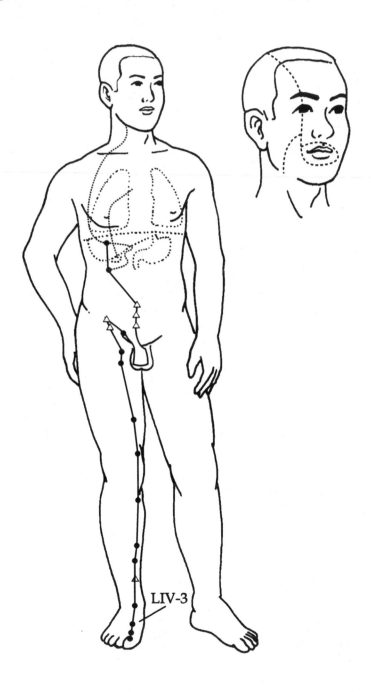

LIV-3

IV. THE ORDER OF THE MOVEMENT OF THE CHANNELS

Just as the proverb goes, "Which came first, the chicken or the egg?" the starting and end point of the movement within these channels cannot be determined. Nevertheless, the channels can be indicated by the mutual relationship between the organs. Establishing the starting point of the channels is like establishing the longitude and the latitude of the Earth. There is no way to answer where the Sun first rises on the Earth's latitude, but the order of the path of sunrise and sunset can be known: 10 degrees west longitude has a faster sunrise time than 100 degrees west longitude, and 10 degrees east longitude has a slower sunrise time than 100 degrees east longitude. Similar to establishing the Greenwich Observatory as the starting point of the Earth's longitude, the reason for establishing the Lung channel as the starting point of the channels is because it is the place where all the channels converge. This is known because the condition of all *Zang Fu* organs manifests as the movement of the radial pulse on the wrist, which is felt along the Lung channel (refer to Chapter 5 on the pulse).

"The movement of the channels starts from the Lung and ends at the Liver. It reunites at the Lung. Because the Lung is the door in which the *Qi* exits, it is called *Qikou*.[10] The Lung is the great gathering place of the vessels thus it presides over the whole body." (*Wu Cao Lu*)

"*Yin* channels are operated by the *Zang* organs and *Yang* channels are operated by the *Fu* organs. *Yin* and *Yang* channels mutually connect like the ring which has no end; the channels start over again without knowing the beginning or the end." (*Li Shi Zhen*)

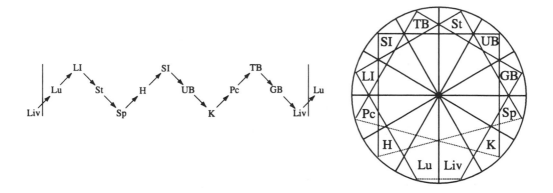

---

10. Qikou literally means "mouth or gate of Qi." In the pulse diagnosis of Oriental medicine, it refers to the radial pulse which is intimately related to the Lung and its channel pathway.

V. YIN–YANG OF CHANNELS AND CONTRACTION AND EXTENSION OF THE MUSCLES

The channels can also be classified into *Yin–Yang*. Channels that belong to *Zang* organs – three Hand *Yin* and three Foot *Yin* channels – are *Yin*; and channels that belong to *Fu* organs – three Hand *Yang* and three Foot *Yang* channels – are *Yang*.

There is a certain relationship between the *Yin–Yang* of these channels and the muscles that each channel passes through; *Yang* channels are all located on the extensor side, and *Yin* channels are all located on the flexor side.[11] Extension is active and flexion is passive. Activeness is *Yang* and passiveness is *Yin*.

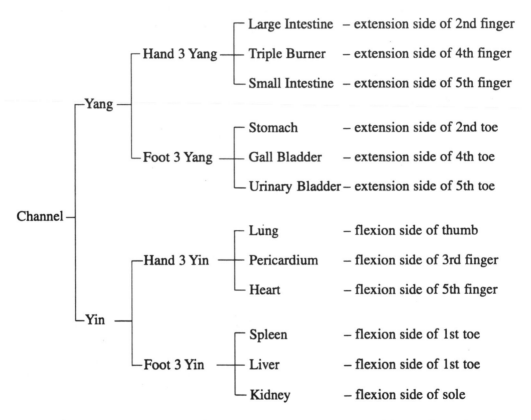

Channel
- Yang
  - Hand 3 Yang
    - Large Intestine – extension side of 2nd finger
    - Triple Burner – extension side of 4th finger
    - Small Intestine – extension side of 5th finger
  - Foot 3 Yang
    - Stomach – extension side of 2nd toe
    - Gall Bladder – extension side of 4th toe
    - Urinary Bladder – extension side of 5th toe
- Yin
  - Hand 3 Yin
    - Lung – flexion side of thumb
    - Pericardium – flexion side of 3rd finger
    - Heart – flexion side of 5th finger
  - Foot 3 Yin
    - Spleen – flexion side of 1st toe
    - Liver – flexion side of 1st toe
    - Kidney – flexion side of sole

There is an easier method of immediately knowing *Yin* and *Yang* channels; when a person feels danger or fear and curls up into a fetal position, for example, the *Yin* channels all·go to the inside, and the *Yang* channels come to the surface.

MORE DEVELOPED EXTENSORS MEAN HIGHER ORDER AMONG ANIMALS

Animals with more developed extensors are higher in order. Among animals, the ones with the most developed extensors are the humans. Humans stand erect since the head

---

11. The author here is referring to the relative location more so than to the actual location.

region and the foot region are vertical. The lower the animal is in the order, the more parallel to the ground its spine is. Among insects, there is no other movement possible other than crawling. Even in humans, babies start out crawling on their stomach when young. Later, according to growth and development, they crawl on four limbs, stand up, and walk. As the vital energy declines in old age, the spine again bends in the shape of a bow. The person cannot stand upright and has to use a cane for support – they essentially start to crawl again. Also, an adult cannot stand erect when ill. Even when there is no illness, the person's head automatically tilts down when he or she is unhappy or gets reprimanded by a superior, so that an upright position cannot be maintained.

VI. CHANNELS AND EMOTIONS, MOVEMENTS, AND SENSE OF TOUCH

CHANGE IN POSTURE WITH PRIDE OR FEAR

When a person has feelings of superiority or feels comfortable, without any feelings of inferiority whatsoever, he or she straightens his or her waist and lifts his or her head so much that the body bends backwards, giving him or her an extremely haughty appearance. When the same person goes before someone superior, his or her head and waist automatically bends forward. When danger occurs, the whole body contracts and shrivels. These facts can be explained through the channel theory. *Yang* channels (Urinary Bladder and Governing channels) are all located in the back region of the body. Because *Yang* is activated at the time of pride the whole body is pulled backwards. Otherwise, the body droops forward because of a reduction in the activity of the muscles of the *Yang* channels. Even more interesting is the fact that the whole body contracts when one feels danger.

When a person gets assaulted by another person, in order to passively reduce injury without resisting, the whole body shrinks to make all the *Yin* channels go inward, and makes only the *Yang* channels come to the surface. This is because as long as one cannot avoid the assault and has to suffer it, it is better to get hit on the *Yang* channels rather than injure the *Yin* channels. Why does the body react in such a way that it is alright to get hit on one region and not on the other? This question fascinated me. It is enough to say that the structure of the human body was originally made like that. Upon a more thorough investigation, it can easily be seen that the reason lies in the relationship between the channels and the *Zang Fu* organs. Then why is it necessary to protect the *Yin* channels more than the *Yang* channels? For the following reasons:

1. Each channel transmits and manifests the state of its attached organ to the exterior and at the same time has the responsibility to reduce and heal the organ's fatigue and the cause of its disease.
2. There are times when all Six *Fu* organs, to which the *Yang* channels are attached, rest without working; accordingly, those channels will be less affected by injuries than the *Yin* channels.
3. The Five *Zang* organs, to which the *Yin* channels belong, never even rest for a moment

until death. So when the *Yin* channels – which are responsible for dispersing and treating fatigue due to the ceaseless activity of the organs – are injured, the overall health will immediately suffer. (Refer to *Yin–Yang* of *Zang Fu* organs in Chapter 1)

4. Important blood vessels are generally situated on the *Yin* channels.

WHY DOES A PERSON FEEL TICKLISH?

I will not try to explain the reason for feeling ticklish by describing how nerves or skin tissues work, physiologically and anatomically. Rather, I am trying to establish what need causes us to have this sense of ticklishness and what reason the body has certain areas that are ticklish and other areas that are not. What kind of a person feels very ticklish?

■ **A virgin feels extremely ticklish.**

Upon inquiring into the degree of feeling ticklish, it is found that more women than men feel ticklish. Among women, virgins feel more ticklish than married women. A thing to think about here is that the person who has the most need to strictly protect and defend her body is the virgin. The virgin, like other people, must naturally avoid bodily injury and taken one step further, having physical contact with others (especially of the opposite sex) is no simple issue. Thus, the virgin has overly sensitive feelings; almost all of her body feels ticklish and sensitive toward a man's body. With this in mind, ticklishness can be seen as a type of special sensation geared for protecting one's body as quickly as possible.

■ **Regions where the most ticklishness is felt.**

In what areas of the body does one feel the most ticklish?

1. front of the neck
2. palms
3. underarms
4. lower abdomen
5. groin
6. soles of feet

These are areas where one feels the most ticklish. Frequently, people say that the area where they feel the most ticklish is where the skin is soft (weak skin). It is interesting to note that the foot feels most ticklish even though it has the thickest skin in the whole body.

■ **Yin channels are very ticklish.**

Even though ticklish areas generally have soft skin, this is not the cause. It is due to the *Yin* channels reaching those areas. Consider the relationship between those regions and the channels:

1. Neck: Conception channel (*Yin* channel of the sexual organs)
        Heart channel
        Lung channel
        Kidney channel

Liver channel

Spleen channel

The six channels mentioned above pass through the neck region.

2. Palms: Heart channel

        Pericardium channel

        Lung channel

The palms are the end of those channels.

3. Underarm: Heart channel

           Spleen channel

4. Lower abdomen and groin: Conception channel

                          Kidney channel

                          Liver channel

                          Spleen channel

These channels wind around in many ways.

5. Soles of the feet: Kidney channel

As this shows, where one feels very ticklish is where many *Yin* channels meet or they are the ends of the extremities. There are no places other than the *Yin* channels where one feels even slightly ticklish.

■ **The reason for feeling ticklish.**

As I have stated above, ticklishness can be explained by the fact that the Five *Zang* organs have no time to rest and there cannot be even the slightest trouble on the *Yin* channels, which must externally manifest and heal the fatigue of the *Zang* organs due to their continual activity. Thus, it can be inferred that in order to protect these channels the quickest, these areas have to be particulary sensitive.

VII. THE REGIONS WHERE REACTIONS OF DISEASES ARE PRONOUNCED

I have already stated that when a disease phenomenon occurs in an organ, the reaction appears on the body surface in the area of its attached channel. Then does the reaction occur uniformly in a fixed degree on the same channel? No, but there is a uniform rule.

REGIONS WHERE STRUCTURES ARE RELATIVELY DEFICIENT AND WEAK

Acupuncture points are the places where needles are inserted and moxibustion is applied. The reason disease reactions are pronounced at an acupuncture point is because when channels are compared to traffic routes or coastlines, the acupuncture point corresponds to the following places:

1. A point of intersection between two streets
2. A railroad station or a pier
3. A bridge
4. A harbor on a coastline

Thus, regions where acupuncture points are located are:

1. between muscles
2. between bones (joint, intercostal spaces, etc.)

When these areas are pressed, they go in deeply and have an extreme pit–like feeling because the structures are looser than other areas. There is no need to talk about how all the changes can be known easily at these places or how all the changes can be put in good order through these places.

THE REACTIONS BECOME PRONOUNCED TOWARD THE ENDS OF THE EXTREMITIES

Pathological reactions clearly show up more toward the ends of the extremities. When the body becomes cooler, the hands and feet get cold first and when the body develops fever, the hands and feet get warm first. Slight physiological or psychological changes appear on the complexion. A headache, a slight flush, and paleness are all examples of this. These phenomena can even be seen in plants so that when growth is flourishing, the ends are fresher and overflow with vital energy. When they wither, the tips are the first to wither. When compared to a scale, the degree of imbalance increases and clearly shows up more towards the end of the beam of the scale. ·

Furthermore, it is known that a force demonstrates its action when it hits an obstacle; the electric heater uses this principle. Like the creation of strong waves when evenly flowing water hits rocks, it can be inferred that the force which reacts to a disease spreads out centrifugally. When this force reaches the end of the extremities – the final obstacle – and cannot go any further, the strongest action of the force is manifested there. One cannot deny these facts for there are too many examples:

■ **When there is an illness in the stomach/intestine:**
1. Headache – end of the branch of the head region of the Stomach channel
2. Dry nose – end of the Stomach and Large Intestine channels
3. Tongue coating – end of the Spleen channel
4. Decay of gums and bad breath – end of the Stomach and Large Intestine channels
5. Joint pain of extremities – pain or slight spasm in the region of the radius on the Large Intestine channel and the region of the tibia on the Stomach channel

■ **In jaundice, yellow tinge or pain first shows up in the following regions:**
1. Eye – end of the Liver channel

2. Thoracic region between the two breasts
3. Headache – obliquely upward from the outer canthus, namely the end of the Gall Bladder channel

■ **Disease of the reproductive system:**

1. Below the knees – women during pregnancy or after delivery sometimes have problems in the lower legs. Syphilis festers and breaks opens on the heels of the feet. The lower legs and heels are the ends of the Urinary Bladder and Kidney channels.
2. Nose region – the end of the Governing channel. There are times when the nose can disappear due to syphilis. Sinusitis and rhinorrhea are also Kidney related diseases that heal well by internal treatment; this becomes the root treatment more so than external surgery.
3. Teeth region – the end of the Conception and Governing channels. There are times when toothache occurs during pregnancy or menstruation. In a sexually weak person, the gums, especially at the site of the incisors, are not firm. When the vital energy of a young person with a loose tooth root improves during adulthood, the root can again become firm. Sometimes, gums ulcerate and decay due to syphilis.
4. Headache – there is pain between the eyebrows, in the eyes or in the occipital region. These areas correspond to the ends of the Governing and Urinary Bladder channels.

SECTION 2 · EXTRAORDINARY CHANNELS
VIII. THE EIGHT EXTRAORDINARY CHANNELS

There are 12 main channels and Eight Extraordinary channels. I have given a general account of the main channels. Among the Extraordinary channels, the names of a couple (the Conception and Governing channels) have been mentioned several times. There are some Oriental doctors who disregard these Eight Extraordinary channels and do not know what these channels are. The reason is that there are insufficient explanations about these channels and accordingly they are not utilized much in practice. It does not mean that the Eight Extraordinary channels are not considered important in Oriental medicine. The Conception and Governing channels can often be observed in the explanation of symptoms. The Penetrating channel is often mentioned in gynecology where there is a common saying, "The uterus is the origin of the Penetrating and the Conception channels." Besides these particular channels, not many books mention the Extraordinary channels. However, these Eight Extraordinary channels are necessary as basic knowledge as well as for clinical practice in Oriental medicine.

YIN LINKING (YINWEI) CHANNEL

This channel starts above the internal malleolus at point K–9 (Kidney channel) and goes up to SP–12 and SP–13 (Spleen channel) in the lower abdomen. It meets the Spleen, Kidney and Stomach channels. Then it goes up and meets the Spleen channel at SP–15 and SP–16 and passes through LIV–14 (Liver channel). Continuing upwards, it meets the Conception channel at REN–22 (upper end of sternum) and REN–23 and ends after reaching the face. Since this channel seems to connect most of the *Yin* channels of the 12 Main channels, it is presumed to preside over the functions (similar to endocrine system) of mutually connecting and regulating the activities of the Five *Zang* organs. For this reason, it can be considered as belonging to those organs.

YANG LINKING (YANGWEI) CHANNEL

This channel starts below the external malleolus at UB–63 (Bladder channel) and passes by GB–35 (Gall Bladder channel). It goes up to the abdominal region and meets the Gall Bladder channel at GB–29 on the way up. It then goes to SI–10 and meets the Triple Burner channel at TB–15 and meets the Triple Burner, Gall Bladder, Large Intestine and Stomach channels at GB–21. Passing by the posterior region of the ear, it meets the Triple Burner, Gall Bladder, Large Intestine and Stomach channels on the forehead at GB–14. This *Yang* Linking channel is presumed to have the function of connecting and regulating the activities of the Six *Fu* organs.

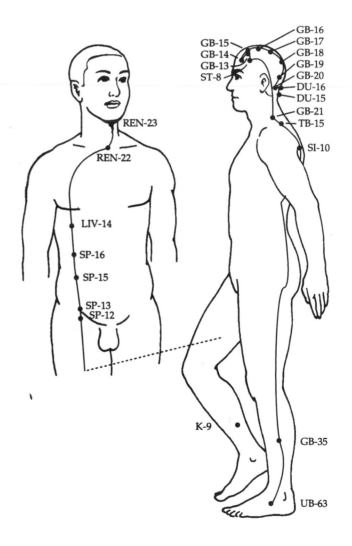

YIN HEEL (YINQIAO) CHANNEL

This channel starts from the posterior region of K–2 of the Kidney channel and goes around K–6 which is below the internal malleolus and passes K–8. Going straight up to the thoracic region, it passes through ST–12 and ST–9 and meets the Penetrating channel after reaching the throat. Then it goes up to the inner canthus and meets the Small Intestine, Urinary Bladder, Stomach and *Yang* Heel channels at UB–1 which is the beginning of the Urinary Bladder channel.

The *Yin* Heel channel is a separate channel that belongs to the Kidney channel and has its foundation in the *Yin* channels and completely connects with the *Yang* channels. The duty of the *Yin* Heel channel is presumed to be the regulation of physiology by making a connection to *Yang* for the benefit of *Yin*.

YANG HEEL (YANGQIAO) CHANNEL

The *Yang* Heel channel starts at UB–62 below the external malleolus, goes around UB–63, and passes UB–59. Then it goes up to the ribs and passes by the scapula and meets with the Small Intestine and the *Yang* Linking channels at SI–14. It then meets the Large Intestine and Triple Burner channels at LI–15. As it continues upwards, it meets with the Heart, Liver and Spleen channels and passes ST–9, meets the Stomach and Conception channels at ST–4 and together with the Stomach channel, passes ST–3 and meets the Conception channel again at ST–1. After reaching the inner canthus, it meets the Small Intestine, Urinary Bladder, Stomach and *Yin* Heel channels again at UB–1 (inner canthus) and again goes up and around the hairline, ending at GB–20 in the posterior region of the ear. The *Yang* Heel channel can be seen as the authority that represents *Yang* for connecting and regulating *Yin–Yang*.

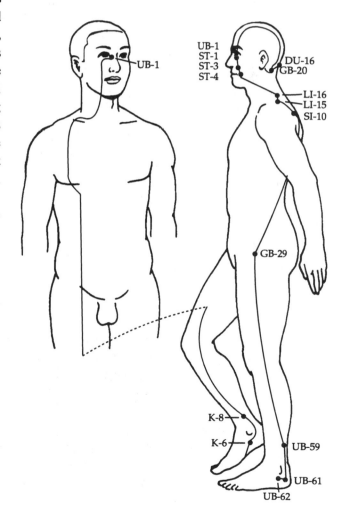

PENETRATING (CHONG) CHANNEL

The Penetrating channel, together with the Conception channel, is a channel that relates to the sexual organs. It is called the "Sea of the channels" or the "Sea of Blood." Appearing on the body surface, it starts from ST–30 (Stomach channel) and ascends bilaterally between the Kidney and Stomach channels. The points that it passes through are generally Kidney channel points. It reunites after reaching the throat region and then separates and surrounds the mouth and lips. It is said that having or not having a mustache or a beard is related to the Penetrating and Conception channels. In the book "*Spiritual Axis*," *Qi Bai*[12] said, "The Penetrating channel is the Sea of the Five *Zang* and Six *Fu* organs." As such, the Penetrating channel can be seen to represent the function of nourishing all the organs.

Even among the acupuncture points, there are many points related to the Penetrating channel such as: TB–1 (*Guanchong*), ST–30 (*Qichong*), ST–42 (*Chongyang*), SP–12 (*Chongmen*), H–9 (*Shaochong*), P–9 (*Zhongchong*), LIV–3 (*Taichong*), etc.[13] The points are mostly on the Stomach, Spleen, and Heart channels which are related to nutrition.

The foundation of the Penetrating channel seems to be the thyroid gland. The enlargement of the thyroid gland with a great increase in appetite can be explained through the intimate relationship between the Penetrating channel and the Stomach channel.

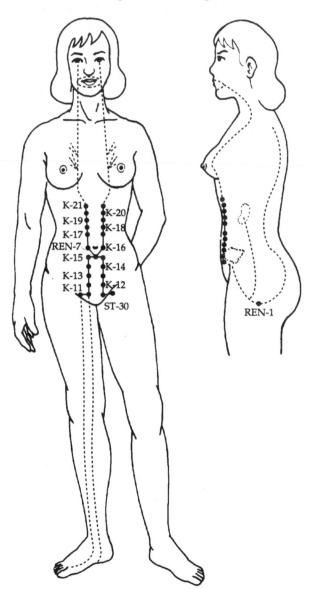

---

12. A minister who served under the legendary emperor Huang Di or Yellow Emperor (2697 – 2597 B.C.).

13. All the acupuncture points mentioned here contain the word "Chong." The Penetrating channel in Chinese is called "Chong channel."

CONCEPTION (REN) CHANNEL

When one imagines a line dividing the front of the body into left and right halves and a line equally dividing lateral aspect of the body into front and back, the crossing point at the top region is DU–20 and the crossing point at the bottom region is REN–1. DU–20 is the highest summit of the body and REN–1 is located midway between the urethra and the anus. The Conception channel starts at REN–1, follows the midline of the front of the body and passes through the center of the umbilicus (REN–8). It then passes the solar plexus (REN–15) and follows the sternum upward and meets with the Large Intestine and Stomach channels at a pit below the lower lip (REN–24). After connecting with the end of the Governing channel, it circles around the mouth region and ends at the eye region.

In the same fashion as the Conception channel, the midline dividing the posterior side of the body is the Governing channel, and the midline of the lateral side of the body is the Gall Bladder channel. The Governing channel is called the "Sea of *Yang* channels," the Conception channel is called the "Sea of *Yin* channels" and the Gall Bladder channel is called "Half Exterior and Half Interior" or "Half *Yin* and Half *Yang*." They are also similar in their functions. Beards and mustaches are located at the end of the Conception and Governing channels. Pubic hair is located at the starting point of the Conception channel. Everyone knows that the growth of beard, mustache and pubic hair is directly related to sexual maturity.

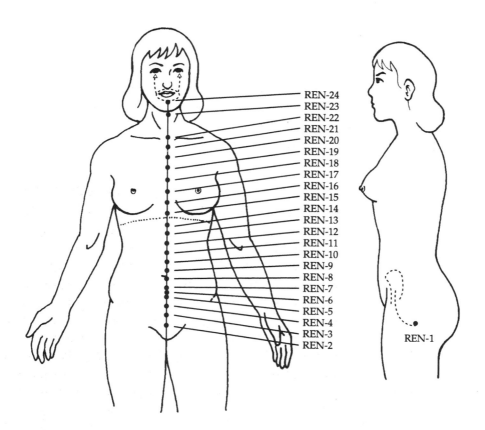

GOVERNING (DU) CHANNEL

The Governing channel is the *Yang* channel of the reproductive system so it starts together with the Conception channel and follows the posterior midline upward, passing over DU–20. It then passes the tip of the nose and connects with the Conception channel after reaching the mouth region. The points of the Governing channel start at the bottom end of the spine at DU–1 and go up to DU–14 below the seventh cervical vertebra (the highest crest when the head is bent forward), DU–15 (in a depression above the posterior hairline), DU–24 (anterior hairline), DU–25 (tip of nose), DU–26, DU–27 (borderline of upper lip) and ends at DU–28 (upper gum).

The Governing channel can also be found in other animals. The cock's comb on top is the end of the Governing channel and the one below is the end of the Conception channel. Depending on the color of a cock's comb, the rise and fall of its sexual function can be known. A cock with exuberant sexual energy has a comb of a deep red color. A hen has a bright red comb at the time it lays eggs and a dark red color from the time of sitting on the eggs to the time of hatching. The horse's mane is also the end of the Governing channel. When a horse becomes angry or runs, its mane stands up.

Everyone agrees that the shape of the nose has a correlation with the shape of a male's sexual organ and the thickness, shape, and color of the labia coincide with the lips and shape of the mouth.

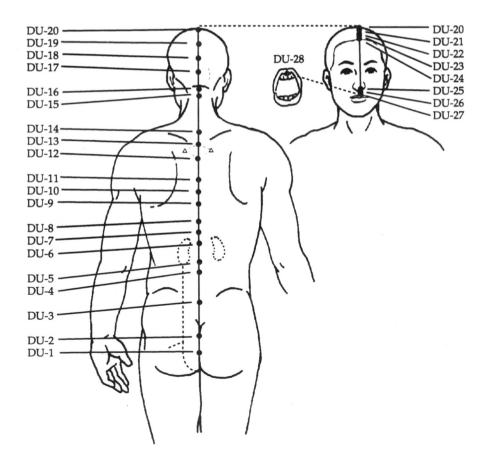

GIRDLE (DAI) CHANNEL

This channel is aptly named because it circles the waist like a belt. It starts at the end of the eleventh rib at LIV–13 and passes GB–26, GB–27 and GB–28. It then circles around the back side to pass GB–26, GB–27, GB–28, and LIV–13 on the opposite side. It goes around the body since the points of the left and the right connect.

Regarding the function of this Girdle channel, it is said that "The Girdle channel completely binds all channels so that they do not move recklessly, much like the belt that binds the clothes of man."[14] Whenever there are statements about diseases of the Girdle channel, examples of the uterine diseases of women are generally given. Since it is extremely vague to consider these examples alone and because I have done careful research on the multiple aspects of this channel, I would like to present the following interpretation, even if it might sound dogmatic: The Girdle channel controls and regulates the extending and contracting movement of all the muscles in the body. The reasons are:

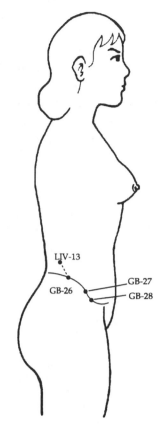

1. The points of the Girdle channel are in common with the points of the Liver and Gall Bladder channels. The Liver is said to control the tendons. In Oriental medicine, diseases of the nervous system are all considered diseases of the Liver channel. Whether it is a mental disease or a stroke, in which there is a breakdown in the central nervous system so that mental functioning is compromised, or contracted muscles cannot be extended, or relaxed (atonic) muscles cannot be contracted, the cause is to be found in the Liver. Physiologically, when there are toxins in the blood, the liver detoxifies them in order to prevent them from injuring the body. However, if this detoxifying function is insufficient so that those toxic substances are sent to the heart and circulated inside the body, a disease phenomenon seems to occur when those toxins finally stimulate and paralyze certain parts of the central nervous system. Thus, it can be presumed that the Girdle channel is in communication with the Liver in an effort to prevent harm to the organs or to the movements of the muscles.

2. It is said in the Chapter 11 of the *Spiritual Axis*, "The Kidney channel exits at the fourteenth vertebra and belongs to the Girdle channel." The acupuncture point of the fourteenth vertebra is the Gate of Life (DU–4) of the Governing channel. Let us take a moment to examine the function of the Gate of Life: Figuratively, the Gate of Life has the function of making the activities of all the organs smooth by providing "machine oil" and supplying

14. Compendium of Materia Medica (appendix) page 1769.

water to prevent inflammation that occurs due to friction. The Pericardium and Triple Burner are channels that belong to this Gate of Life. The pericardium is the envelope surrounding the heart and the Triple Burner is presumed to be the general name for the pleura, diaphragm, peritoneum, mesentery, endometrium, etc. We saw that the Girdle channel passes through the point of the Gate of Life, which functions to smooth out the activities of all the organs. As such, it can be deduced that the Girdle channel, which increases or decreases the extending and contracting movements of the organs, has a connection with the Gate of Life.

3. In Oriental medical textbooks, the following information concerning the Girdle channel can be found:

(a) In the *Inner Classic*, there is a statement that says: "Evil dew in women follows the Girdle channel and descends, thus it is called *Dai Xia*." In Oriental medicine, the term for leukorrhea is "*Dai Xia*" or "Below the girdle" and is originally related to the Girdle channel.[15]

(b) In the Atrophy Syndrome chapter of *Simple Questions*, it says: "The Stomach and the Penetrating channels both belong to the Girdle channel and connects with the Governing channel. Thus, when the Stomach channel becomes deficient, Muscle channels that gather in the groin will be relaxed and the Girdle channel will be unable to pull them together. As a result, a person will suffer from paralysis of the feet and will not be able to walk."

(c) In the book *Introduction to Oriental Medicine*, it says: "When there is a disease in the Girdle channel, the abdomen becomes distended and full and the waist is slack."

4. I, myself, have frequently seen women with the following complaints:

(a) "Lower abdomen feels so hollow that I can't stand it."
(b) "The wind is blowing briskly in the waist."
(c) "Ribs on both sides feel weighed down and oppressed."
(d) "Ribs on both sides often feel like splitting apart."

I can still remember one case that I saw in Seoul last year:

• female patient about 50 years old
• never been pregnant
• with an extremely delicate physical constitution

Symptoms:

(a) Abdomen, like water inside a rubber balloon, comes down when she stands up. She can barely move about even after wrapping the whole abdomen with a

---

15. The Girdle channel in Chinese is called the "Dai channel."

bandage. When she lies down straight, water fills both sides. When she lies sideways, her abdomen droops forward.

(b) There is no elasticity in the whole body.

(c) Ribs on both sides seem to often split apart.

(d) Physiological functioning is not active by any standard, but there are no particular symptoms of a disease.

(e) Even after having major surgery at Seoul University hospital, it is just like before, and the hospital doctor said there is no problem ....

This is a typical Girdle channel disease.

IX. THE COMMUNICATING RELATIONSHIP BETWEEN THE EXTRAORDINARY CHANNELS AND THE MAIN CHANNELS

After simply comparing the functions of the Eight Extraordinary channels, I am now going to chart their relationship to the Main channels:

1. Governing channel controls *Yang*.
2. Conception channel unites *Yin*.
3. *Yang* Linking channel connects *Yang*.
4. *Yin* Linking channel connects *Yin*.
5. *Yang* Heel channel connects with *Yin* from *Yang*.
6. *Yin* Heel channel connects with *Yang* from *Yin*.
7. Girdle channel regulates movement (extension and contraction of muscles).
8. Penetrating channel regulates nutrition.

A Chart of Relationships between Channels

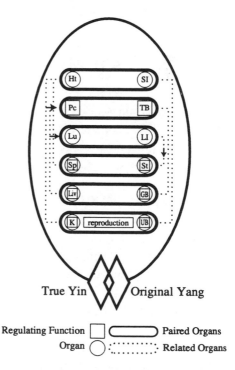

The Eight Extraordinary channels regulate all physiological functions while being controlled by the Original *Yang* and True *Yin*, and because of this, they all belong to *Yin* in comparison to the Main channels. The reason for this is that it is not possible to anatomically or tangibly show a certain organ which is represented by the Eight Extraordinary channels – only a certain function is expressed.

To understand the Eight Extraordinary

channels, it is best to recollect the functions of nerves and hormones. Even with the degree of knowledge of modern times, the subtle physiological regulation that is provided by the reciprocal action between nerves and hormones can only be imagined as vague, subtle, and complicated. It would not be inappropriate to view the Eight Extraordinary channels as that which represents this incredibly subtle regulating function. The Original *Yang* and True *Yin* here imply life force, i.e., the Original *Qi*. When the Original *Qi* is exuberant, all physiological regulations run smoothly so that a perfect state of health can be maintained.

A Chart of Relationships between
Main and Extraordinary Channels

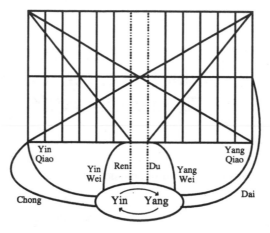

Ren = Conception, Du = Governing, Yangwei = Yang Linking, Yinwei = Yin Linking, Yangqiao = Yang Heel, Yinqiao = Yin Heel, Dai = Girdle, Chong = Penetrating

X. CHANNELS AND CLINICAL SYNDROMES

Channels, in addition to being akin to a public notification place or a bulletin board for the presence of a disease, are also places where the disease is treated and made to disappear. For this reason, it is not necessary to elaborate about the importance of the channels in the diagnosis of diseases.

SHANG HAN AND CHANNELS

According to Oriental medicine, the term *Shang Han* has a wide meaning.[16] Wind pathogen, Cold pathogen, common cold, Invasion by Pathogenic Cold, Invasion by External pathogen, epidemic pathogen, etc. imply *Shang Han*. In modern medical terminology, even infectious diseases such as influenza, epidemic meningitis, typhoid fever, etc. all belong to the category of *Shang Han*. Therefore, *Shang Han* is considered the most important category in Oriental medicine and is, accordingly, the most highly developed.

---

16. Shang Han literally means "injury due to cold."

The great scholar of this *Shang Han* Theory is *Zhang Zhong Jing.*[17] The Six Channel Syndromes in the *Shang Han* Theory are classified according to the channels. They are divided into syndromes of *Taiyang* (Greater *Yang*), *Yangming* (Bright or Extreme *Yang*), *Shaoyang* (Lesser *Yang*), *Taiyin* (Greater *Yin*), *Shaoyin* (Lesser *Yin*) and *Jueyin* (Declining *Yin*) according to the symptoms that manifest on the channels. Thus, the methods of treatment are different depending on individual syndromes. The symptoms of common cold are truly complex and so it is not appropriate to use diaphoretic (sweat–inducing) formulas indiscriminately. I am going to avoid explaining the whole *Shang Han* Theory here, but I will record those features that relate to the channels.

SIX CHANNEL SYNDROMES

1. "In *Taiyang* channel syndrome, there are headaches, neck pain, stiffness of the lower back and spine, fever, chill, body ache, absence of sweating, and a superficial and tight pulse. These symptoms occur because *Taiyang* channel travels along the whole spine. *Taiyang* is the Exterior of the three *Yang* channels." *Complete Works of Jing Yue*

The diseases of the *Taiyang* channel are the diseases of the Urinary Bladder channel. Thus, one feels chilly as if water was poured down the back. There is fever and headache, or it may not be possible to turn the head easily due to pain in the nape of neck, or to move well due to pain in the waist. In the *Taiyang* Syndrome, the area just behind and below the external malleolus and calf is extremely painful with just light touch.

It is the Urinary Bladder channel which occupies the largest area on the body surface. The Stomach channel (*Yangming*) occupies the next largest area. The Urinary Bladder channel completely occupies the posterior half of the body and the Stomach channel occupies most of the anterior half. The small area on the lateral side of the body is the domain of the Gall Bladder channel (*Shaoyang*). Therefore, in *Shang Han*, the *Taiyang* Syndrome is the most common, *Yangming* is next and *Shaoyang* follows that.

I have discovered an interesting phenomenon on the state of distribution of these channels. The greatest issue in the biological world is the breeding of offspring and the preservation of the individual. No one will deny that sex and food are the two greatest issues in human life. Roughly speaking, it is sufficient for an organism to merely eat and breed offspring. All effort and strife are for the purpose of solving these two problems. So-called social position, fame, and power are ultimately the means to acquire the best of these two things. The Urinary Bladder channel, which is related to the sexual organs, occupies almost half of the body surface. In addition, the combination of the Governing, Kidney and Conception channels, which are all related to reproduction, occupy almost all of the body. Next, the Stomach channel, which presides over nutrition, occupies most of

---

17. Zhang Zhong Jing (142 – 220 A.D.) was a distinguished medical scholar. He created the Shang Han Theory and wrote the book, which was later divided into "Shang Han Lun" (A treatise on febrile diseases caused by cold) and "Jin Kui Yao Lue Fang Lun" (Synopsis of prescriptions of the golden chamber). He established the Oriental prescription therapy, invented treatment principles and founded "differentiation of syndromes" and the "discussion on the treatment."

the rest of body. A little left over spot is occupied by the Gall Bladder channel. The Gall Bladder is seen as the organ which supplies strength for combat. Through this, we can understand that sexual issues in the biological world have such a great importance that even sacrificing one's life is not as precious. In the animal world, there is the occasional loss of one's life after reaching the goal of reproduction. Even in human society, murder may occur in connection with a love affair or suicide due to disappointment in love. Both prove how important sexual issues are. This might sound like a digression from our topic, but this fact must always be remembered when studying Oriental medicine.

This is the reason for conflicting principles such as, "Tonifying the Spleen (digestive organ) is not better than tonifying the Kidney (sexual organ)" and "Tonifying the Kidney is not better than tonifying the Spleen."

> 2. "In *Yangming* channel syndrome, there is fever, pain in the eyes, dryness in nose, insomnia, and a flooding and big pulse. These symptoms occur because *Yangming* controls the muscles. Its channel runs beside the nose with a collateral to the eye. *Yangming* is the Interior of Three *Yang* channels." *Complete Works of Jing Yue*

In addition to the above symptoms, there are other symptoms such as headaches and joint pain in the extremities.

> 3. "In *Shaoyang* channel syndrome, there is chest and hypochondriac pain, deafness, alternating chills and fever, vomiting, bitter taste in the mouth, dry throat, dizziness, and a wiry and rapid pulse. These symptoms occur because the *Shaoyang* channel circulates in the hypochondriac region with a collateral to the ear, and is between three *Yang* and three *Yin* channels. From there it gradually enters Three *Yin*; therefore, it is called the channel of Half Exterior – Half Interior." *Complete Works of Jing Yue*

> 4. "In *Taiyin* (Spleen) channel syndrome, there is abdominal fullness, vomiting, indigestion, dry throat, spontaneous heat of hands and feet, or at times diarrhea with abdominal pain, and a deep and thready pulse. These symptoms occur because the *Taiyin* channel is distributed in the Stomach with a collateral to the throat." *Complete Works of Jing Yue*

> 5. "In *Shaoyin* (Kidney) channel disease, there is dry tongue, dry mouth, diarrhea, thirst, dry retching, desire to wear clothing, desire to lie in a curled position, or irritability with a desire to sleep. The pulse is deep. These symptoms occur because the *Shaoyin* channel passes through the Kidney with a collateral to the Lung and connects to the root of the tongue." *Complete Works of Jing Yue*

> 6. "In *Jueyin* (Liver) channel disease, there is irritability with fullness of chest, constricted testicles, upward rising of *Qi* penetrating the Heart, pain and heat in the Heart, or hunger without a desire to eat and a deep and wiry pulse. These symptoms occur because the *Jueyin* channel circulates around the sexual organs with a collateral to the Liver." *Complete Works of Jing Yue*

With the above statements, the reader should be able to realize the importance of the channels in diagnosing *Shang Han* diseases. As far as the other diseases are concerned, I believe that no matter what the disease is, there is no way to be sure of the diagnosis without these channels.

CHANNELS AND THE GENERAL DIAGNOSIS OF A DISEASE

A. Chronic Headaches and Channels

Since the ends of all the channels reach the head region, regardless of which organ has trouble, there are many instances of headaches occuring concurrently. Hence, with only a patient's complaint of having a headache, the method on how to manage that headache will not be known. Even for the same headache, the painful region will be different according to the location of its cause.

According to my observation, the chronic headache, for example, is a *Yangming* channel headache for the most part. The cause of that headache is in poor digestion. It is a symptom commonly seen especially when there is an inflammation in the stomach (Stomach Fire). Let me explain this in a somewhat detailed manner:

1. The Yangming headache is caused by incomplete digestive function. This is due to any of a variety of stomach problems. For instance:

    (a) When food gets stagnated and ferments in the stomach because of insufficient expansion and contraction of the stomach (stomach dilation).
    (b) When the stomach wall is injured by excess acid (catarrh of the stomach, stomach ulcer, etc.).
    (c) Other stomach diseases.

2. Signs and symptoms

    (a) The stomach feels uncomfortable and the patient demands water, especially cold drinks.
    (b) The headache becomes even more extreme two to three hours after meals and lessens when the stomach is empty.
    (c) It usually occurs with constipation.
    (d) The tongue coating is thick.

3. Changes on the channel

    (a) ST–8: It is a region where headaches occur, a place where headache ointment is commonly rubbed. It is the upper end of the Stomach channel.
    (b) LI–4: It is the region of thickest muscle between the thumb and the index finger and is the end of the Large Intestine channel.
    (c) REN–17: It is located between the two nipples on top of the sternum and is the region closest to the stomach.
    (d) ST–43 & ST–44: These are at the lower end of the Stomach channel, in the crevice between the bones of the second and third toes.

A hypersensitivity occurs at all of the above points so that one feels pain with the slightest touch and when very severe, numbness occurs.

B. Intercostal Neuralgia and the Channels

In Oriental medicine, intercostal neuralgia is called chest and hypochondriac pain. Most Oriental doctors consider this chest and hypochondriac pain merely as "Phlegm" and use Phlegm dissolving formulas. However, Phlegm is not the original cause of the disease; rather it is the result of the disease. In order to be a good doctor, one must govern Phlegm without using Phlegm dissolving formulas. The saying in Oriental medicine, "Do not treat Phlegm after seeing Phlegm, and do not treat cough after seeing cough" implies just that. At the time when all Oriental medical doctors were shouting "Phlegm is the cause for nine out of ten diseases," it was *Zhang Jing Yue* who single–handedly advocated the theory "Phlegm is not the cause of a disease; rather Phlegm is produced as a result of a disease." In this age, we can only praise this foresight. Phlegm indicates pathological substances that are stagnated in the tissues. Thus, the mucus that we spit out is a Phlegm and having a stitch (sideache) on the side is also Phlegm. When unhealthy blood accumulates in a certain region because of poor circulation, the pain due to the stimulation on the nerves of that region by toxins is namely "Phlegm pain." I will discuss Phlegm at a later opportunity. Speaking of the regions according to the channels on the subject of intercostal neuralgia, the body can generally be divided into three sections:

1. The section centered around the line of the sternum.
2. The section centered around the vertical line that passes through the breast.
3. The section covered with the arms when a person stands straight.

The cause of neuralgia of the first section is in the reproductive system; the cause for the second section is in the digestive system; the cause for the third section is in the Liver and Gall Bladder.

Imagining lines that vertically divide the body into eight sections, the line that separates the front region passes through the Conception and Governing channels, the line on the lateral side passes through the Gall Bladder channel and the oblique line passes through the Stomach channel. Thus, the thickness of the thoracic cavity can be known from the front side by the position of the breast. Intercostal neuralgia of the first section is frequently seen in sexually weak men with spermatorrhea, nocturnal emission, premature ejaculation, etc. Intercostal neuralgia of the second region is accompanied by indigestion, and pain in the third section occurs frequently from emotional problems. One can frequently see women who immediately get pain on the sides when they get extremely angry.

Even though this neuralgia subjectively appears between the ribs, according to its cause, there must be a sensitive region in the foot area. So if we examine that region, we can understand even more clearly.

C. Examples of Examining Diseases According to the Channels

1. A conversation with an elderly man in Seoul

- Man: "My right arm has been hurting recently, so that I can't lift it and when I answer the telephone, it is extremely uncomfortable and I can't bear it."

- Author: "Have you gone to the hospital?"
- Man: "The Western doctor said that it is neuralgia and the Oriental doctor said that it is Phlegm."
- Author: "Those disease names are probably correct, but the cause seems to be related to the large intestine. Do you have severe constipation?"
- Man: "Yes! My stools are extremely dry so I always take laxatives. I have an errand boy who goes to the pharmacist. I only have a bowel movement once every two to three days or once in three to four days.
- Author: "Then, the pain in your arm is due to your constipation, so you should eat more foods that will lubricate the intestines."

2. A woman in Tokyo (wife of a friend)
- Woman: "I have dryness and frequent boils inside the nose that are unbearable."
- Author: "Do you ever get boils around the mouth?"
- Woman: "Of course! When I have menstruation, the nose is worse and I get sores around the mouth. Why is that?"
- Author: "Is your period the same as an average person?"
- Woman: "The quantity is quite small and my period is not exactly on time."
- Author: "All your symptoms are due to weakness in the Uterus. After tonifying the Blood and your period gets regular, the dryness in your nose will totally disappear."

3. A man
- Man: "Look at my hands. It has been exactly eight years since I got this thick layer of sores on my palms. It doesn't heal and I can't use them. They look so terrible that I can't stand them."
- Author: "How did you leave it like that for eight years without treatment?"
- Man: "No treatment? I've seen many doctors and I don't know how much medicine I have taken. I steamed them many times because I was afraid that it might be leprosy and also got many shots at the hospital because I thought it might be syphilis, but they didn't heal at all."

(After thinking about it for a while, I asked the following)

- Author: "Wasn't the place where you got the sores the very first time on the line of the little finger?"
- Man: "Yes! It was here the very first time." (pointing to a place on the line of the Heart channel)
- Author: "Wasn't the first time you got the sores in May or June?
- Man: "Surely, it was around June."
- Author: "Does your body feel much more comfortable at night than in the daytime?"
- Man: "Yes, indeed. It is useless to plan to do something the next morning. I can't wake up in the morning at all. The day either has to be cloudy or it has to be after sunset before my energy comes up a bit."
- Author: "Doesn't your heart beat fast like when you are very scared?" (palpitations)
- Man: "How do you know all that?"
- Author: "You drink a lot of cold water?"

- Man: "Yes!"
- Author: "You have a good appetite?"
- Man: "I eat all my share."

Because the above statements are all related to the heart and blood circulation, it was inferred according to the channels, but the statements were so correct that I was almost mistaken for a fortune teller. Six months later he was completely cured.

4. Mental illness

While writing this book, I was told that a distant relative had lost her mind. When I visited her, she had lost all mental function and the only thing she was doing was putting anything she could get her hands on like socks, pieces of newpaper, towels, rags, etc. on top of her foot and wrapping it a foot high. Sometimes she rubbed her nostrils and areas around the mouth with two fingers and touched the area in front of her ears. I discovered the following after observing her for 20 to 30 minutes.

(a) The area covered on top of the foot is the lower end of Stomach channel.
(b) The nostrils and the sides of the mouth are the upper end of the Stomach channel.
(c) The front of the ear is the end of the upper end branch of the Stomach channel.
(d) At times, she had slight vomiting.
(e) It is a *Yang* Syndrome since the symptoms are less severe in the early morning and worse in the afternoon.

When all of the above are synthesized, we know for sure that it is a mental derangement due to a breakdown in the digestive system. Under my guidance, the woman easily recovered her mental faculties by the next morning and the symptoms did not reoccur.

There are many examples aside from these, but these alone will be sufficient to show that diseases can be examined according to the channels.

C H A P T E R

THE STUDY OF PULSE

I. WHAT IS A PULSE (MAI)[1]?

There are many meanings to a pulse, but in medical terms they can be usually divided into three types:

1. Channels (mainly in Oriental medicine)
    The pulse represents the channels such as the Liver channel, the Large Intestine channel and the Eight Extraordinary channels – Governing, Conception, Penetrating, Girdle, *Yang* Linking, etc.
2. Blood vessels (mainly Western medicine)
    It refers to the blood vessels such as the arteries, veins, aorta, pulmonary vein, portal vein, etc.
3. Pulse beat
    It denotes the movement of the blood within its vessels that we can feel due to the heart beat.

Since the state of a person's health can be known by observing the state of the pulse, great importance is attached to the pulse in medicine. In Oriental medicine, so much importance is attached to the pulse that examining the pulse is sometimes misunderstood as the complete way of diagnosing a disease. Obviously, the study of the pulse is one of the most important categories in the study of Oriental medicine, however, there is a lot of room for development in the future.

II. DIAGNOSIS OF DISEASE AND THE PULSE

DO DISEASES APPEAR ON THE PULSE?

When the heart stops, it is the end of a person's life. This is why we should always pay

---

1. The word for "pulse" in Oriental medicine is "mai," which has three meanings as mentioned in this chapter.

attention to the movement of the heart and the condition of the heart can be observed through the pulse.

Traditionally, doctors have considered the pulse an important element of diagnosis. Hence, the statement: "diagnosing the pulse like a Spirit" has become a metaphor for a famous doctor.[2] If the eyes are the window of the Heart, then the pulse can be considered the key to life. Each beat of the pulse has an intimate connection to life itself.

When a doctor palpates the pulse of a patient, he looks for the size, strength and speed of the pulse. The size of the pulse indicates the differences in thickness of the blood vessel when the pulse is beating and not beating. The strength of the pulse indicates the force with which the blood moves. The speed of the pulse indicates the time between pulse beats. An average adult has an approximate pulse rate of 70 beats per minute, but if it speeds up to 100 or 140, it is a warning of danger. The occurences of abnormalities in the pulse are all indications of a disease and of where the danger is. Taking it one step further, the pulse is not only something that gives indications about a disease or a danger, but even slight psychological or physiological changes are inevitably manifested on the pulse. At the time of joy, a specific pulse can felt and the complexion changes accordingly. At the time of anger or fear, a unique pulse can be felt and a unique complexion can be seen.

CAN DISEASES BE DIAGNOSED BY THE PULSE?

It is a fact that diseases, without fail, manifest in the pulse. Conversely, it is certainly possible to diagnose a disease with the pulse, but the issue here is one of degree. The question is, to what degree can a disease be diagnosed with the pulse? This is where we can see a difference in opinions between Western and Oriental doctors.

Even in Western medicine, there is a lot of research done on the pulse. It is frequently used in diagnosing a disease by observing the strength, speed, size and regularity of the beat. Through experiments, there is a determination as to what kind of a pulse state can be seen in particular kinds of diseases. Unlike Oriental medicine, it does not specify which organ is affected or what disease is present. I will state the results of many years of research regarding how much practical and theoretical accuracy there is in being able to diagnose all types of diseases with the pulse in Oriental medicine.

CRITICISMS OF THE PULSE STUDIES OF ORIENTAL MEDICINE

An Oriental medical doctor taking the pulse and knowing where the disease is – among Five *Zang* and Six *Fu* organs – is considered to be unreliable by Western medical doctors, as well as by almost all newly educated groups who sneer and look down on it. I was also among them, but the thing we must consider here is that whenever we observe a certain matter, we must always face it with a cool head and without prejudices or emotions. One must not unconditionally deny the validity of pulse diagnosis in Oriental medicine just because Oriental medicine does not have the same basis for arguments that Western medicine has. This is an attitude that a scholar should not take. It is an irresponsible act especially for the students of medicine who handle human lives.

---

2. This is a metaphor for a doctor who is so good at pulse taking that he or she can correctly diagnose the condition of the patient's disease just by taking the pulse.

I have established the order and plan of study regarding Oriental pulse diagnosis and established the steps for its criticism and examination as follows:

1. Logically, is it possible to observe all the physiological phenomena taking place in a person's body through the pulse?

The emotions of a person, without fail, appear on the complexion. In regards to the mysterious and complicated expressions that are manifested on the face, we have not yet arrived (even with analytical science) at a conclusion of how much of a certain pigment and what muscle movement is needed to differentiate emotions. However, with our eyes only, we can sufficiently and correctly observe a person's emotions by taking a brief look at his or her face. Similarly, physiological changes in a person always manifest on the pulse. Theoretically, the physiological changes in a person can also be judged with the pulse. Furthermore, I have carefully observed the pulses of many people and regardless of their state of health, I have felt many people's pulses upon meeting them. I have also felt the pulses of the people that I see often whenever I met them. I have even felt my own pulse countless times in a day. It is obvious that each person has different states of pulse, but I found out that even in the same person, the pulse differs during an illness, before and after meals, during ordinary times and at times of anger, joy or depression. This is indeed strong evidence that a disease can be diagnosed through the pulse.

2. Does the Pulse Theory of Oriental medicine agree with actual practice?

For the second step, in order to test whether Oriental pulse theory agrees with actual practice, I observed the pulses of patients who had already received a diagnosis by a Western doctor from the hospital, with the name of a disease already determined. For example, I observed the Spleen pulse of a patient with a disease of the digestive organs and the Kidney pulse of a patient with a disease of the reproductive organs in order to examine the existence of an abnormality. Except for an extremely small number of unclear cases, the results all agreed with the Oriental pulse theory. In such a manner, the rationality of the Oriental pulse theory was investigated inductively.

3. Deductive experiments on the Pulse Theory

For the third step, the following topics were studied deductively through feeling the pulses of different people without getting any information from them:

(a) Whether or not there is a doctor's diagnosis and a name for the determined disease
(b) Channels
(c) Emotion
(d) Taste preference
(e) Other symptoms of disease

[Example 1]: When the Liver pulse (left second position) is excessively strong, I sought to determine:

(a) Whether the patient had gotten a diagnosis by Western doctors as having a disturbance in the liver

(b) (While giving acupressure on the Liver channel) whether the patient is hypersensitive to pressure on these points

(c) Whether the patient gets easily angered

(d) Whether the patient likes sour or bland foods

(e) Whether the patient has a hypochondriac pain (intercostal neuralgia) or abnormalities in the eye region

[Example 2]: When the Kidney pulse (left third position) is weak, I sought to determine:

(a) Whether the patient had ever gotten a diagnosis of kidney disease in the hospital

(b) (While giving acupressure on the Bladder channel) whether the patient is hypersensitive to pressure on these points

(c) Whether the patient gets afraid easily or becomes extremely scared at night

(d) Whether the patient likes pungent or toasted (sesame seeds, burned rice) foods

(e) Whether the patient has any symptoms such as incontinence, enuresis, frequent urination, nocturnal emission, spermatorrhea, premature ejaculation or diarrhea

After synthesizing this data, I have found that the results of the examinations are in complete agreement.

4. Practical usage of the pulse study.

After confirming the rationality of the Oriental pulse study as we saw above, pulse study was applied in practice as the fourth step in order to modernize and popularize it. As a result of this, one thing that can be considered as a benefit is that the condition of a woman's reproductive system (Kidney) can be known in a fairly detailed manner through the pulse. To explain this in concrete terms, the following are conditions which can be judged through the pulse:

(a) pregnancy

(b) metritis

(c) abnormality in the position of the uterus.

(d) incomplete development or functional debility of the uterus.

These too were experimentally confirmed through the inductive and the deductive methods by me.

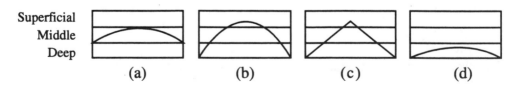

(a) Pregnancy Pulse (left third position).

The pulse beat cannot be felt simply by applying the finger tips lightly on the left third position. A very soft, harmonious and smooth moving pulse similar to a fish drinking water is felt when a slight pressure is applied. It disappears upon firm pressure.

(b) Metritis (left third position).

As in the second chart, this pulse is extremely strong. It beats strongly even when deeply pressed. However, this pulse beat has many differences according to the degree of illness. The pulse that does not signal an extreme degree of illness can easily be mistaken because of its similarity to the pulse of pregnancy, but the pulse of metritis has a stronger reactionary force, however small, when compared to the pulse of pregnancy. This pulse also has differences in the superficial, middle and deep positions. The variations will probably be unlimited when minutely subdivided. I believe that Blood stagnation, inflammation, boils, cancer, etc. can all be distinguished by their degrees of variation.

(c) Retroflexion of the uterus (left third position).

This pulse feels like getting poked by something sharp like a stylus.

(d) Incomplete development or functional debility (left third position).

This pulse is extremely weak and feels like it is there and then not there. In some people, this pulse cannot be felt at all. Among these pulses, the one that can be clearly judged in terms of its correctness is the pregnancy pulse. In my experience, I have never failed to identify the pregnancy pulse, even at the onset of pregnancy. Therefore, I began to give high praise to and started trusting the principles of Oriental pulse diagnosis.

III. LOCATIONS OF THE PULSES

There are broad and narrow meanings to the location of the pulses. In a broad sense, it implies feeling the pulse beat anywhere in the body. However, the locations where the pulses can be felt all have the following conditions:

1. The arteries are thicker.
2. The locations of the arteries are closer to the skin surface.
3. The muscles that surround the arteries are soft.

PULSE POSITION IN THE BROAD SENSE

When a pulse diagnosis is performed, whether it is in Oriental or Western medicine, it customarily involves observing the movement of blood within the radial artery at the flexion side of the thumb. However, there are many locations other than the radial pulse in Oriental medicine:

1. *Taichong* (Liv–3) pulse
    This is a point on the Liver channel, but I could not feel the pulse in that region. In my humble opinion, perhaps it has been mistaken for the pulse of the point ST–43.
2. *Fuyang* (*Chongyang*) (ST–42) pulse
    This pulse can be felt in the deep depression in front of the ankle.
3. *Taixi* (K–3) pulse
    This pulse can be felt fairly clearly in the deep region in front of the Achilles tendon behind the internal malleolus.

4. The *Xuli* (Cardiac Apex) pulse

    This pulse can be felt below the left breast. It is on the course of the Stomach channel in the region of the heart. In a healthy person, it cannot particularly be felt even by touching, but in some people, there are times when this pulse beats so strongly that it can be seen through their clothing even when they sit quietly. This is due to the weakness in the *Zong* or Pectoral *Qi*.

5. *Shaoyin* (H–7) pulse

    This is the ulnar pulse. I have seen a person whose radial pulse could not be felt at all, but his ulnar pulse was as strong as a normal radial pulse. This person had weak lungs with an extremely excited heart, but the cause had not yet been identified. Some people call the pulse behind the tibial bone the *Shaoyin* pulse. This is the Foot *Shaoyin* (Kidney) pulse.

6. *Renying* (ST–9) pulse

    This is the pulse on both sides of the Adam's apple, namely the carotid pulse. The region is ST–9 of the Stomach channel. This is an important pulse so it will be discussed separately at a later time.

7. *Qikou* (LU–9) pulse

    This is the radial pulse of both hands and belongs to the Lung channel. This is the genuine pulse position so the explanations in this chapter are all related to the radial pulse.

THREE POSITIONS: CUN (first), GUAN (second), CHI(third)

In general, diagnosing the pulse implies diagnosing the radial pulse. The radial pulse is divided into *Cun*, *Guan* and *Chi* which are the pulse positions in a narrow sense.

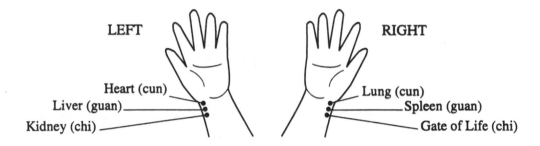

The condition of the Heart is observed at the left Cun (1st) position.
The condition of the Liver is observed at the left Guan (2nd) position.
The condition of the Kidney is observed at the left Chi (3rd) position.
The condition of the Lung is observed at the right Cun (1st) position.
The condition of the Spleen is observed at the right Guan (2nd) position.
The condition of the Gate of Life is observed at the right Chi (3rd) position.

Upon quick reflection, a person might think that it is not possible to observe the conditions of the Five *Zang* organs at these left and right radial pulses. However, this can actually be felt and is proven by facts. If there are any doubts, think of a baseball pitcher.

When you first think about it, it seems impossible for the baseball to change its course after approaching the hitter by the so–called incurve, outcurve or drop, but in reality, it can be done voluntarily through the throwing method of the pitcher.

It is not impossible for the conditions of the Five *Zang* and Six *Fu* organs to influence the waves of the pulses. It is certain that the states of the pulses in the first, second and third positions vary according to the rise and fall of those waves.

When palpating the pulse in practice, it is difficult to locate the different positions. Thus, there is a method of determining accurate positions without measuring them. At the end of radial bone near the wrist, there is a small projection near the wrist which anyone can easily feel by palpating. It is the styloid process of the radial bone and at the tip end of it is the second position. The second position can be determined by putting the middle finger on top of this projection and with the index and ring fingers, the first and third positions are determined.

THE REGION OF PULSE MANIFESTATION OF THE ZANG ORGANS

There are several theories regarding the pulse location of the Five *Zang* organs, but of those, the following is the most universally accepted:

- **The Correct Position**

Left wrist		**Right wrist**	
First position	Heart	First position	Lung
Second position	Liver	Second position	Spleen
Third position	Kidney	Third position	Gate of Life

The reasons for deciding on these regions are as follows:

1. First, whether or not the positions concur with the *Zang* organs must be validated through actual applications – their validity was assured through the inductive and deductive experimental method explained earlier in this chapter. For example, the change in the pulse of the left second position can be felt in a person with a liver disease. Conversely, noticing a change in the left second pulse first and then examining a person for the existence of a liver disease generally produced results consistent with expectations. Thus, each pulse position stood up to the same medical scrutiny.

2. It agrees with the mutual generating and controlling relationships between the *Zang* organs:

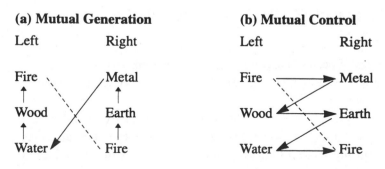

(a) Mutual Generation

Left	Right
Fire	Metal
Wood	Earth
Water	Fire

(b) Mutual Control

Left	Right
Fire	Metal
Wood	Earth
Water	Fire

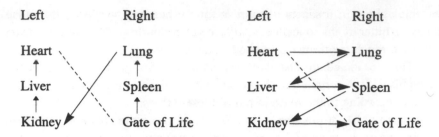

* The Fire of the right third position is the "Ministerial Fire."

When looking at the relationships between these positions, we see that the vertical line is Mutual Generation and the horizontal line is the Mutual Control so the rules are quite systematic.

(a) Gate of Life (Ministerial Fire) generates Spleen (Earth)
   Spleen (Earth) generates Lung (Metal)
   Lung (Metal) generates Kidney (Water)
   Kidney (Water) generates Liver (Wood)
   Liver (Wood) generates Heart (Monarch Fire)
   Heart (Monarch Fire) connects with Gate of Life (Ministerial Fire)

(b) Heart (Fire) controls Lung (Metal)
   Lung (Metal) controls Liver (Wood)
   Liver (Wood) controls Spleen (Earth)
   Spleen (Earth) controls Kidney (Water)
   Kidney (Water) controls Gate of Life (Ministerial Fire) and Heart (Monarch Fire)

3. The left and right sides have functional classifications so that in the right, oxygen is supplied by the Lungs, nutrients by the Spleen and Essence (hormones) by the Gate of Life. On the left side, distribution is done by the Heart, detoxification and storage by the Liver and waste elimination by the Kidney. The left side is active and the right side is passive. The right side supplies the raw materials and the left utilizes them. Therefore, the right side is *Yin* and the left is *Yang*.

IV. THE PRINCIPLES OF THE PULSE

When referring to the types of pulses, one person said that there are 16 types of pulses and another person said that there are 24 types. Yet another said there are 27 types and some said there are even more than that.

The differentiations of pulse types are unlimited. The states of the pulses are as different as human faces. There are slight changes each moment, even in the same person; thus, there is probably no limit when all the variations are taken into account. Therefore, by holistically knowing the principles of pulse diagnosis – rather than studying pulses with an analytical attitude – the applications will be unrestricted so that there will be no difficulty in determining the various types of pulses.

LONGITUDE AND LATITUDE IN THE STUDY OF THE PULSE

Although there are many types of textiles in the world, it is a sure fact that all are woven through longitudes and latitudes of threads. Similarly, although each person has different states of pulses, it is clear that all have developed from the mixture of upper, middle and lower positions (longitude) and superficial, middle and deep positions (latitude).

A. Upper, Middle and Lower

I have already explained a great deal about this in the last section. The so–called three positions in the pulse studies are namely upper, middle and lower positions. It is through the three positions of the pulses that the region where the cause of the disease exists is identified.

High/Low	Pulse Position	Yin and Yang	Body Regions	Organs
Upper	Cun (first)	Yang	chest to head	Heart, Pericardium, Lung
Middle	Guan (second)	Half Yin – Half Yang	chest to umbilicus	Stomach, Spleen, Pancreas, Liver, Gall Bladder
Lower	Chi (third)	Yin	umbilicus to foot	Kidney, Urinary Bladder, Small Intestine, Large Intestine, Reproductive organs

In practice, I have often experienced that when there is a disease in the upper or lower region of the body, there are corresponding changes in the first or third positions of the pulse. This has been explained in the preceding sections.

B. Superficial, Middle and Deep

Superficial, middle and deep indicate regions where the pulse can be felt. So–called *Renying* (carotid artery), *Qikou* (radial artery), *Cun* (first position) or *Chi* (third position) refer to the regions of the pulse beat. In each of these regions, there are different depths where the beat can be felt. So there are distinctions of superficial, middle and deep pulses in all of these regions.

- Superficial Pulse: it is felt with just a light touch and can be seen with the naked eye when the beat is strong (touching).
- Middle pulse: it is felt with slight pressure (searching).
- Deep pulse: it is felt with strong pressure (pressing).

"Touching" is the method used to take the superficial pulse. "Searching" is the method used to take the middle pulse and "Pressing" is the method used to take the deep pulse.

Traditional opinions regarding superficial, middle and deep positions are generally in agreement:

> "The superficial position controls the skin and manifests the conditions of the exterior region of the body and of the *Fu* organs." *Complete Works of Jing Yue*

> "The middle position controls the flesh and manifests the state of Stomach *Qi*." *Complete Works of Jing Yue*

> "The deep position controls the tendons and bones and manifests the state of the interior region of the body and of the *Zang* organs." *Complete Works of Jing Yue*

In my observations, there are superficial and deep pulses in External diseases (skin, flesh, bone and tendon), Superficial Syndromes and Deficient Syndromes. So in all, it seems reasonable to say that *Yang* Syndromes have a superficial pulse and *Yin* Syndromes have a deep pulse. Undoubtedly, there are unclear points and a few exceptions to the rule.

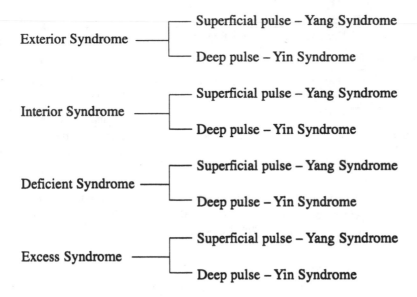

C. Three Regions and Nine Manifestations

There are broad and narrow meanings to the "Three Regions and the Nine Manifestations." In a narrow sense, we talk about the three regions and the nine manifestations of the radial pulse and in a broad sense, we talk about the three regions and the nine manifestations of the whole body.

1. In a narrow sense – it is the three regions and the nine manifestations in general, so the three regions are *Cun* (first), *Guan* (second) and *Chi* (third). Each region has superficial, middle and deep positions, making nine manifestations.
2. In a broad sense – it is dividing the body into upper, middle and lower regions. The state of the pulses at three separate places in each of the upper, middle and lower regions are observed.

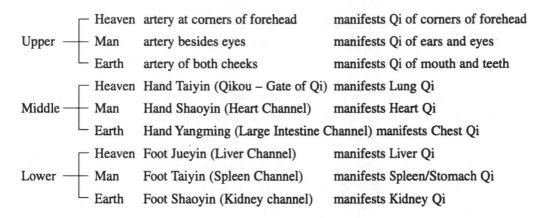

Upper	Heaven	artery at corners of forehead	manifests Qi of corners of forehead
	Man	artery besides eyes	manifests Qi of ears and eyes
	Earth	artery of both cheeks	manifests Qi of mouth and teeth
Middle	Heaven	Hand Taiyin (Qikou – Gate of Qi)	manifests Lung Qi
	Man	Hand Shaoyin (Heart Channel)	manifests Heart Qi
	Earth	Hand Yangming (Large Intestine Channel)	manifests Chest Qi
Lower	Heaven	Foot Jueyin (Liver Channel)	manifests Liver Qi
	Man	Foot Taiyin (Spleen Channel)	manifests Spleen/Stomach Qi
	Earth	Foot Shaoyin (Kidney channel)	manifests Kidney Qi

I have not gathered enough information to comment on these. I have recorded them only as a reference.

THE FIVE ESSENTIAL FACTORS IN THE PULSE BEAT

The changes in pulse beats are ceaseless and the primary factors that bring about these changes can be generally seen as the five types which become the five basic standards of pulse diagnosis.

1. Depth of positions where the pulses are felt – superficial, middle, deep
2. Time between pulses – slow, fast, irregular
3. Difference in the expansion/contraction of blood vessels – large, small
4. Smoothness of the state of blood circulation – slippery, choppy
5. Strength of the heartbeat – empty, full

All sorts of pulse states appear as a result of mixing these five primary factors. For example:

- Flooding pulse = superficial + large + full
- Minute pulse = small + empty
- Wiry pulse = middle + large + full
- Hollow pulse = superficial + large + empty
- Tight pulse = deep + large + full
- Knotted pulse = deep + irregular

HEALTHY PULSE (NORMAL PULSE)

A healthy pulse is an appropriate pulse that is neither excessive nor deficient when compared to the five standards above. It probably cannot exist in actual practice, but an ideally healthy pulse is:

1. Neither superficial nor deep
2. Neither slow nor fast, but regular and moderate (approximately 70 per minute in an average adult)

3. Neither excessively large nor small
4. The pulse is neither excessively slippery nor choppy. It is bad for the blood to pass through blood vessels too easily and it is also bad for blood circulation to stagnate due to roughness.
5. The force of the heart beat is neither excessively strong nor weak. An excessively strong heart beat is proof that there is trouble in the body. It indicates the stagnation of waste matter in the body or an extraordinary effort by the heart to eliminate other abnormalities. The force of the beat also becomes stronger when the elasticity is decreased due to the hardening of the blood vessels. When the force of the heart beat is extremely weak, separation and transportation of useful substances as well as elimination of waste matter become inadequate.

DISEASED PULSE

The essentials of pulse study consist of determining the diseased pulse. To do so, it is imperative to know what a healthy pulse is like, just as a bank teller must sufficiently know genuine dollar bills in order to identify counterfeit ones. A person who is constantly handling genuine dollar bills will be able to immediately identify counterfeit money because "it simply feels different."

The first requisite in pulse study is to be able to know that a pulse is not a normal pulse. In a strict sense, pulses that are not normal are all diseased pulses. However, because a perfectly healthy pulse cannot actually exist, what we commonly call a diseased pulse is one which has a fairly high degree of deviation from the normal pulse.

1. Twelve Original Pulses

Like the multitude of colors that occur as a result of mixing three basic colors (adding white and black makes five colors), a multitude of pulses also can be seen as a result of mixing the 12 original pulses.

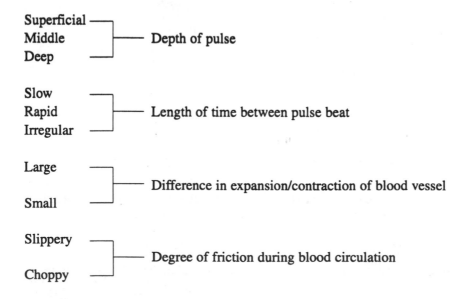

Superficial
Middle ——— Depth of pulse
Deep

Slow
Rapid ——— Length of time between pulse beat
Irregular

Large ——— Difference in expansion/contraction of blood vessel
Small

Slippery ——— Degree of friction during blood circulation
Choppy

Empty ─┐
        ├─── Strength of force of heart beat (blood pressure)
Full ──┘

2. Complex pulses – 359 pulses

From the 12 original pulses, the following complex pulses can be synthesized.

superficial–slow
superficial–minute
superficial–slippery
superficial–empty
superficial–slow–minute
superficial–slow–slippery
superficial–slow–empty
superficial–irregular–minute
superficial–knotted–choppy
superficial–irregular–full
superficial–rapid–large
superficial–rapid–choppy
superficial–rapid–full
superficial–irregular
superficial–large
superficial–choppy
superficial–full
superficial–slow–large
superficial–slow–choppy
superficial–slow–full
superficial–irregular–minute
superficial–irregular–empty
superficial–rapid–minute
superficial–rapid–slippery
superficial–rapid–empty

superficial–slow–minute–slippery
superficial–slow–minute–choppy
superficial–slow–minute–empty
superficial–irregular–minute–slippery
superficial–irregular–minute–choppy
superficial–irregular–minute–empty
superficial–irregular–minute–full
superficial–rapid–minute–slippery
superficial–rapid–minute–choppy
superficial–rapid–minute–empty
superficial–rapid–minute–full
superficial–slow–large–slippery
superficial–slow–large–choppy
superficial–slow–large–empty
superficial–slow–large–full
superficial–irregular–large–slippery
superficial–irregular–large–choppy
superficial–irregular–large–empty

superficial–irregular–large–full
superficial–rapid–large–slippery
superficial–rapid–large–choppy
superficial–rapid–large–empty
superficial–rapid–large–full
superficial–slow–minute–slippery–empty
superficial–slow–minute–slippery–full
superficial–irregular–minute–slippery–empty
superficial–irregular–minute–slippery–full
superficial–rapid–minute–slippery–empty
superficial–rapid–minute–slippery–full

superficial–slow–large–slippery–empty
superficial–slow–large–slippery–empty
superficial–irregular–large–slippery–empty
superficial–irregular–large–slippery–full
superficial–rapid–large–slippery–empty
superficial–rapid–large–slippery–full
superficial–slow–minute–choppy–empty
superficial–slow–minute–choppy–full
superficial–irregular–minute–choppy–empty
superficial–irregular–minute–choppy–full
superficial–rapid–minute–choppy–empty
superficial–rapid–minute–choppy–full
superficial–slow–large–choppy–empty
superficial–slow–large–choppy–full
superficial–irregular–large–choppy–empty
superficial–irregular–large–choppy–full
superficial–rapid–large–choppy–empty
superficial–rapid–large–choppy–full
superficial–minute–slippery
superficial–minute–choppy
superficial–minute–empty
superficial–minute–full
superficial–large–slippery
superficial–large–choppy
superficial–large–empty
superficial–large–full
superficial–minute–slippery–empty
superficial–minute–slippery–full
superficial–large–slippery–empty
superficial–large–slippery–full
superficial–minute–choppy–empty
superficial–minute–choppy–full

superficial–large–choppy–empty
superficial–large–choppy–full
superficial–slippery–empty
superficial–slippery–full
superficial–choppy–empty
superficial–choppy–full

There is a total of 95 pulses

Middle position – 95 pulses
Deep position – 95 pulses

That is a total of 285 pulses.

slow–minute
slow–large
slow–slippery
slow–empty
slow–full
irregular–full
irregular–minute
irregular–large
irregular–slippery
irregular–choppy
irregular–empty

rapid–minute
rapid–slippery
rapid–empty
rapid–large
rapid–choppy
rapid–full
slow–minute–slippery
slow–minute–empty
slow–minute–choppy
slow–minute–full

irregular–minute–slippery
irregular–minute–choppy
irregular–minute–empty
irregular–minute–full
rapid–minute–slippery
rapid–minute–choppy
rapid–minute–empty
rapid–minute–full
slow–large–slippery
slow–large–choppy
slow–large–empty
slow–large–full
irregular–large–slippery

irregular–large–choppy
irregular–large–empty
irregular–large–full
rapid–large–slippery
rapid–large–choppy
rapid–large–empty
rapid–large–full
slow–slippery–empty
slow–slippery–full

irregular–slippery–empty
irregular–slippery–full
rapid–slippery–empty
rapid–slippery–full
slow–choppy–empty
slow–choppy–full
irregular–choppy–empty
irregular–choppy–full
rapid–choppy–empty
rapid–choppy–full

50 pulses

minute–slippery
minute–choppy
minute–empty
minute–full
large–slippery
large–choppy
large–empty
large–full
minute–slippery–empty
minute–slippery–full
large–slippery–empty
large–slippery–full
minute–choppy–empty
minute–choppy–full
large–choppy–empty
large–choppy–full

16 pulses

slippery–empty
slippery–full
choppy–empty
choppy–full

4 pulses

Grand Total: 359 pulses

3. Traditional names of the pulses and their complex contents

Although there are approximately 30 names for traditional pulses, if we exclude the 12 original pulses, the remaining pulses are nothing more than a combination of the 12 original pulses. There are instances where the contents of the pulses are different even though the names are the same and there are times when the pulse name is different, even though the contents are the same. Here, I have selected contents that are relatively common among all schools in order to compare them with the complex pulses described above:

- Long pulse: large + moderate (not slow nor fast) + full, or full + large + slippery
- Short pulse: small + empty + choppy
- Flooding pulse: large + full, or superficial + large + full, or large + slippery, or full + large + rapid
- Minute pulse: middle + small + empty
- Tight pulse: deep + slippery + rapid + full, or deep + large + full, or deep + small + slippery + full
- Moderate pulse: neither fast nor slow, 4 beats per breath
- Hollow pulse: superficial + empty or superficial + large + empty
- Wiry pulse: middle + large + full, or slippery + rapid + full
- Leather pulse: superficial + large + slippery + rapid + empty (wiry + hollow)
- Firm pulse: deep + full + large
- Soft pulse: superficial + small + empty
- Weak pulse: deep + small + empty
- Scattered pulse: extremely empty, or empty + irregular
- Thin pulse: deep + small
- Hidden pulse: extremely deep
- Moving pulse: middle + small + full + choppy
- Hurried pulse: superficial + rapid + irregular
- Knotted pulse: deep + slow + irregular
- Intermittent pulse: middle + empty + irregular, or suddenly large or suddenly small, or momentarily slow or momentarily fast
- Swift pulse: extremely rapid

I have already explained the *Yin–Yang* of the pulses in the *Yin–Yang* chapter. As a quick reminder, *Yin–Yang* are relative. Rather than explaining the *Yin–Yang* of the pulses one by one, I believe that it would be more practical for the readers to learn to use the *Yin–Yang* relationship of the original pulses as the standard in order to determine the *Yin–Yang* for the rest of the complex pulses.

YANG	superficial	rapid	large	slippery	full
YIN	deep	slow	small	choppy	empty

V. PULSE DIAGNOSIS

ESTABLISHING A PERSONAL VIEWPOINT

In making the diagnosis of diseases by using the pulse in actual practice, one must acquire personal views about the pulse more than anything else. Establishing personal views does not mean doing whatever one pleases. Rather, it implies developing one's own exclusive gauge of measuring the pulse by having a sufficient understanding of the principles of pulse studies, and by examining in practice the pulses of many people. Otherwise, trying to mechanically diagnose a disease by remembering the pulses individually and reciting the symptoms related to those pulses is not possible even by a memory expert. Even if one could do that, since the symptoms of diseases recorded in the pulse theory section of medical textbooks do not cover all diseases, how can one judge the differences in the constitution of individuals in the variances of diseases from person to person and in the changes in symptoms over time? Even if the names of the pulses are the same, their descriptions are different according to the different schools. Thus, there are many times when one does not know which descriptions he or she should refer to. The study of the pulse is a difficult thing to hand down. This idea is implied by the statement of *Zhang Jing Yue*: "It is difficult to talk about, but it has a deep significance. It is difficult to picture, but it is truly profound."

FOUR STEPS IN THE PULSE DIAGNOSIS

In diagnosing a pulse, do not try to immediately find out which organ has which disease, but rather, set the order to gradually make a detailed observation; it is the same in any matter or study.

A. Distinguish Yin–Yang.

Distinguish *Yang* with superficial, large, slippery and rapid pulses and distinguish *Yin* with deep, slow, small and choppy pulses. At this time, it is not necessary to distinguish first, second and third positions. The pulse should be observed in its totality. The main focus should be on whether it is a *Yin* pulse or a *Yang* pulse. In actual practice, it does not show up simply as a *Yin* or *Yang* pulse, but rather there are many times when *Yin* pulses and *Yang* pulses mutually cross and mix, confusing the person making the diagnosis. However, by identifying which one is more or less distinct, the status of *Yin–Yang* of that pulse can be determined.

B. Determine Deficiency and Excess

After distinguishing *Yin* and *Yang* pulses, the second step is to determine excess and deficiency by feeling the strength of the pulse. When making a pulse diagnosis in practice, carelessness can cause one to easily mistake superficial, slippery or large pulses as having strength and deep or small pulses as having no strength. Even in superficial, large and slippery pulses, there are deficient ones and deep and small pulses can be excess pulses. Statements such as, "There is Deficiency within Excess" or "There is Excess within Deficiency" all express how complicated the deficiency–excess state of the pulse is. The cause of a Deficient Syndrome lies within the weakness of the body and the cause of an Excess Syndrome comes from the outside, for example, from extreme changes in weather or from an infection due to epidemic germs. In "Excess within Deficiency," the internal cause is greater than the external cause and in "Deficiency within Excess" the external cause is greater than the internal cause.

C. Identify the Position and Region of the Cause of a Disease.

As a third step, the region of the cause of a disease should be discerned. The region of the symptoms of a disease is known subjectively. For example, headaches, abdominal pain and knee pain are easily located, but in order to know the region of the cause of a disease, pulse diagnosis is necessary. Through the state of the pulse on the first, second and third positions, one must find out whether the cause of a disease is in the chest region, the diaphragm region or the abdominal region. To give an example, the main cause of a headache lies in the Stomach (*Yangming* headache), next is the Urinary Bladder channel (*Taiyang* headache) and the Gall Bladder channel (*Shaoyang* headache) follows that.[3] Although the disease is in the head region in a *Yangming* headache, its cause is in the middle region of the body, so the abnormal pulse occurs in the second position and in a *Taiyang* headache, the cause is in the lower region so the abnormal pulse will occur in the third position.

One thing to be cautious about here is that according to the principle of "mutual generation and control cycle" in Oriental medicine, when one organ gets diseased, another organ also shows disease phenomena as a result of the influence of the first one. Consequently, there will be a slight change in each pulse position. So without subtle observation, it will be difficult to distinguish where the region of the cause of a disease is or where the region that received its influence is.

D. Look for the System of the Organ Where the Cause of a Disease Exists.

After discovering the region of the cause of a disease, the fourth step consists in identifying the system to which the diseased organ belongs.

- **Upper region (thoracic region) pulse corresponds to *Cun* (first position).**
  1. Heart system (blood circulating function) left *Cun*
  2. Lung system (breathing function) right *Cun*
- **Middle region (diaphragm region) pulse corresponds to *Guan* (second position).**
  3. Spleen system (digestive function) right *Guan*
  4. Liver system (detoxifying function) left *Guan*

---

3. The headache that occurs in the front part of the head is called "Yangming headache," or frontal headache and usually occurs due to problems in the digestive system. The Taiyang channel (Urinary Bladder) runs up the back of the head. Headaches occuring on the back of the head are called "Taiyang headaches" or occipital headaches. It generally occurs from the disharmony in the genitourinary system or an imbalance in the Urinary Bladder channel from an illness such as the common cold. Shaoyang headaches correspond to temporal headaches and generally occur due to an imbalance in the Liver and the Gall Bladder.

■ **Lower region (abdominal region) pulse corresponds to *Chi* (third position).**
   5. Kidney system (eliminating function) left *Chi* (urine, feces, semen)
   6. Endocrine system (regulating function) right *Chi* (Source *Yang* and True *Yin* of Gate of Life)

These alone are sufficient for treatment. It will be up to the individual's abilities and experiences to know more details. As I have already said earlier in the last section, not only will it be difficult to find out more about the condition of the patient with the pulse, but it is not necessary to know more. We can expect accuracy of a diagnosis only after the results of this pulse diagnosis and other symptoms are compared and synthesized.

PULSE DIAGNOSIS IS ONLY A PART OF THE DIAGNOSIS OF A DISEASE

There is a tendency to think of pulse diagnosis as the whole of Oriental diagnosis, but this is a misunderstanding. I think the reason for this is that only pulse diagnosis gives the patient a feeling of actually being diagnosed when the patient and the doctor meet directly. The other symptoms can be diagnosed by listening. The bodily shape and facial color can be examined by looking – these do not give the patient the feeling of being diagnosed. They usually request pulse diagnosis again and again. According to Oriental medicine, the Four Methods of Diagnosis (looking, listening/smelling, asking and palpating) are considered the four essential factors in the diagnosis of diseases. Pulse diagnosis (palpating) represents only one of four factors and so it is not enough to perform only the pulse diagnosis.

The order of diagnosis in Oriental medicine is looking (observing the shape and looking at the color), listening (patient's complaints), asking (questioning the symptoms) and palpating (pulse diagnosis).

The pulse diagnosis is done in order to assess whether the diagnosis made from looking, listening and asking is accurate or not.

■ **The Seven Essential Factors of a Diagnosis**

In order to make an accurate diagnosis, observation should be made in the following seven areas.

1. Physical constitution (refer to the *Yin–Yang* chapter) – distinguish the *Yin–Yang* of the physical constitution by observing the relationship between the weather and the state of health and usual likes and dislikes of food, etc.
2. Symptoms (refer to the *Yin–Yang* and the Syndrome chapters) – each symptom should be minutely observed to discern *Yin–Yang*, Excess–Deficiency, Exterior–Interior and Upper–Lower of a diseased organ.
3. State of pulse (refer to the Pulse chapter) – discern *Yin–Yang*, Excess–Deficiency and Upper–Lower of the diseased organ through the pulse.
4. Channels (refer to the Channel chapter) – discern the diseased organ by examining the regions based on the channel that developed a change in sensation.
5. Emotion (refer to the Syndrome chapter) – discern the diseased organ and its Deficiency –Excess by emotions.

6. Color (refer to the Syndrome chapter) – discern the diseased organ and its Excess – Deficiency by looking at the color.
7. Speech and movement (refer to the *Yin–Yang* chapter)–discern *Yin–Yang* and Excess– Deficiency by speech, voice, behavior and movement.

If the diagnosis is not made holistically like this, there will be instances when one will make the same mistake as "the three blind men describing an elephant." The method described above gives the utmost effort in the diagnosis of a disease that is most difficult to discern. This does not imply that a diagnosis must always be made according to this method. In general, a diagnosis can be made well with the symptoms only and when combined with the pulse, the diagnosis will almost be complete.

VI. PULSE SYNDROMES

Commenting individually on the pulse syndrome is not possible since the scope is too broad, so I have left my own opinions out. Next, I will be quoting the pulse methods of various schools as a reference.

STATE OF THE BEAT OF EACH PULSE AND INDICATIONS

1. Superficial pulse (Yang)
It feels strong upon light pressure, but deficient upon heavy pressure. The superficial pulse is *Yang*; flooding, large, hollow and leather pulses all belong to this category.

Indications: Middle *Qi* Deficiency,[4] *Yin* Deficiency, Wind, Summer Heat, distention and fullness in the abdomen, anorexia, Exterior Heat and asthmatic breathing.

2. Deep pulse (Yin)
It cannot be felt upon light pressure, but it is felt upon heavy pressure. The deep pulse is *Yin*; thready, small and hidden pulses all belong to this category.
The deep pulse moves between the tendons.
The hidden pulse moves above the bones.
A deep pulse, which is large with strength, is called a firm pulse.
A deep pulse, which is thready without strength, is called a weak pulse.

Indications: Cold, Damp–Phlegm, *Qi* stagnation, Retention of Fluid, a mass in the lower abdomen, excessive distention in the abdomen, syncope and diarrhea.

3. Slow pulse (Yin)
It is less than four beats per breath and comes and goes extremely slowly. This pulse

---

4. Middle Qi Deficiency refers to weakness in the digestive system.

does not come on time because *Yang* is unable to control *Yin*. The slow pulse is *Yin*; intermittent, moderate, knotted and choppy pulses all belong to this category. This pulse indicates Exuberance of *Yin* and Decline of *Yang*.

A slow pulse that has strength is a moderate pulse.

A slow pulse that has no strength is a choppy pulse.

An extemely slow pulse is a defeated pulse.

Indications: Cold and Deficiency.

4. Rapid pulse (Yang)

It has more than five to six beats per breath. The rapid pulse usually beats six times per breath. *Yin* is deficient and *Yang* is exuberant. It indicates extreme irritability. Rapid, swift, urgent and hurried pulses all belong to this category.

A rapid pulse that is wiry and urgent is a tight pulse.

A rapid pulse that is flowing smoothly is a slippery pulse.

A rapid pulse that has pauses is a hurried pulse.

A rapid pulse that is severe is an extreme pulse.

Indications: chills and fever, Consumption,[5] External Pathogen, carbuncles and furuncles.

5. Slippery pulse (Yin within Yang)

It flows smoothly like feeling a pearl between the fingers. Flooding, large, hollow and excess pulses all belong to this category. It indicates Excess *Qi* and the obstruction of Blood.

Indications: Rebellious Phlegm,[6] food stagnation, vomiting, fullness and discomfort of chest and abdomen and Blood stagnation.

6. Choppy pulse (Yin)

It flows with difficulty and movement is not smooth. It is similar to scraping bamboo with a knife. Empty, thready, minute and slow pulses all belong to this category. It indicates Deficiency of both *Qi* and Blood.

Indications: lack of energy, anxiety, arthritic pain, spasm, numbness, absence of sweating, Coldness in the Spleen, anorexia, Coldness in the Stomach, vomiting, irregular bowel movements, cold extremities, Injury to Essence in a man, loss of Blood in a woman, infertility and irregular menstruation.

---

5. Consumption is a general term that implies a variety of disorders that manifest due to weakness in Qi and Zang Fu organs. It is caused by constitutional weakness, improper living and dietary habits, malnutrition due to chronic illness, overstraining, inability to recover from chronic illness, etc.

6. Rebellious Phlegm indicates phlegm that we cough up or vomit.

7. **Empty pulse (Yin) – has aspects of both Yin and Yang**

It indicates Deficiency of *Zheng Qi* (Upright *Qi*), lack of energy and lack of vitality. It is slow, large and soft. There is no strength when heavily pressed and feels hollow at the center when lightly pressed.

Indications: fever, Injury due to Summer Heat,[7] spontaneous sweating, severe palpitations, palpitations due to fright and *Yin* Deficiency.

8. **Full pulse (Yang) – has aspects of both Yin and Yang**

It feels strong at all three levels and indicates excess Pathogenic *Qi*. It beats with strength and feels large and long at both superficial and deep levels. Wiry, flooding, tight and slippery pulses all belong to this category. It indicates an obstruction of the Triple Burner.

Indications: Mania due to the stagnation of Fire, delirious speech, vomiting, *Yang* toxins, Injury due to food, constipation and *Qi* pain.[8]

9. **Flooding pulse (Yang)**

It is large and excessive and feels excessive at both superficial and deep levels. It is extremely large under pressure; comes on strong and goes weakly; comes on large and goes on long. Superficial, hollow, excess and large pulses all belong to this category. It indicates the scorching of *Qi* and Blood and great Heat. It also indicates Excess *Yang* and Deficient *Yin*; Excess *Qi* and Deficient Blood.

Indications: High Fever (*Yangming* and *Qi* Level Syndromes),[9] Excess Heat in the *Zang Fu* organs, chronic diseases, *Yin* Deficiency and carbuncles in the lungs or intestines.

10. **Minute pulse (Yin)**

It is a fine, spiritless pulse which is extremely soft and weak. When heavily pressed, it seems ready to disappear, fading in and out. Thready, small, empty and soft pulses all belong to this category. It indicates Deficiency of both *Qi* and Blood.

Indications: Intolerance to Cold, fear, timidity, lack of energy, Coldness in the Middle Burner, distention and fullness in the abdomen, vomiting, sneezing, diarrhea, Defi-

---

7. Symptoms such as weakness and loss of energy result from Injury due to Summer Heat.

8. In Oriental medicine, mania is caused by Phlegm–Fire which occurs due to extreme stress and improper dietary practices including excess amount of alcohol and spicy and greasy foods. Yang toxins cause symptoms of inflammation such as pain, redness, swelling and heat. Qi pain is due to the obstruction in the movement of Qi. Its symptoms are distending pain and a palpable mass that is movable and disappears at times.

9. Both Yangming and Qi Level Syndromes includes symptoms such as high fever, profuse sweating, great thirst and big and flooding pulse.

cient sweating, indigestion, low back and abdominal pain, Injury to Essence, loss of Blood, dizziness and vertigo, syncope, metrorrhagia and leukorrhea.[10]

11. Wiry pulse (Yin within Yang or Hidden Yin within Yang)

It does not move when pressed, but whips like a bowstring; the edges are straight and long like an extended bowstring. Slippery, large and tight pulses all belong to this category. The Wiry pulse is superficial and tight; the firm pulse is deep and tight.

Indications: disharmony between Blood and *Qi*, *Qi* rebellion,[11] Exuberance of Pathogens, Liver Excess/Spleen Deficiency, alternating chills and fever, Phlegm–Damp, food stagnation, abdominal mass, distention and fullness of the abdomen, Consumption, pain, spasm, malaria, chest and hypochondriac pain.

12. Hollow pulse (Yin within Yang; Yang)

It is superficial, large and hollow in the middle, like a green onion when pressed. It feels strong on the outside but empty in the middle. Superficial, wiry and flooding pulses all belong to this category. It indicates isolated *Yang* with exhaustion of *Yin*.

Indications: Loss of Blood, Exhaustion of Blood (thus *Qi* does not have a place to return and *Yang* does not have a place to attach to), *Yin* Deficiency fever, dizziness and vertigo, fright palpitations or severe palpitations, asthmatic breathing and night sweats.

Although a hollow pulse belongs to the *Yang* pulse, it is a *Yang* excess without root and indicates a great Deficiency of *Yin*, Blood or Essence.

13. Tight pulse (Yang; or more Yin, less Yang)

It is urgent and rapid with strength and beats firmly, resisting the finger like a twisted rope. Wiry and rapid pulses both belong to this category. It manifests *Yin* pathogen beating violently. It is a pulse of Heat binding the Cold.

Indications: pain and coldness.

14. Moderate pulse (Yin; but has aspects of both Yin and Yang)

It is harmonious and moderate and is not tight. It has four beats per breath and is elegant and relaxed like the image of willows moving with the wind in the early spring. The moderate pulse has aspects of both *Yin* and *Yang*. It is the normal pulse of an average person.

---

10. Spirit of the pulse indicates a pulse that is soft, but has strength. Coldness in the Middle Burner shows symptoms of digestive problems such as pain that is relieved by heat, poor appetite, indigestion, loose stools, etc. Injury to Essence indicates loss of vital essence due to a cause such as excessive sexual activity.

11. Qi rebellion refers to the rising of energy in the stomach (as in vomiting and nausea) and in the lungs (as in cough and asthma).

Moderate, slippery and large indicates Excess Heat.
Moderate, slow and thready indicates Deficient Cold.

15. Knotted pulse (Yin; but has aspects of both Yin and Yang)

It comes and goes moderately and at times stops and then returns again. Knotted pulse indicates Coldness and Extreme *Yin*, especially of the Heart (*Qi* or *Yang* Deficiency).

Indications: *Qi* stagnation, Blood stagnation, food stagnation, Phlegm stagnation, abdominal mass, stagnation of seven emotions, *Qi* and Blood Deficiency and weakness in *Zang Fu* organs.

16. Hurried pulse (Yang)

It is rapid, but pauses at times; this is extreme *Yang* with near collapse of *Yin*. The Fire that is stagnated in the Triple Burner is burning exuberantly. The prognosis is poor if there is gradual increase in the pauses, but the prognosis is favorable if the pauses disappear.

Indications: cough and asthma, Phlegm accumulation, mania, toxic furuncle.

17. Intermittent pulse (Yin)

It beats with pauses in between, unable to return on its own. When seen in an ill person, it indicates favorable prognosis; when it is seen in a healthy person, it is greatly inauspicious. It indicates the death of a *Zang* organ with the Collapse of *Qi*.
The hurried pulse is rapid with irregularly missed beats.
The knotted pulse is moderate with irregularly missed beats.
The intermittent pulse is slow with regularly missed beats.

The cause of the intermittent pulse is a weakness in the *Qi* of a *Zang* organ. It indicates a weakness of the Original *Qi* causing abdominal pain and diarrhea or a disease of the Middle *Qi* causing vomiting and diarrhea. It can be seen in a woman in her third month of pregnancy. Since Fetal *Qi*[12] causes obstruction in the third month of pregnancy, there is no harm to an intermittent pulse during this time.

18. Hidden pulse (Yin)

It can only be felt when pressed heavily to the bone and the pulse moves below the tendons. Whether or not the beat is distinct, it can only be felt next to the bone. This is a sinking of *Yin–Yang*, indicating blockage and obstruction. It can also indicate obstruction of Fire, Cold or *Qi*.

Indications: extreme pain, Sudden Turmoil Syndrome, Hernial disorders, loss of consciousness, *Qi* rebellion, food stagnation, anger, syncope, edema, Phlegm–Damp and a mass in the upper abdomen.

---

12. Fetal Qi is the vital energy of the fetus.

19. Long pulse (Yang)

It is neither large nor small. It is long and passes beyond the first and third positions. The Long pulse indicates diseases of Excess.

Indications: *Yang* toxins, epilepsy and *Yangming* Heat.

20. Short pulse (Yin)

It does not reach nor fill all positions. The short pulse indicates diseases of Deficiency.

Indications: Injury due to alcoholic drinks, Blood Deficiency, headache and abdominal pain.

21. Leather pulse (Yin)

It is knotted and flooding and feels like pressing on a drum skin. *Zhang Zhong Jing* said;

"A knotted pulse indicates Coldness and a hollow pulse indicates Deficiency. When there are both Deficiency and Coldness, it is called a leather pulse. In a man, it occurs when there is a collapse of the Blood and loss of Essence, and in a woman, it occurs when there is a miscarriage with continuous uterine bleeding."

Indications: metrorrhagia after miscarriage, collapse of Blood, loss of Essence, Deficiency of *Ying Qi*, Windstroke[13] with Dampness.

22. Firm pulse (Yang within Yin)

Similar to a deep and hidden pulses, it is full, large, long and slightly wiry.
The position of a firm pulse is usually between a deep pulse and a hidden pulse.

Indications: Coldness and pain in the epigastric region, Liver overacting on Spleen, Hernial disorders, and a mass in the lower abdomen.

23. Soft pulse (Yin)

It is extremely weak, superficial and thready like silk inside water. It is felt with a light touch and disappears with heavy pressure.

Indications: Collapse of Blood, *Yin* Deficiency, continuous Deficient sweating, steaming bone heat sensation,[14] *Qi* Deficiency, Injury due to Dampness, Cold *Bi*,[15] diarrhea immediately after meals, heaviness of body, tidal fever, weakness of legs and difficult urination.

---

13. Windstroke is the equivalent to apoplexy in Western medicine.

14. Steaming bone heat sensation occurs due to extreme Yin Deficiency. The patient feels heat generating from deep inside the bone.

15. The Cold Bi is a form of arthritis in which there is a severe and fixed pain with a dislike of cold.

24. Weak pulse (Yin)

It is extremely feeble, deep and thready. It can be felt when heavily pressed but disappears with a light touch.

Indications: *Yang* Deficiency, chills and fever, atrophy of tendons and bones, severe fright, profuse sweating, weakness in the Spleen and Stomach, Blood Deficiency, spasm and pain in the tendons, asthma, weakness in walking, and facial edema due to an invasion of Wind after delivery of a child.

25. Scattered pulse (Yin)

It is large, scattered, and exists superficially, but not deeply. It is dispersed and not gathered like the image of a dispersing willow. The scattered pulse indicates Deficiency of both *Qi* and Blood. It is a pulse of the collapse of the Original *Qi*. When this pulse occurs in a pregnant woman ready to deliver a child, it means birth is going to occur, but when this pulse occurs in a pregnant woman not ready to deliver, it indicates that a miscarriage is going to occur.

Indications: severe palpitations, sweating, superficial edema[16] and edema of the lower limbs.

26. Thready pulse (Yin)

It is small to minute and beats continuously. It feels thready and weak, like a fine thread, upon palpation.

Indications: all types of Deficiency and Consumption, Injury due to the seven emotions, Injury due to Dampness, profuse sweating, spermatorrhea, diarrhea and dysentery due to Coldness, vomiting, abdominal distention, Stomach Deficiency, prolapsed uterus, abdominal mass with severe pain, atrophy, and pain and coldness in lower leg.

27. Moving pulse (Yang)

It can be felt above the second position. Shaped like a round bean, a moving pulse is short and just rises from the center without a head and a tail. It is called a moving pulse since it spins and vibrates under the finger. It occurs when the *Yin* and the *Yang* fight with each other; when the *Yang* moves, sweating occurs and when the *Yin* moves, fever occurs.

Indications: sweating due to fright, Cold pain, Phlegm pain, contraction and spasm of the four limbs, Consumption, bloody dysentery, metrorrhagia and spermatorrhea.

28. Large pulse (Yang)

It flows like a bubbling spring well. A large pulse indicates the progression of an illness; a superficial and large pulse indicates an External disease and a deep and large

---

16. This is edema of the skin.

pulse indicates an Internal disease. It also indicates a Deficiency of Blood with Exuberance of the *Qi*. A moderate and large pulse in the middle position indicates a normal pulse.

Indications: headache, dizziness, fullness in the chest with shortness of breath, etc.

29. Small pulse (Yin)

It feels extremely small when searched for and disappears on light pressure. It is neither fast nor slow. It is slightly bigger than the minute pulse.

30. Swift pulse (Yang)

It moves extremely rapidly under the fingers. It has seven to eight beats per breath. It is a pulse of utmost speed and indicates extreme heat.

31. Extreme pulse (Yang)

It is extremely rapid. A rapid pulse has six beats per breath and an extreme pulse has seven beats per breath; or a swift pulse has seven beats per breath, an extreme pulse has eight beats per breath, and a collapsed pulse has nine beats per breath.

32. Defeated pulse (Yin)

It is extremely slow. A slow pulse has three beats per breath and a defeated pulse has two beats per breath; or an injured pulse has two beats per breath and a defeated pulse has one beat per breath.

33. Injured pulse (Yin)

It has two beats per breath.

34. Collapsed pulse (Yang within Yin)

It has nine beats per breath.

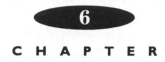

PHARMACOLOGY

(Theory of Herbology)

𝒯he study of herbal properties and the study of syndromes in Oriental medicine are like the two wings of a bird. Correctly identifying the syndrome and applying the appropriate herbs will allow the treatment to come about naturally, but the study of herbs is troublesome for the students of Oriental medicine. Even though the theory is simple, the practical application is complicated. When one tries to use the herbs in actual treatment, there are many occasions when it is impossible to pick which herb to use for which disease.

Over 1,800 varieties of herbs are recorded in the *Li Shi Zhen's Compendium of Materia Medica* and over 900 herbs are listed in *Zhao Xue Min's*[1] *A Supplement to the Compendium of Materia Medica,* totalling nearly 3,000 herbs. As such, it is impossible for a person to remember the properties of all these herbs nor is it necessary.

The following is an example of various categories of herbs for different treatment indications:

1. Herbs from *Shang Han* Theory:
   Diaphoretics: 32 types, Purgatives: 14 types, Harmonizing herbs: 133 types, Warming channels: 28 types, Recovery from fatigue after meals: 21 types.
2. Herbs for the Spleen and Stomach (herbs for the diseases of digestive system):
   Consumption:[2] 159 types, Deficient Cold: 26 types, Food Stagnation: 100 types, Alcohol intoxication: 100 types.
3. Herbs for Diarrhea:
   Damp–heat: 24 types, Deficient Cold: 79 types, Accumulation: 8 types, External treatment: 9 types.

---

1. Zhao Xue Min (1719 – 1805 A.D.) was a physician and famous pharmacist in the Qing Dynasty (1644 – 1911 A.D.).

2. See note 5 in Chapter 5.

As one can see, there are many treatment herbs even for a single disease. The question is which herb or herbs among many should one use? Could the disease be cured by just using any herb? Not necessarily, because among the herbs that are mentioned above, the particular herb chosen must match the patient's constitution and syndrome. This is why it is necessary to know the properties of each herb.

I. SELECTION OF MEDICINE

EMPIRICAL METHODOLOGY

According to the empirical methodology, one must depend on multiple statistics to confirm that a certain medicine has a certain effect on a particular disease. When the result of a certain treatment that was administered to many people is found to be beneficial as compared to another treatment technique, the medicinal substance used in that treatment can generally be recognized as being efficacious. In Western medicine, however, there are discrepancies in selecting a medicinal substance according to this empirical methodology. In selecting this methodology, an observer has to carefully examine the progression and the changes in a disease, then predict the future symptoms. The problem is that this prediction is frequently influenced by one's biased opinion. Consequently, it can easily become inaccurate and since it is difficult to know what type of action the selected medicinal substance has in influencing the progression of the disease (e.g., it could worsen), it is obvious that students of modern science try to avoid using empirical methodology. Furthermore, Western medicinal substances, unlike Oriental herbs, cannot be used without having concrete scientific proof. This methodology is avoided morally and ethically because there is a concern that the health will greatly worsen if inappropriate medicine is used.

EXPERIMENTAL METHODOLOGY

In experimental methodology, animals closely resembling the anatomical structure of a human being are selected and minutely observed to determine which medicine has what effect on their health and illness. Based on the results, it is deduced that a given medicinal substance has the function of healing or reducing the severity of a certain disease or symptoms. A certain disease or the symptoms that are connected with it are transmitted to the experimental animals, to observe whether or not a medicinal substance really is effective on that disease or symptoms. After confirming its efficacy, it is finally applied to a patient to accumulate more data and statistics upon which to base the effectiveness of the medicine. This is the rational experimental procedure for selecting medicinal substances.

This experimental method of choosing a medicine is based on Western pharmacology, but whether it is a theory that fits Oriental herbology (the study of herbal properties) is another question.

THE METHOD OF SELECTING ORIENTAL HERBS

A. Are the Oriental Herbs Medicinal Substances?

Though substances that treat diseases can all be considered medicines in a broad sense, it is appropriate to consider a large portion of Oriental herbs as foods rather than as medicinal substances in a strict sense. Oriental herbs can be divided into two types. One is the food type and the other is the medicinal type. In actuality, only the food types are recognized as true Oriental herbs. Consequently, medicinal type Oriental herbs are not prescribed as a fundamental rule by a wise Oriental medical doctor.

In Oriental herbology, there are minerals or inorganic substances and animals and plants which are organic substances. True Oriental herbal medicine should be composed of organic substances. Historically, the beginning of Oriental herbology is said to have started when *Shen Nung*[3] tasted a variety of plants and established them as medicinal substances.

Therefore, treating diseases using food is the most natural approach. It is a common phenomenon in the animal world for an animal to select whether a food is injurious or beneficial through its sense of taste. In this way, it ingests foods that are necessary for the physiological regulation of itself based on likes and dislikes.

There probably are times when the disease must be treated by major surgery and a strong or toxic medication, but it is also true that they can have unwanted side effects or even endanger the life of an individual.

The following is a chart that illustrates how Oriental herbs are divided into food and medicinal types.

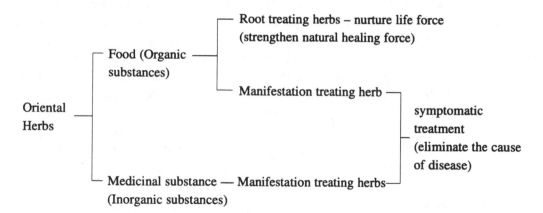

It is often asked where the dividing line between a food and medicine should be drawn? I have chosen to divide it in the following manner:

1. A food, while giving a healing effect on a sick person, is a substance beneficial even to a healthy body. Medicinal substances, on the other hand, need not be taken if a person

---

3. Shen Nung (2836-2698 B.C.) is one of three legendary emperors of China. He is called "Divine Husbandman" and is considered as the founder of Oriental herbal medicine.

is not sick and can be harmful when taken by a healthy person.

2. To use an analogy, a food substance could be likened to payment for work and a medicinal substance likened to a loan. A loan is necessary in unavoidable circumstances, but one must be prepared for the disadvantage of paying "interest." Thus, not only is a payment for the work good to earn at any time, but it also makes a person more economically sufficient.

3. Similar to the high or low interest on a loan and receiving compensation from hard or easy work, there is a different ratio of benefits and consequences in using medicinal substances. It is a fundamental rule in the selection of medicinal substances to select those that have maximum effectiveness with minimum side effects. In keeping with this, organic medicinal substances are selected rather than inorganic medicinal substances. Even in the compensation for labor, if the fundamental rule of economics is in trying to receive maximum pay by selecting the most appropriate work through personal talent and ability, then it is a fundamental rule in selecting our food to ingest the most appropriate food for the personal constitution to get the maximum effectiveness in maintaining or improving health. This is the chief aim in the study of herbology.

From the above statements, I believe one can conclude that there are many differences between the use of herbal medicines according to Oriental herbology and medicinal substances according to Western pharmacology.

B. Discovery of the Principles of Herbology

The distinctive feature of Oriental herbology is "The Principle of Pharmacology" or "The General Summary of Pharmacology." The properties of all herbs can be analyzed according to this principle, so it is sufficient to comprehend this principle in studying Oriental herbology. The principle is extremely simple: the properties of substances are determined by the taste, *Qi* and color. I will elaborate on this *Qi*–Taste–Color Theory later. First of all, I wish to give a few examples. Mustard or black pepper promotes heat with a pungent taste, whereas pear or watermelon cools the heat with a bland taste. This theory was discovered inductively through the following method:

- When one eats a lot of mustard seed, the body becomes hot and sweats profusely.
- It is the same with red pepper, black pepper, fresh ginger, cinnamon bark and garlic.
- Therefore, the temperatures of mustard seed, red pepper, black pepper, fresh ginger, cinnamon bark and garlic all are warm.
- The taste of mustard seed is pungent and so are red pepper, black pepper, fresh ginger, cinnamon bark and garlic.
- The common taste is pungent.
- Mustard seed has an aromatic fragrance and so does red pepper, black pepper (in slight amounts), fresh ginger, cinnamon bark and garlic.
- They commonly contain volatile oil.

The common characteristic that can be found in the above six substances are: (1) heat promoting property, (2) pungent property, (3) aromatic property and (4) dispersing property (they promote sweating and eliminate gas). In addition, they have the power of digestion – they increase appetite (only in *Yang* Deficiency constitution). Thus, substances with pungent properties tend to increase body temperature and aromatic properties eliminate gas in the body. The carbon dioxide inside the tissues is eliminated through the skin pores and lungs and the harmful gas developed inside the digestive organs is eliminated upward and downward.

Treated dried ginger "Warms the Middle"[4] and does not disperse as a result of eliminating volatile oil from fresh ginger. Peppermint, agastache and perilla leaves have a slight pungent taste and a lot of fragrance. As a result, they do not increase the heat much, but disperse greatly. Through a method of observation similar to this, properties such as bitter–cools, sweet–tonifies, salty–softens, sour–astringes, bland–promotes urination, etc. can be discovered.

C. Practical Application of the Principle

After the discovery of such principles and applying those principles in practice to examine their accuracy, the efficacy of an herb is determined. In selecting medicinal substances, theoretical knowledge and thorough clinical experiments are necessary, and especially in the empirical method, a large number of statistics are required. Oriental herbal medicine, based on the simple principles that even a child can understand, is a synthesis of experiences which all people have had, ever since humans came into existence. Hence, there is no room to doubt the practical effects of Oriental herbs. For example, after deciding that a pungent property promotes heat, no matter which one among the pungent substances a person ingests, body temperature can be increased. That is why pungent taste and warm temperature follow each other.

White atractylodes is a pungent and warm herb. So is dried ginger, cinnamon bark, aconite, psoralea and pinellia. These herbs share the common effect of promoting heat because they all have a pungent taste. At the same time, they have individually unique tastes and have individually peculiar effects in other areas (refer to the section on *Qi*–Taste Theory).

D. Experiments on the Drastic and Toxic Herbs

Although it is appropriate to eliminate harsh and toxic herbs from Oriental herbal medicine, let us put that view aside since Oriental herbal medicine up to now has included harsh and toxic herbs. How were the herbal effects known and how were dangerous experiments performed? I have not yet been able to gather textual records on that method, but it can be generally presumed to have been discovered in the following ways:

1. Examining the effects of disinfection (detoxification) on the external diseases.
2. Sometimes the effects of toxic herbs are recognized accidently due to an unexpected outcome. For example, there are cases in which a poverty stricken person gets an incurable disease and after taking drastic or toxic medicine for the purpose of

---

4. Warming the Middle means warming up the digestive organs, which are in the Middle Burner (between the diaphragm and the umbilicus).

committing suicide, unexpectedly gets completely cured. In this way, it is discovered that a certain type of toxic herb is actually effective for curing a certain type of a disease.

3. For the very toxic herbs, the strength of the toxins can be determined by experimenting with the herbs on domestic animals.

4. The temperature (*Qi*) and taste of toxic herbs can be observed to the degree that the herbs will not actually harm human life and one can approximately infer the herbal properties through the principles of Oriental herbology.

5. After herbal properties are inferred, as a last resort, the herbs can be tested on a patient who has given up all hope of surviving.

6. In ancient times, there were cases where criminals who were to be executed were used to experiment with the effects of medicines.

In modern times, this field should be handed over to Western pharmacology. Performing experiments on medicinal substances which are not Oriental herbs through such primitive and crude methods must absolutely be avoided.

II. RESEARCH METHOD OF HERBAL MEDICINE

Recently, the desire to research herbal medicine has greatly increased. This is a fortunate circumstance for mankind, but we must inquire into its research methods, so I will discuss which among the following research methods are appropriate for current students of Oriental medicine to select.

There are two main types of research methods. One is a method of analyzing scientifically and the other is a method of observing holistically. The former is a Western method and the latter is an Oriental method.

THE METHOD OF ANALYZING SCIENTIFICALLY

This is the research method used by modern medical students studying Oriental herbs. A certain effective ingredient in Oriental herbs is extracted in order to investigate the pharmacological effects using the experimental method. This might be a good research approach for a scientist, but it has many discrepancies when it comes to the goal of looking for herbal substances that clearly produce effective treatment.

A. Organic Chemistry is Still in an Infantile Stage

No matter how much modern science has developed, where organic chemistry is concerned, it is still at an infantile stage. So with current organic chemistry, there is no ability to adequately analyze and experiment on Oriental herbs, which are organic substances, by the chemical method. This is due in part to the complexity of a single herb which can have dozens or even hundreds of active compounds. Furthermore, since herbs are rarely used individually, but rather in combination with many other herbs, the number of potential interactions between active compounds rises exponentially.

B. The Problem with Analysis

Although analysis is the distinctive characteristic and strong point of modern science, there are times when it becomes the weak point. This is illustrated in the following examples:

1. A diamond is made out of carbon. Lead, coal and charcoal all have carbon as their ingredient. Should a diamond be considered the same as charcoal? It might be good to know that carbon is an ingredient of a diamond, but one must not ignore its solidity, brilliance and value as a precious stone. The fault of the analysis is in frequently losing the original nature.

2. Water is made out of hydrogen and oxygen. Yet water does not combust while its elements, hydrogen and oxygen, both combust. Hence, the water will not combust even if the amount of oxygen and hydrogen is supplied by numerical proportion when one uses the water. So, even if an inorganic compound is like this, it is nothing but an unreasonable act to observe pharmacological action by analyzing and extracting the ingredients of an herb, which is much more of an organic substance. Moreover, because current organic chemistry is still in its infancy, it will not be able to sufficiently analyze all the ingredients in an herb.

Function of water ≠ function of hydrogen + function of oxygen

Even though ice, vapor, cold water and hot water all have the same elements as regular water, they are all different.

3. A desk is made out of wood. So is a chair, a door and a cotton gin. An analytical breakdown will reveal the same basic atomical structure whether the object is a desk, a chair, a door or a cotton gin. Nevertheless, the desk and cotton gin cannot be seen as identical objects. No matter how much one researches a piece of wood, one will not be able to grasp the concept of a chair or a cotton gin. Accordingly, there will be no way to know their effective uses.

C. The Faulty Logic in Extracting Organic Ingredients

Extracting effective ingredients from Oriental herbs to research their herbal properties invites inadequate understanding as exemplified in the following:

Let us call ginseng [A] and its ingredients [a b c d e ...]. Now suppose that from ginseng ingredient [a] is extracted and its pharmacological effect is discovered by an experiment. Discussing the effects of ginseng based on this knowledge alone would yield only partial understanding of what it is. The effect of [a] which is an ingredient of ginseng is but an isolated pharmacological action of [a] when examined by itself and cannot be seen as the whole pharmacological action of ginseng.

Though [a] might be an ingredient of ginseng, the function of [a] cannot necessarily characterize what can be observed as ginseng's function. There might be times when it can, but there are also times it cannot. Likewise, although oxygen is an element of water, the function of oxygen cannot be seen as a part of the function of water.

If we consider Function of [a] = Function of [A],

then a = A − [b, c, d],

thus we get a conclusion like A = A − [b, c, d].

Taking a step further, even if we knew all the ingredients of ginseng, we cannot see the combined results of experiments with its individual ingredients as the total function of ginseng. Thus, if we view ginseng as [A], the function of ginseng as [A'] and the ingredients of ginseng as [a b c d e] and their functions as [a' b' c' d' e']:

A = [abcde] ≠ a + b + c + d + e
A' = [a'b'c'd'e'] ≠ a' + b' + c' + d' + e'

This logic can be seen as appropriate and its reason is because:

$(H_2O)' \neq H_2' + 0'$ Function of water ≠ function of hydrogen + function of oxygen

Another problem is that even if we knew all the ingredients of ginseng, the mechanics of the human body are subtle and complicated beyond descriptions. Thus, it will not be possible to know the pharmacological effects of the whole herb itself, which is an organically synthesized system, through synthesizing experiments performed on one body part with one extracted ingredient of the herb. This is because an herb acts through mutual interrelation and holistically toward each tissue and organ of the human body, which is also an organically synthesized system. No matter how much modern science develops, it will not likely be able to sufficiently experiment on each part of the human body.

We can observe problems in isolating a specific ingredient from the herbs in the modern medical experiments. The more purely extracted morphine is, the more extremely violent action it has, but when morphine is used in its natural state, which is unripened poppy fruit, with milk–like liquid components, then its side effect is reduced. Santonin has extremely violent side effects, however chewing the bark of its raw material has no side effect. Recently I heard that epimedium, said to have a strong aphrodisiac effect, was researched by using a pure extract of its active ingredient, but it had little effect. Researchers ultimately came to the conclusion that the extract is not as effective as ingesting the decoction of the whole plant and stopped the research. This is a very interesting topic and proves how unique effects of organic herbs can be obtained by not destroying their original integrated function.

THE METHOD OF OBSERVING HOLISTICALLY

Holistic observation is the method used in Oriental herbology. For example, when studying the properties of ginseng, the method is a process of studying the characteristic of ginseng as it is without analyzing its ingredients and holistically observing its effect on the body. The following are the properties and functions of ginseng from a holistic observation:

Taste: slightly sweet – nourishment – Spleen
fragrant – regulates breathing and sweat dispersing function of skin, eliminates gas inside the digestive organs.

slightly bitter – calms Heart (recovery from fatigue)

Temperature: slightly warm – promotes physiological function

Color: yellow (noticeable on fresh ginseng) – digestive organ – sweet
white (white ginseng) – respiratory organ – fragrant
red (red ginseng) – blood circulation – bitter

The physiological phenomena and disease symptoms in humans also must be holistically observed in order to treat fundamentally, so it will be difficult to hit the mark with partial observation. There cannot be a fixed "treatment indication" for ginseng but only the "treatment constitution." The suitable constitution for ginseng is a person with a totally weak or debilitated physiological function including the following:

1. Insufficient function of the digestive organs
2. Insufficient function of the respiratory organs
3. Insufficient function of the circulatory organs
4. Undernourishment
5. Fatigue of the Heart (whole body fatigue)

For the disease of a person with such a constitution, regardless of what the type and name of the disease is, ginseng will be an appropriate medicine. The herbal medicines that promote physiological action and increase body temperature are generally pungent and warm herbs that have stimulating properties, but only ginseng includes a bitter taste which settles the excitement of the Heart, relieves fatigue and supports nourishment for the fundamental strengthening of the life force. In this regard, it is unparalleled among all the herbs. This is the unique reason why ginseng is a miraculous medicine.

The reason why the main treatment disease of ginseng cannot be pointed out can be known by the following functions and treatment indications:

• Tonifies Five *Zang* organs, calms Spirit, settles *Hun* and *Po*, stops fright palpitations, eliminates Pathogenic *Qi*, brightens eyes, opens Heart (orifice) and benefits wisdom. If taken for a long time, it can make the body light and give longevity. *Ben Jing*[5]

• Treats Coldness in Stomach and Intestines, epigastric pain, chest and hypochondriac fullness and Sudden Turmoil. It regulates Middle, stops Wasting and Thirsting Syndrome and opens Blood Vessels. If taken for a long time, ginseng can improve memory. (*Bie Lu*)[6]

---

5. "Ben Jing" is the oldest materia medica, said to be written by a legendary emperor Shen Nung (2836 – 2698 B.C.). It is also called "Shen Nung's Herbal." This book enumerates 365 types of herbs which are divided into three classes: superior, common and inferior.

6. Coldness in the stomach and intestine manifests as abdominal pain, diarrhea, liking for heat, poor appetite, poor digestion and absence of thirst. Regulating the Middle means regulating the digestive system. Wasting and Thirsting Syndrome refers to diabetes. Opening the Blood Vessels means improving blood circulation. Ming Yi Bie Lu or Transactions of Famous Physicians is a book on pharmacology and was compiled by Tao Hong Jing (452 - 536 A.D.), based on Shen Nung's Herbal.

- Controls Five Strains and Seven Emotions, emaciation and weakness, tonifies Five *Zang* and Six Fu organs, protects Middle, settles Spirit, disperses Phlegm in the chest, treats pulmonary collapse and epilepsy, Cold *Qi* surging upward, Injury due to Cold and anorexia. It is applicable for a person with weakness, much dreaming and confusion. (*Zhen Quan*)[7]

- Stops irritability and sour taste in the mouth. (*Li Xun*)[8]

- Digests food, improves appetite, regulates Middle *Qi*, eliminates the toxins of herbs from mineral source. (*Da Ming*)[9]

- Treats insufficient *Yang Qi* of Lung and Stomach, shortness of breath due to Lung *Qi* Deficiency, feeble breathing, tonifies Deficiency of Middle *Qi*, relaxes Middle, sedates Pathogenic Fire of Heart, Lung, Spleen and Stomach, stops thirst and produces body fluid.[10] (*Yuan Su*)[11]

- Treats the entire Deficiency Syndrome of men or women, fever, spontaneous sweating, dizziness and vertigo, headache, vomiting, malaria, diarrhea, chronic dysentery, frequent urination, painful urination, Consumption, Windstroke, Summer Heat, Atrophy and Painful Obstruction Syndromes,[12] vomiting blood, coughing up blood, blood in the stool, bloody urine, metrorrhagia, all diseases during pregnancy and after delivery. (*Li Shi Zhen*)

- Tonifies both *Qi* and Blood Deficiency, recovers a person with *Yang Qi* Deficiency and stops metrorrhagia. It can treat various conditions that arise due to Deficiency such as fever, spontaneous sweating, dizziness and vertigo, fatigue, fright, seminal emission, diarrhea and dysentery, headache, gall bladder pain, indigestion, stagnation and exuberance of Phlegm–fluid, coughing up blood, vomiting blood, painful urination, constipation, vomiting, irritability, blood in the stool and bodily weakness with inability to assimilate nutrients. (*Zhang Jing Yue*)

---

7. Five strains are as follows: prolonged use of the eyes injures the blood, prolonged lying down injures Qi, prolonged sitting injures the muscles, prolonged standing injures bones and prolonged walking injures tendons. Seven emotions refer to joy, anger, anxiety, rumination, grief, fear and fright. Settling the Spirit implies calming the mind down. Cold Qi surging upward includes symptoms such as nausea, vomiting, hiccup or belching that are caused by Cold pathogens. Zhen Quan (about 540 – 643 A.D.) was a physician in the Tang Dynasty. He was a great exponent in acupuncture therapy and authored "Needling Prescription" and "Figures of the Human Body."

8. Li Xun (approximately 855 – 930 A.D.) was an herbalist in later Tang Dynasty (618 –960 A.D.).

9. Da Ming was a medical scholar of Southern Song Dynasty (1127 – 1279 A.D.).

10. Insufficiency of Yang Qi of the Lung includes symptoms such as cough, shortness of breath, feeble breathing, spontaneous sweating and weak voice. Insufficiency of Yang Qi of the stomach includes poor appetite, loose stool, indigestion and fatigue. Pathogenic Fire of the Heart includes symptoms such as irritability, thirst, insomnia, tongue ulcer, dark and painful urination. Fire of the Lung includes symptoms such as cough with thick yellow sputum, chest pain and difficult breathing. Fire in the Spleen and Stomach includes symptoms such as thirst, swelling/pain/bleeding gums, bad breath and excessive hunger.

11. Zhang Yuan Su, also called Zhang Jie Gu, was a physician in the 13th century. He is responsible for breaking away from the traditional method of treatment, discarding obsolete traditional formulas. Most of the doctors in the Jin–Yuan Dynasty (1115 – 1368 A.D.) were influenced by his theory.

12. Atrophy (Wei) Syndrome can be seen in the following Western diseases: acute myelitis, progressive myotrophy, myasthenia gravis, periodic paralysis, hysterical paralysis, multiple neuritis, sequelae of poliomyelitis, traumatic paraplegia, etc. Painful Obstruction (Bi) Syndrome includes Western diseases such as rheumatic fever, rheumatic arthritis, rheumatoid arthritis, fibrositis, neuralgia and gout.

It is not possible to know among these descriptions which is the main indicated disease of ginseng. This is merely a record of how entire syndromes in weak persons can be treated through the use of ginseng. For more details, look at the following section on *Qi*–Taste Theory, and the chapter on prescriptions (Chapter 7).

III. CLASSIFICATION OF HERBAL MEDICINE

There are many types of herbs. For this reason they must be classified systematically in order to make a general survey easier and to make the research convenient. There are many types of traditional methods in the classification of herbs.

CHEMICAL CLASSIFICATION METHOD

Due to the recent advancement in pharmacology and chemistry, we have gradually found that in a certain pharmacological property, there is a certain chemical element or a certain chemical structure that accompanies it. That is, we can see phenomena such as the fact that fat molecules generally have anesthetic effects, fragrant properties have antiseptic power, organic compounds that contain kalium or kalium compound cause heart attacks and substances that contain NH_2 excite the hypothalamus. As this research progresses, there might be a time when pharmacological action can all be detected through chemistry. At that time, the *Qi*–Taste–Color Theory of Oriental herbology will be proven chemically, but for now the classification method based on pure chemistry has inadequacies as follows:

1. Since the substances that have no common function cannot be considered as belonging to the same category, the chemical system cannot be truly seen as a pharmacological system.
2. There are herbs that have not yet been chemically clarified as to their properties.
    Oriental herbs, for the most part, have not yet been closely examined for their properties chemically. It is hard to know when the time for applying this classification method to Oriental herbs will come about.

CLASSIFICATION METHOD BY THE ORGANS

This is a classification method determined by the effects of medicines on two to three organs that are especially necessary for life. It is divided into the medicines that act on the brain, medicines that act on the spinal cord and medicines that act on the heart; namely cerebrospinal medicine and heart medicine. However, most of the medicines do not act only on one organ, rather they act on a great number of organs simultaneously. Even on one organ, the function is different according to the individual medicine, so even this classification method is not suitable. Moreover, the organ is difficult to classify as far as Oriental herbs are concerned. Ginseng is said to tonify the Five *Zang* and Six *Fu* organs; epimedium is a medicine for Hand *Yangming* (Large Intestine), Foot *Yangming* (Stomach), Hand *Shaoyin* (Heart), Foot *Shaoyin* (Kidney), Triple Burner and the Gate of Life.

Anemarrhena is said to enter Hand *Taiyin* (Lung), Hand *Shaoyin* (Heart), Foot *Yangming* (Stomach), Foot *Jueyin* (Liver) and Foot *Shaoyin* (Kidney). Thus, it is difficult to specify which organ medicine an herb represents.

CLASSIFICATION METHOD ACCORDING TO CLINICAL PRACTICE

This is a classification method determined according to the results of the efficacies of medicinal substances that can be clinically observed. For example, categories include purgatives, diuretics, anti–phlegmatics, anti–fungals, etc. This is the most frequently used classification method in herbology and there are times when herbs are divided into Sweat–promoting formulas, Mediating formulas, Tonifying formulas, Purging formulas, Astringing formulas, Dispelling–Wind formulas, Clearing–Heat formulas, Dispelling–Damp formulas, Moistening–Dry formulas, Dispelling–Cold formulas, etc. However, because the clinical results of medicinal substances are numerous, this classification method in actual practice is extremely vague. Moreover, that tendency is even more extreme on Oriental herbs.

CLASSIFICATION METHOD ACCORDING TO NATURAL SCIENCE

Similar to other natural sciences, the pharmacological actions of many substances are individually examined and according to the similarities in their properties, they are gathered into one genus. The medicinal substance that is especially prominent is fixed as representative of that genus and the rest of the medicinal substances are added and incorporated into the same genus.

This method was created by Buchheim and completed by Schmiedeberg and is recognized as the most logical method according to Western pharmacology. According to this method, a medicinal substance that newly appears in the future is incorporated into an appropriate genus by its function or a new subcategory is established to avoid complication such as changing the system that has been formed up to now. When studying pharmacology, knowing all of the pharmacological actions of the representative medicinal substance has the added convenience of enabling one to roughly infer the functions of other medicinal substances in that genus (this classification method has many similarities to the classification method according to the *Qi*–Taste Theory in Oriental herbology).

However, this method too is not without flaws because in all raw medicines or unprocessed substances, there are many without clearly effective ingredients. Moreover, in quite a few medicinal substances, the type of function they perform in the living body is completely unknown or incompletely known. Thus, it is a confession of modern pharmacologists that it is very difficult to differentiate which genus these medicinal substances should be added or how the order should be arranged.

In truth, almost all Oriental herbs are unclear in regard to their effective ingredients and how they act on the organism according to modern pharmacology. Consequently, this classification method is inappropriate for Oriental herbs.

CLASSIFICATION METHOD ACCORDING TO QI–TASTE THEORY

This is a classification method based on *Qi* and Taste and is suitable for the principle of herbology. Keep in mind that the classification method according to *Qi*–Taste Theory is a classification based on herbal properties or herbal constituents and not of the herb (e.g., genera and species as would be used in botany). After classifying the herbal properties by *Qi*–Taste Theory, its properties are classified according to the herb and the medicinal effect or value of that herb is noted.

A. Presumption of Herbal Constituents

In understanding the properties of Oriental herbs, it is necessary to make presumptions about the existence of herbal constituents. Thus, there might be an extreme sense of insufficiency from the viewpoint of modern science, but there is no alternative with the present situation.

For example, the way a constituent of an herb is determined is to presume that there are heat promoting constituents in herbs which increase heat and sweat promoting constituents in the herbs which promote sweating. It is a simple statement, but all theories of Oriental medicine are like that – truth is found within simplicity. However, these constituents indicate their existence to us in three ways. They are *Qi*, taste and color. Similar to knowing the volume of all objects by width, length and height, the properties of all substances can be discerned by *Qi*, taste and color. Even in the experiments of modern physics and chemistry, the criterion of observation does not go beyond this *Qi*, taste and color. Specific gravity, vapor, liquid, solid, acid–alkaline base and color reaction, etc. are all observed through the criterion of *Qi*, taste and color.

B. Classifications

When making observations according to the aspect of *Qi*, there are names assigned to the formulas such as Ascending formula, Descending formula, Heat formula, Cold formula, Tonifying formula, Sedating formula, Exterior formula, Interior formula, Dispersing formula, Astringing formula, Aromatic formula and Bland formula. When observing with respect to the aspect of taste, there are names assigned to the formulas such as Bitter formula, Pungent formula, Sour formula, Sweet formula, Salty formula, Aromatic formula and Bland formula.

This classification method by the *Qi* and Taste governs and includes every classification method mentioned thus far. Since bitter taste acts on the Heart and sour taste acts on the Liver, Hand *Shaoyin* (Heart) channel medicine, Foot *Jueyin* (Liver) channel medicine, Spleen–Stomach medicine, etc. are classified according to the organs. The pungent–fragrant natured herbs are said to promote sweat and detoxify. Using cinnamon, fresh ginger and agastache for *Taiyang* Syndrome or epidemic disease is mutually compatible with classification according to chemistry. Since bitter taste purges, pungent taste promotes sweat and sweet taste tonifies, this is a method according to clinical practice. Agastache, saussurea, clove, fennel, aquilaria and cyperus are gas eliminating and *Qi* regulating herbs that have similar *Qi* and taste and have common pharmacological actions. Therefore, they are regarded as being in the same category and are commonly used together in a formula. Because the herbs coptis, scutellaria, phellodendron and raw rehmannia, which contain bitter-descending properties, have the function of cooling Blood, producing Blood, tonifying Blood and descending Heat, they too are commonly used together. This coincides with the classification method according to natural science.

C. An Oriental Herb is a Complex Body of Many Medicinal Constituents

An Oriental herb, as a single medicine, contains many types of medicinal constituents. Oriental herbs are classified by many methods in the *Compendium of Materia Medica* for the sake of convenience. In actuality, it makes no difference whether the herbs are classified or not because one herb can belong to different categories. Oriental herbs are a type of holistic medicine that has been prescribed by and manufactured in nature. To make an analogy, when compared to construction work, each individual medicinal constituent is a carpenter, landscaper, architect, stone cutter, etc., and the herb itself is a construction contractor. Even among the contractors, there is one who is experienced in roads and bridges or one who mainly works with wooden structures or one who is proficient in brick and stone construction. There are differences in proficiency as to the construction of a small building, large building, family homes, public halls, schools, etc. so the construction cannot be assigned to any one specialist such as a carpenter, landscaper, stone cutter, designer or draftsmen. Just as a contractor should be observed holistically as to his strong points as a contractor, attention should be paid especially to the strong points of an herb while observing the functional influence on the body holistically.

IV. QI, TASTE AND COLOR THEORY

QI

According to Oriental medicine, the word "*Qi*" has a vast number of meanings. Some of the meanings of *Qi* are listed below:

1. Breathing such as *Hu Qi* (exhalation), *Xi Qi* (inhalation), *Duan Qi* (shortness of breath), and *Qi Chuan* (asthmatic breathing).
2. Emotions such as "*Qi* is not spreading out", *Nu Qi* (anger), and *Xi Qi* (joy).
3. Dynamic force or life force of the human body as in *Qi* Deficiency, *Qi* power, and Original *Qi*.
4. Weather and temperature as in Cold *Qi*, Warm *Qi*, and Damp *Qi*.
5. Gas produced in the stomach and intestines as in *Qi* rebellion, *Qi* stagnation, and *Qi* abdominal mass.
6. Epidemic germs as in *Zhang Qi* (endemic disease) or *Li Qi* (epidemic disease).
7. Physiological changes or pathological reactions such as *Jiao Qi* (beriberi), *Shan Qi* (Hernial disorders), and Fetal *Qi*.

There might be many more implications aside from these. According to the study of herbal properties, *Qi* can be divided into the following two types: the herbal reactions and the stimulation of the sense of smell.

A. Herbal Reactions (herbal properties in the narrow sense)

1. Ascending – Descending

When the reaction and function of an herb is greater in the upper part of body, that herb has what are called ascending properties and when the reaction is greater in the lower part of the body, it has what are called descending properties. Astragalus, cimicifuga, cnidium, bupleurum, polygala and peppermint have strong ascending properties. Coptis, achyranthis, peony and evodia have strong descending properties. White atractylodes, licorice, Chinese angelica and pinellia contain both ascending and descending properties. According to the herb, there are a great number of varieties in the combination of ascending and descending properties.

2. Cold – Heat

Warm, Cool, Cold and Hot are the "Four Qi" or "Four Temperatures" in herbal properties. They all relate to the actions of herbs influencing the body temperature. In herbology, there are distinctions such as warm, greatly warm, hot, greatly hot, cold, greatly cold, slightly cold and neutral. Aconite and cinnamon bark are hot herbs. Coptis and rhubarb are cold herbs. Peppermint and mountan bark are cool herbs. Poria and schizandra are neutral herbs. Even among hot herbs, there are those referred to as "stimulating type of promoting heat"[13] and "strengthening type of promoting heat."[14] Even in cold herbs, there are those known as "suppressing type of descending heat"[15] and "recovering type of descending heat."[16]

3. Tonifying – Sedating

It is the basic principle of Oriental medicine to tonify what is deficient and sedate what is excess. Tonifying herbs are root treating herbs so they are good to take for a long time in accordance with the constitution. However, sedating herbs are manifestation treating herbs or symptomatic herbs, so they must be stopped when the cause of a disease is eliminated. Ginseng, astragalus, white atractylodes, cooked rehmannia and Chinese angelica are tonifying herbs and bupleurum, ephedra, rhubarb and magnolia are sedating herbs.[17]

---

13. The herbs in this category are pungent and hot herbs such as aconite, cinnamon and fennel.

14. The herbs in this category are Yang tonics such as antler horn, epimedium, psoralea, cistanche and walnut.

15. The herbs in this category are Heat clearing herbs such as gypsum, rhubarb, gardenia, scutellaria and coptis.

16. The herbs in this category are Yin tonics such as glehnia, American ginseng and ophiopogon.

17. Tonifying herbs are mild herbs that help treat the root cause of the problem which is basically the person's constitution. These herbs help slowly build up the body's immune system, for example, so that the body can resist or recuperate from an illness quickly. Sedating herbs only treat the manifestation or symptoms of the diseases and are harsh in nature so that once the disease disappears, they must be stopped or else they will weaken the person's constitution.

4. Exterior – Interior

The herbs that react on the exterior of a body are Exterior herbs so the herbs that promote sweating and relieve heat all belong in this category. Bupleurum, cinnamon twig, ephedra and pueraria all are herbs that have strong Exterior–releasing properties. Rhubarb, peach seed, immature bitter orange, sparganium and zedoaria are Interior-attacking herbs. Astragalus and peony are tonifying herbs that prevent excess sweating, while dioscorea, euryale and dolichos are tonifying herbs that prevent excessive diarrhea.

5. Dispersing – Astringing

In the category of Dispersing herbs, there are Sweat–promoting herbs such as schizonepeta, siler, bupleurum, asarum and perilla leaf and Gas–eliminating herbs that dispel the gas of digestive organs such as agastache, saussurea and lindera. In the category of Astringent herbs, there are herbs to stop sweating, stop diarrhea, stop cough and to consolidate Essence[18] – schizandra, zizyphus, peony and cornus.

B. Stimulation of the Sense of Smell

1. Light – Heavy

Peppermint and musk have Light Qi, asafoetida and immature bitter orange have Heavy Qi. The herb ascends when it has Light Qi and descends when it has Heavy Qi.

2. Clear – Turbid

This property of herbs is similar to the ideas of Light – Heavy in that the herb ascends when it is Clear and descends when it is Turbid.

3. Thick – Thin

When Qi is thick, the function is strong and active and when Qi is thin, the function is weak and passive. White atractylodes, magnolia, rhubarb and aconite have Thick Qi; poria, coptis, agastache, forsythia and peony have Thin Qi.

4. Fragrance – Odor

Fragrance is a property of the sense of smell that is aromatic and refreshing. Odor is the sense of smell that is unpleasant. There are many fragrant herbs in Oriental medicine such as agastache, saussurea, cnidium, nutmeg, cardamon, peppermint, elsholtzia, fresh ginger, white mustard seed, etc. The list is too long to mention all of them. In general, aromatic fragrant herbs have the function of promoting sweat, eliminating gas, disinfecting, eliminating parasites and harmonizing the Stomach. Substances that have a foul odor are not used much in Oriental herbology, but among them there are relatively foul smelling herbs such as asafoetida, torreya, quisqualis and areca seed. These especially have a great effect as anti–parasitic herbs which eliminate parasites. Generally, aromatic fragrance functions to stimulate the nerves while foul odor functions to calm the nerves.

---

18. Essence is stored in the Kidneys and is roughly equivalent to the hormones in Western medicine. Here consolidating Essence implies preventing seminal emission, spermatorrhea or excessive urination.

C. The Method of Stimulating the Olfactory Nerve

When the sensory receptivity as well as motor excitability of the nervous system are abnormally accelerated, sometimes various kinds of plant substances that contain foul odor are used to stimulate the olfactory nerve in order to calm the nervous system by reflex action. They are used frequently for hysteria patients and the reason for their efficacy is said to be by the reflex action and not by the assimilation of the substance itself.

Asafoetida is used as foul odor nerve stimulant. Aside from that, ammonia, formic acid, acetic acid, ether, mustard seed oil, etc. are applied as smelling–drugs for fainting, coma and collapse. They are effective because they cause a reflex action in the central nerves, especially in the medulla oblongata, by stimulating the end of the olfactory nerve or the end of sensory nerve (the trigeminal nerve). When the strongly stimulating gas or vapor is applied to the mucous membrane of the nose, it closes the glottis by reflex and at same time, urges spastic breathing. In addition, by exciting the nerve center of the heart restraining branch of the vagus nerve as well as the motor center of the blood vessel, a slowing down of the heart beat and a rise in the blood pressure are said to occur.

D. Yin–Yang of Qi

When the *Yin–Yang* of *Qi* and taste is divided, *Qi* is *Yang* and taste is *Yin*. *Yin–Yang* of *Qi* can be divided as described by the chart on the right.

YIN	YANG
cold	heat
descend	ascend
interior	exterior
sedate	tonify
astringe	disperse
heavy	light
turbid	clear
thin	thick
odor	fragrance

TASTE

Since the principles and theories regarding taste have been generally explained in the Taste section of the Syndrome chapter, they will not be reiterated here, so please refer to that section.

A. Sense of Taste and Physiological Management

1. Pungent Taste

When one feels hot by eating pungent food, one opens the mouth widely and lifts the tongue to increase the surface area that contacts the air and tries to blow out air in order to quickly disperse it. The body becomes hot at this time and one feels a sensation of heat in the upper body (ascending), sweats profusely (disperses sweat) and the breathing becomes deepened (lung). Therefore, pungent taste, warm temperature, ascending property and dispersing property follow together and for this reason it is said, "Pungent taste first enters the Lung."[19]

2. Bitter Taste

When one experiences a bitter taste, one frequently swallows saliva. Pungent taste excites while bitter taste settles. Therefore, purgatives all have bitter taste. Bitter taste, cold temperature, descending property and purging property are all mutually related, so it is a basic rule to use bitter tasting substances for the purpose of descending heat, settling down[20] and purging.

3. Sweet Taste

When one experiences a sweet taste, all the muscles in the mouth become relaxed and move to chew and taste the food well. Sweet tasting substances are used for tonifying and relaxing the body. Licorice is greatly used in Oriental medicine and as an analogy, a person who does not miss out on any affair but always participates in every activity is called "The licorice of the pharmacy." The reason for using licorice a lot is that it contains harmonizing and relaxing properties. Try giving sweets to a young child. See how his facial expression becomes harmoniously relaxed and satisfied. Among the properties of licorice, the following has been said:

"Licorice detoxifies myriads of herbs. It calms and harmonizes 72 types of minerals and 1,200 types of plants." *Bie Lu*

"Its properties can moderate urgency and conciliate all herbs so that they do not conflict. Thus, when used with hot herbs, it can moderate the heat. When used with cold herbs, it moderates coldness. When used on a person with a mixture of hot and cold, it brings about harmony." (*Li Dong Yuan*)[21]

4. Sour Taste

All the muscles in the mouth contract when one experiences sour taste. Both sides of the mouth become even more contracted. Sour taste functions as an astringent. So sour

---

19. Inner Classic, Su Wen (Simple Questions), Chapter 23.

20. Settling down here implies descending of energy (Qi). The bitter taste can calm the mind or it can bring down the energy that rises in the lungs with symptoms such as cough and asthma; or in the stomach with symptoms such as nausea, vomiting and belching; or in the Liver with symptoms such as dizziness, severe headache, red eyes, getting easily angered, flushed face, etc.

21. Li Dong Yuan (1180 – 1251 A.D.) was the founder of the "Tonify Earth" school of thought. He said that all diseases arise from the disharmony in the digestion. Thus, he used the formulas that strengthen and clear Spleen and Stomach. He is the creator of the formula Bu Zhong Yi Qi Tang (Tonify the Middle and Augment the Qi Decoction) mentioned in the Chapter 7 on the Prescriptions.

substances are used for profuse sweating, cough, diarrhea, spermatorrhea, incontinence, etc. This is because sour herbs generally have contracting properties which tightly compress air pores, sweat pores or sphincters.

5. Salty Taste

The tongue surface and palate makes a motion to rub and soften things in the mouth when one experiences salty taste. Hence, salty substances have the function of "softening the hard." A fresh vegetable shrivels up when the salt is added to it. Ingesting salt during vomiting or coughing up blood calms down the condition because salt slows down the vigorous circulation of the blood (blood congeals when salt is added). Quieting of an epileptic seizure from ingesting salt can be seen as the result of salt softening up the spasm and contraction of the muscles.

6. Bland Taste

A pure taste that does not have a distinctive taste is called a bland taste. Although bland taste does not cause unusual changes in the mouth, it is not altogether without a taste. It is actually a sense of taste that is contrary to a salty taste and an experience of taste contrary to a fragrance. The explanation was made in Chapter 3 (Syndromes) on the five tastes that bland taste also belongs to the Kidneys. Since more than one taste belongs to the Kidneys, including bland, we can see that the Kidneys are different from other organs. There are many organs, channels and types of taste that belong to the Kidneys.

7. Fragrant Taste

Fragrance falls under the category of *Qi*, but it also affects the sense of taste and experience of taste. Fragrant taste is in opposition to bland taste. Fragrant substances have the function of eliminating gas and spreading *Qi*, while bland substances have the function of calming and harmonizing the Blood. The function of fragrance is active and that of bland is considered passive. Fragrance is *Yang* and bland is *Yin*. Since fragrance is said to act on "Stomach *Qi*" and "harmonizes Stomach" and "neutralizes *Qi*," it is related to the Spleen while bland is related to the Kidneys.

B. Experience of Taste

There are experiences of taste aside from the senses of taste and these can be generally viewed as the senses of taste that are related to the *Qi*.

1. Clear – Turbid

This is in common with the Clear–Turbid dimension of *Qi*; a Clear tasting property ascends and a Turbid tasting property descends.

2. Thick – Thin

If a taste is Thick, the *Yin* function is strong and if a taste is Thin, the *Yin* function is weak. However, there are many occasions when Thick–Thin of *Qi* and taste do not coincide. Rehmannia, peony, coptis, apricot seed and gardenia have Thick taste and Thin

Qi. Cnidium, schizonepeta and cluster have Thin taste and Thick *Qi.* There are herbs with both Thick *Qi* and taste such as rhubarb, white atractylodes, magnolia and immature bitter orange. There are also ones with both Thin *Qi* and taste such as eucommia and morus bark.

3. Light – Heavy

A taste that gives a refreshing experience has an ascending property and a taste that is deep and heavy has a descending property. Lycium, Chinese angelica, scutellaria and platycodon have Heavy taste and astragalus, peppermint, bupleurum and glehnia have Light taste. Chinese angelica and platycodon have Light *Qi* and Heavy taste. Bupleurum and peppermint possess both Light *Qi* and taste.

4. Astringent – Relaxed

Since an astringent taste is a puckery taste, there is a feeling of constriction in the tongue and whole oral cavity. Torreya, areca, rosa and cornus all have astringent tastes and are often used in astringent formulas. Frequently, astringent taste accompanies sour taste. A relaxed taste is an experience of taste that is felt in sweet or bland substances. It is the experience of taste in licorice, poria and lily.

C. Yin–Yang of Taste

YIN	YANG
bitter	pungent
sour	sweet
salty	bland
bland	fragrant
turbid	clear
heavy	light
thick	thin
astringent	relaxed

Since *Yin* and *Yang* are completely relative, sweet taste is *Yang* in comparison to sour taste, but is *Yin* in comparison to pungent taste. Sour taste is *Yin* in comparison to sweet taste, but is *Yang* in comparison to bitter taste. Bland taste is *Yang* in comparsion to salty taste, but is *Yin* in comparsion to fragrant taste. Bland taste, in comparison to fragrant taste, can be considered as a "pure taste" in order to avoid repetition in the above chart, but since they are of the same property, it is easier to understand by keeping it as the bland taste. This bland taste being repeated in the above chart also expresses, in one aspect, the complexity of the Kidneys.

D. Distribution of Gustatory Nerves; Five Zang Organs and Channels

Observing the distribution of the gustatory nerves, the nerve that senses pungent taste is at the tip of tongue, the nerve that senses bitter taste is in the posterior section of tongue, sweet taste in the center, sour taste is greatly distributed on both sides and salty taste is distributed along the whole surface.

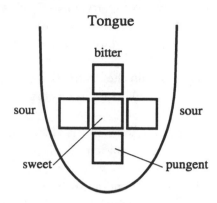

Salty taste in the whole surface
Bland taste in the whole surface
Fragrant taste in the center and upper end

The chart illustrates the tastes that are especially noticeable in those areas and does not imply that they are not distributed in other areas at all. In the center, all of the gustatory nerves are evenly represented.

When I spoke of the relationship between the Five tastes and Five *Zang* organs in the Syndrome chapter, I explained the relationship of pungent to Lung, bitter to Heart, sweet to Spleen, sour to Liver and salty to Kidney. Thus, the theoretical basis will not be reiterated, but one thing that needs review is the Heart and bitter taste. Since the Heart is located in the upper part of the body and belongs to *Yang* among the Five *Zang* organs, in relation to taste it should connect with the gustatory nerve at the tip of the tongue and the pungent taste should belong to the Heart. Obviously it is not that pungent taste does not belong to the Heart since the pungent property stimulates the Heart to invigorate blood circulation, but because the action on the Lung is even more notable, pungent taste was assigned to the Lung. Since "The tongue is the mirror of the Heart," the whole tongue belongs to the Heart and since the Heart is the Monarch organ, it governs everything. Accordingly, it is the same for the other tastes.

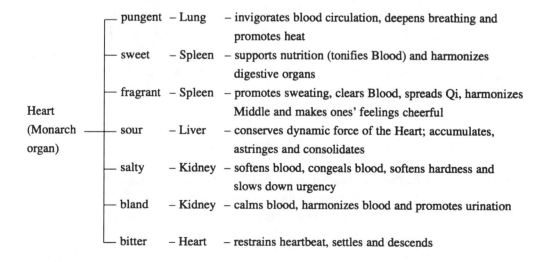

The tastes are distributed in the Five *Zang* organs as in the example above. Bitter taste can be observed to act heavily even on the Kidneys – bitter is "*Yin* within *Yin* taste" and Kidney is the "*Yin* within *Yin Zang* organ." A bitter property is frequently used in diuretic and purgative formulas – urination and defecation both belong to the duty of Kidneys.

The following can be observed when the distribution of the gustatory nerves is compared with the distribution state of the channels (refer to the Liver in the Channel chapter and in the *Zang–Fu* chapter):

1. The Liver and Gall Bladder channels are distributed on the lateral aspect of body. The nerve of sour taste is distributed on the lateral aspect of the tongue. Sour taste is a taste that belongs to the Liver.
2. In the distribution of the channels, the reproductive system (Kidney) has the most number of channels, covering most of the body surface. Next is the digestive system and the Liver channel system follows that. Even in the distribution of the taste nerves, the salty–bland–bitter region is the widest, next is the region of sweet–fragrant taste and next is the region of sour taste. This agrees with the distribution state of the channels.

COLOR

A. The Reason for adding Color to the Qi–Taste Theory.

Color is observed greatly in the study of syndromes. A commonly used phrase in Oriental diagnosis is "Observing the shape and watching the color." In the study of herbal properties, however, color is not emphasized as much. Accordingly, among the herbal properties, one usually speaks of *Qi* and Taste, but I have felt a great need for the observation of color in the study of herbal properties. As a result of having always paid attention to the observation of color, I have found some things which will not only be referred to in the current study of herbal properties, but the observation of color will eventually become one of the most important topics in the study of herbology. Thus, I am adding color to the *Qi*–Taste Theory and will discuss this theory in this next section.

Even in modern chemical experiments, a great importance is put on the observation of color. Looking at phenomena in nature, the reason for colors varying in all matters is that their properties and constituents are all different. Even in the same plant, the changing of pigment in relation to the light, nutrition and seasons is due to the changes in its constituents. Accordingly, there is also a change in the properties.

B. The Relationship between Herbal Properties and Color.

1. Yellow colored herbs and the Spleen – "Spleen controls muscles"

The following substances have been used effectively on the site of inflammation long before the invention of iodine tincture (anti–inflammatory). Even now, these substances are used as a folk medicine when iodine tincture is not available.

(a) Rhubarb is ground with vinegar and rubbed on the site of inflammation.

(b) Ox gallstone is ground and rubbed on the site of inflammation.

(c) Raw rehmannia root is pounded and attached to the site of inflammation.

(d) Gardenia fruit is soaked and pounded in vinegar and attached to the site of inflammation.

(e) Egg yolk is attached to the site of inflammation.

These substances all have some effects in reducing inflammation and we can discover a similarity in the color. The sites of inflammation where where the medicines were attached all become deep yellow in color so that one cannot in any way differentiate whether iodine tincture was rubbed or raw rehmannia root was attached or ox gallstone or rhubarb was rubbed. Accordingly, we can infer that there is an inseparable relationship between the property that disperses inflammation of the skin and the deep yellow color. There are more remedies aside from the above examples. Coptis, which is yellow, is used as an eyewash for the inflammation of the eye lid. Turmeric, which is also yellow, is held in the mouth for swelling and pain of the gum. Scutellaria is cooked and drunk for the swelling and pain of throat. These remedies all have a common color pigment and are used effectively for eliminating inflammation.

2. White colored herbs and the Lungs

As a cough medicine pinellia, white atractylodes, morus bark, apricot seed, lily, ophiopogon, platycodon, glehnia, fritillary and coix are most important. All of these herbs are white colored. As discussed in the *Zang–Fu* chapter, the color white is related to the Lungs. Herbs that stop cough and dispel phlegm generally contain white color. So we can infer the relationship between herbal properties which act on the Lungs and the color white.

3. Black colored herbs and the Kidneys

(a) Cooked rehmannia

"Fills the bone, produces Essence and Blood — treats Five strains and Seven injuries[22] in man; injury to Middle and bleeding during pregnancy, irregular menstruation and all diseases after pregnancy in woman." (*Li Shi Zhen*)

"Tonifies Blood and *Qi*, tonifies Kidney Water and True *Yin*." (*Yuan Su*)

(b) Scrophularia

"The King herb for the Kidney channel." (*Yuan Su*)

"Tonifies Kidney *Qi* and brightens eyes." *Ben Jing*

---

22. Seven Injuries are – (1) overeating injures Spleen, (2) great anger injures Liver, (3) excessive strain in lifting heavy objects and prolonged sitting in damp place injures Kidneys, (4) cold weather and cold drinks injures Lungs, (5) anxiety, melancholy and rumination injures Heart, (6) wind, rain, cold and summer heat injures the body and (7) great fear that is unregulated injures Will.

"Tonifies *Yin*, descends Fire,[23] promote urination and eliminates Blood stagnation." (*Li Shi Zhen*)

(c) Cistanche

"Treats Five Strains and Seven Injuries, Cold and Heat pain in the male genitals, strengthens *Yin* and augments Vital *Qi*." *Ben Jing*

"Used for impotence and blood in urine in man and infertility, leukorrhea and genital pain in woman." (*Da Ming*)

"Patients with Deficiency of the Fire in the Gate of Life can be tonified with this herb; it is a Kidney channel Blood level herb." (*Wang Hao Gu*)[24]

"Supports Ministerial Fire, tonifies Essence and stimulates *Yang*. It can treat infertility due to Blood Deficiency in women." (*Zhang Jing Yue*)

(d) Black Ink

"Stops bleeding, treats post–delivery vertigo due to Blood Deficiency, metrorrhagia and sudden blood in stool – grind with vinegar and take it." (*Kai Bao*)

"Promotes urination and menstruation." (*Li Shi Zhen*)

Grinding and drinking black ink at the time of vomiting of blood or blood in the stool has a miraculous effect. The carbon has the power to absorb toxins, so it is also used widely for colonic. However, this is a chemical explanation. Speaking in terms of color, black ink has the color of the Water Element and the Kidney is the organ of the Water Element. Heart is the organ of the Fire Element and blood belongs to the Heart. Thus, by the basic principle of Water controlling Fire, black colored carbon can be interpreted as having the property to stop bleeding.

(e) Iron

"Its color is black and belongs to the Water Element. Its property can suppress the Wood Element, thus it is suitable for treating epilepsy."[25] (*Li Shi Zhen*)

"Kidney tonics should not be stored in iron containers." (*Li Shi Zhen*)

---

23. Descending Fire refers to the lowering of high fever. It also refers to the lowering of the heat in the upper part of the body in which there are such symptoms as a flushed face, headache, red eyes, thirst for cold drinks, angering easily, etc.

24. A famous medical scholar in the 13th century. He compiled the book titled "Materia Medica for Decoction."

25. Epilepsy in Oriental medicine is caused by rising of Wind which belongs to the Wood Element. By strengthening the Water Element, Wind can be brought down and extinguished.

(f) Magnetite

"Nourishes Kidney *Qi* and fills up Essence and Marrow:[26] It can be used for all patients with deafness and dizziness due to Kidney Deficiency." (*Zong Shi*)

"Magnetite has black color of Water Element and enters Kidneys; that is the reason for using it to treat all conditions of the Kidneys." (*Li Shi Zhen*)

4. Blue–Green colored herbs and the Liver

(a) Green tangerine peel

"Its sour taste enters the Liver. It eliminates hypochondriac pain and relieves stagnated anger. It eliminates Hernial disorders and has the function of decongesting the Liver." (*Zhang Jing Yue*)

"It enters *Jueyin* (Liver) and *Shaoyang* (Gall Bladder) channels and treats diseases of Liver and Gall Bladder." (*Yuan Su*)

"Green tangerine peel is a conductant herb for the Liver channel." (*Li Dong Yuan*)

(b) Sweet wormwood

"Because it received the *Qi* of Spring–Wood (Liver) and *Shaoyang* (Gall Bladder) energy, its treatment symptoms are all *Shaoyang* and *Jueyin* diseases in the Blood Level." (*Li Shi Zhen*)

"It treats chill and fever of malaria." (*Li Shi Zhen*)

"It treats the Blood Level diseases of Liver, Kidney and Triple Burner." (*Zhang Jing Yue*)

(c) Prunella Spike

"It is said in the *Materia Medica* that prunella can best treat scrofula, disperses Knotted *Qi* and has the effect of tonifying the blood vessels of the *Jueyin*, but there is no discussion on its ability to eliminate the Cold and Heat." (*Zhu Dan Xi*)

"It is able to clear Liver Fire and Blood Heat. Thus, it treats red eyes, cataract and pterygium. It can suppress the Liver and improve hearing and vision." (*Zhang Jing Yue*)

Those enumerated here are especially notable ones; all medicines from the plants have a blue–green color to some extent.

(d) Copper

"This is the consolidated liquid of copper. It has a sour taste and is slightly toxic and enters

---

26. Marrow is the substance that is made from the Essence in the Kidneys. It is said that "Brain is the Sea of Marrow." See Chapter 2 on Zang Fu organs for further detail.

the Liver and Gall Bladder. Therefore, it eliminates the Wind–Phlegm through vomiting or diarrhea, brightens the eyes and eliminates Childhood Nutritional Impairment."[27] (*Li Shi Zhen*)

(e) Azurite (Gong Qing)

"It has blue–green color and governs the Liver." (*Han Bao Sheng*)[28]

"It treats glaucoma and deafness. It brightens the eyes, benefits the nine orifices,[29] opens the Blood vessels, nourishes the Spirit and augments the Liver *Qi*." *Ben Jing*

(f) Scorpion

"It has a blue–green color which belongs to Wood Element and is a Liver channel herb. Thus, it treats Windstroke and all types of disorders due to Wind. It opens Wind–Phlegm obstruction, deviation of eyes and mouth, hemiplegia, difficult speech, malaria, deafness, Hernial disorders, Wind boil, urticaria, Wind–Phlegm[30] in infants and epileptic seizure. This too is an important herb in the treatment of Wind." (*Zhang Jing Yue*)

"Treats all diseases of *Jueyin*. It treats dizziness and convulsion due to Wind, chills and fever of malaria, tinnitus, deafness – these symptoms all belong to the category of *Jueyin*–Wind–Wood. Thus, *Li Dong Yuan* has said, "Hernial disorders and leukorrhea both belong to Wind and scorpion is an important medicine to treat Wind." (*Li Shi Zhen*)

5. Red colored herbs and the Heart

(a) Salvia

"It is red in color and has a bitter taste, neutral temperature and descending property. It is *Yang* within *Yin* and enters the Heart and Pericardium channels. It is a Blood Level herb for those two channels. *Si Wu Tang* (Four Substance Decoction)[31] treats all women's diseases, whether they are before or after delivery or whether menstrual flow is excessive or deficient. These disorders can all be treated equally effectively with a decoction of salvia alone. Salvia breaks up stagnated Blood, produces new Blood, calms the fetus, facilitates the removal of a dead fetus, stops metrorrhagia and leukorrhea and regulates channels. It is very effective and is in the category of Chinese angelica, cooked rehmannia, cnidium and peony." (*Li Shi Zhen*)

"It nourishes and regulates Blood, produces new Blood and moves stagnated Blood. Thus, it

---

27. A group of disorders that occur in small children. It is characterized by sallow complexion, weakness, abdominal distention and chronic indigestion. Other clinical manifestions include failure to grow properly, thin hair, poor temper, sucking the fingers, pica and diarrhea with sour odor. The causes for this order are early stopping of breast feeding, improper diet, chronic illness, parasites, etc. These causes lead to the weakening of Spleen and Stomach that results in malnutrition. If left untreated, this disorder can injure other organs as well.

28. A medical scholar of later Shu Dynasty (221 – 263 A.D.).

29. Nine orifices refers to the orifices of the eyes, ears, nose, mouth, urethra and anus.

30. Wind–Phlegm is a form of phlegm which causes symptoms such as dizziness, seizures, epilepsy, paralysis, numbness, deviation of eyes and mouth, etc. It is commonly seen in stroke patients.

31. Four Substance Decoction consists of cooked rehmannia, Chinese angelica, peony and cnidium.

can calm the fetus, facilitate removal of a dead fetus and stop metrorrhagia and leukorrhea. It regulates imbalances in the channels. It is a Blood Level medicine of the Heart, Spleen, Liver and Kidney." (*Zhang Jing Yue*)

"It nourishes the Spirit, settles the Will, stops irritability due to pathogens in the Blood, eliminates pus, stops pain, produces new flesh and makes muscles grow." (*Da Ming*)

(b) Carthamus

"It breaks up stagnated Blood in large doses, but nourishes Blood in small doses." (*Zhu Dan Xi*)

"It enters the Heart and nourishes the Blood, assists Chinese angelica and governs new Blood. (*Zhang Yuan Su*)

"It has a pungent, sweet, bitter taste and warm temperature. It is a Blood Level herb of the Liver channel." (*Wang Hao Gu*)

"It activates Blood, moistens dryness, stops pain, dispels swelling and opens channels." (*Li Shi Zhen*)

(c) Rubia root

"It has red color, warm temperature and slightly sour and salty tastes. It enters the Nutritive Level[32] due to the red color, and moves stagnation due to its warm temperature. Also, it enters the Liver due to its sour taste and goes into the Blood due to its salty taste. It is a Blood Level herb of the Pericardium and Liver channels. It circulates and activates the Blood." (*Li Shi Zhen*)

"It has a bitter taste, thus it is able to move stagnated Blood and it has a cool temperature, thus it is able to stop bleeding. It treats vomiting of blood and nose bleeding due to excess strain and continuous metrorrhagia. It also opens stagnation in the channels." (*Zhang Jing Yue*)

(d) Sappan wood

"It is a Blood Level herb of the three *Yin* channels (Heart, Liver and Spleen). It harmonizes Blood when used in a small amount, but breaks up Blood when used in large amounts." (*Li Shi Zhen*)

"Indications for sappan wood include irregular menstruation in women, epigastric pain, Blood and *Qi* stagnation in the abdomen, distention and discomfort due to Blood stagnation after delivery. Also, it disperses carbuncles and dead Blood, it eliminates pus, stops pain and eliminates blood stagnation due to trauma." (*Zhang Jing Yue*)

---

32. Nutritive Level is the third energetic layer of the body. From the superficial to deep energetic layers are as follows: Protective Level, Qi Level, Nutritive Level and Blood Level.

(e) Cinnabar

"It has a red color and governs Heart." (*Han Bao Sheng*)

"It is the main herb for the Blood Level of the Heart channel." (*Wang Hao Gu*)

"Its color belongs to the Fire Element. It enters the Heart and can calm the Spirit and goes into the Blood Vessels." (*Zhang Jing Yue*)

The relationship between the yellow colored herbs and the Spleen was not exemplified, but there is a definite correlation between the yellow color and the herbal properties. *Han Bao Sheng* has said "realgar belongs to the Earth Element. Thus, it has a yellow color and controls the Spleen." Polygonatum has a yellow color and *Li Shi Zhen* has said, "it received pure *Qi* of *Wu Ji*[33] (Spleen–Earth), thus it is a superior herb for tonifying the Spleen. Earth is also the mother of all things." On the property of chicken, *Li Shi Zhen* said, "the yellow rooster belongs to the Earth Element so it is suitable for the Spleen and Stomach." Also, tonics generally contain a yellow color – ginseng contains a yellow color and so does licorice, astragalus and white atractylodes.

With the above mentioned examples, though vague, one can guess that there is a certain relationship between the color and property of an herb. As we advance this study, I firmly believe that we can make herbology even more complete. Among the above examples, there might be points that differ from practice, but the purpose of recording them here is to show proof that among the practitioners of herbology up to now, there have been many who observed the color. Among them were *Li Shi Zhen*, *Han Bao Sheng* and *Zhang Jing Yue*.

THE COMPOSITION OF HERBAL PROPERTIES AND THE MUTUAL RELATIONSHIP BETWEEN ORGANS

Having a complex of many pharmacologically active constituents within a single herb is a strong point with Oriental herbology, but at the same time, it becomes the reason for being theoretically ambiguous.

As a subject of study in analytical science, an Oriental herb might be a difficult matter, but as a pharmacologically active body that serves as a mediator for recovering health, there is no equal. The reason is that there is a mutual relationship between each organ and structure in the body. Thus, it is most natural and effective to eliminate the physiological

---

33. A third pair of Ten Celestial Stems, which are ancient devices used to denote time. Wu and Ji are the Yang and Yin of the Earth Element, respectively.

5 Element	Yang	Yin
Wood	Jia	Yi
Fire	Bing	Ding
Earth	Wu	Ji
Metal	Geng	Xin
Water	Ren	Gui

abnormality or pathological phenomenon by organically connecting, regulating and organizing the function of each organ with a single medicinal substance. This substance is an Oriental herb which contains constituents that will act upon each organ and structure.

To give an example, hawthorn fruit has a sweet and sour taste, neutral temperature and light *Qi*. Yet, hawthorn fruit is an effective herb for acid regurgitation, namely hyperchlorhydria. Having excessive acid is a disease. Then why does the disease lessen in severity by ingesting a sour tasting substance? In modern medicine, bicarbonate of soda would be used to neutralize the secreted acid, but the treatment method in Oriental medicine is to reduce the acid secretion at the source. This is done by sending a message to the origin of the acid digestive juices.

Acid regurgitation is referred to in Oriental medicine as: "Liver pathogen overacting on the Spleen." That is, it implies a Wood Element overacting on an Earth Element. Ultimately, it means that acid bile secreted by the liver is greater in quantity than alkaline pancreatic juice secreted by the pancreas. After ingesting this herb, acid regurgitation disappears because hawthorn fruit, which has a sweet and sour taste, sends a messenger to both the liver and the pancreas (Spleen) to adjust the imbalance in the amount of the secretion of digestive juices (refer to *Yin–Yang* chapter). Furthermore, since the *Qi* of hawthorn fruit is light, it eliminates harmful gas inside the digestive organs which harmonizes the Stomach and help digestion.

There is much more to discuss on the treatment indications of the hawthorn fruit according to its properties. Since its color is composed of both red and yellow, one can infer that it acts on the Heart and blood, Spleen–Stomach and nutrition. The following are the functions and treatment indications of hawthorn fruit: It treats low back pain, disperses food stagnation, tonifies Spleen, treats Small Intestine, Hernial disorders and ulcerated rash in children, strengthens the Stomach, circulates Accumulation of *Qi*, treats abdominal pain in women after delivery and leukorrhea, disperses meat stagnation and abdominal mass, Phlegm–Damp,[34] Focal Distention,[35] acid regurgitation, pain and distention of Blood stagnation, dissolves Blood and *Qi* mass, activates Blood, etc. It seems difficult to imagine all of the various functions and indications, but this is only a partial list. In short, it is enough to understand the basic properties of hawthorn fruit. No matter what the symptoms are, it will fundamentally be the result of the imbalance in the function of the Liver and Spleen and assimilation of toxic gas developed in the digestive organs. So for this condition, hawthorn fruit will be effective.

Just as in the repair of a big building, rather than individually hiring a carpenter, stone cutter, landscaper, etc. one can save time and effort and have the repair done most efficiently by hiring a contractor who then organizes all these separate activities. Similarly, the hawthorn fruit is the contractor of health improvement for the symptoms and condition mentioned.

---

34. A form of disorder of water metabolism. There is a stagnation of water in the stomach and intestines with symptoms such as poor appetite, chest and hypochondriac distention, dizziness, palpitations, shortness of breath and vomiting thick white clear sputum.

35. It is a subjective feeling of fullness and distress in the epigastric region. The cause of focal distention is pathogenic Heat, Qi Deficiency or Qi Stagnation in the epigastric region.

(ADDENDUM) ANIMAL ORGAN EXTRACTS AND THEIR MEDICINAL EFFECT ON THE HUMAN BODY

A. Animal organs tonify each corresponding organ in the human body. For example, a person with weak lungs likes to ingest the lung of an animal and a person with a weak brain likes to eat the brain of an animal. I have always observed when eating meat with several people that the person whom I thought had weak lungs through my observation or a lung disease patient without fail likes a piece of lung meat in the beef soup and a person with a weak liver likes a piece of cooked or raw liver. I myself enjoy eating stomach meat or raw stomach and cooked heart, but do not like lung or liver at all. Some people enjoy eating ox brain because of the tastiness and others enjoy ingesting raw blood. These are all responses in taste towards foods that are most effective in treating the particular physiological needs of the body. The following animal organs and their respective functions or indications can be found in Oriental herbology:

Chicken:

- **Brain** – Treats childhood convulsion and difficult labor in women. (*Su Gong*)
- **Liver** – Treats dimmed vision due to Liver Deficiency. (*Li Shi Zhen*)

The eye is said to belong to the Liver, so the cause of eye disorders is said to be in the Liver. It is well documented and experienced in folk medicine that eating chicken liver for night blindness has a miraculous effect.

- **Gizzard** – Treats Food Malaria[36] in children and stomach disorder in adults. (*Li Shi Zhen*)

Ox:

- **Marrow** – Tonifies the digestive system and fills out the bone marrow. *Ben Jing*
- **Brain** – Treats dizziness and Wasting and Thirsting Syndrome. (*Su Gong*)

Ox brain is eaten frequently for feelings of emptiness in the head with dizziness and vertigo.

- **Heart** – Treats forgetfulness and tonifies the Heart. *Bie Lu*
- **Spleen** –Tonifies the Spleen. (*Chen Zhang Qi*)
        Disperses focal mass. (*Li Shi Zhen*)

Note: Focal mass implies enlargement of the spleen.

---

36. Food Malaria is a type of malaria in which the patient first has food stagnation and then gets affected by an External pathogen. Its symptoms are alternating chills and fever, belching, anorexia, vomiting immediately upon eating, abdominal distention and epigastric distress, etc.

- **Lung** – Tonifies the Lung. (*Chen Zhang Qi*)
- **Liver** – Tonifies the Liver and brightens eyes. *Bie Lu*
- **Kidney** – Tonifies the Kidney *Qi* and augments the Essence. *Bie Lu*
- **Stomach** – Tonifies the digestive system, augments *Qi*, detoxifies and nourishes Spleen–Stomach. (*Li Shi Zhen*)

B. I have already said that in the medicines collected from plants, the organ of our body that they act on is determined by the taste and color, but there is also a definite relationship between the parts of the plants and their properties. I have listed them below along with some examples of specific herbs.

Roots – The function of roots is related to their original function of absorbing nutrients from the ground. They are frequently used for supporting nutrition and the Original *Qi* of the human body.

- **Licorice** – Treats the Five *Zang* and Six *Fu* organs, eliminates Cold and Heat Pathogenic *Qi*, strengthens tendons and bones, promotes the growth of muscles and increases energy.
- **Astragalus** – Assists *Qi*, strengthens tendons and bones and tonifies the Blood.
- **Ginseng** – Treats all Deficient Syndromes in men and women.

Thus, not only are most tonics and nutritional herbs collected from the roots, but also a majority of the herbs in the Oriental medicine are from the roots: rehmannia, Chinese angelica, white atractylodes, glehnia, platycodon, polygonatum, anemarrhena, polygala, scrophularia, sanguisorba, salvia, coptis, scutellaria, bupleurum, pubescent angelica, peucedanum, cimicifuga, fritillary, gentiana, asarum, cnidium, peony, moutan, saussurea, fresh ginger, etc. – to mention a few.

Fruits/Seeds – due to their original nature, they act mostly on the reproductive system, namely the Kidney channel.

- **Plantago** – Promotes urination.
- **Rubus** – Augments the Kidney and astringes the urine.
- **Rosa fruit** – Treats nocturnal emission, spermatorrhea, excess uterine bleeding, leukorrhea and incontinence.
- **Cardamon** – Enters the Lung, Kidney and Urinary Bladder channels; treats incontinence and metrorrhagia in women.
- **Black cardamon** – Governs Deficient Cold in the Lower Burner, warms the Kidney Qi, treats spermatorrhea, dribbling of urine, nocturnal emission, red and white turbid leukorrhea, and frequent urination at night. Thus, it is an appropriate herb for a person with weakness of *Yang Qi* of Triple Burner and the Gate of Life.
- **Schizandra** – Enters the Lung and Kidney channels, nourishes the Kidney Water, tonifies Original *Yang*, strengthens the tendons and muscles and assists the Gate of Life.

- **Lycium** – Nourishes *Yin* and assists *Yang*; increases Essence, consolidates the Marrow, strengthens bones and tendons.
- **Euryale** – Enters both the Spleen and Kidney channels, tonifies Kidney and consolidates Essence, treats incontinence, spermatorrhea and white turbid leukorrhea.
- **Coix** – Eliminates Dampness, promotes urination and treat Heat *Lin* Syndrome.
- **Cuscuta** – Enters the Liver, Spleen and Kidney channels, tonifies the marrow, increases Essence, assists *Yang*, consolidates diarrhea, astringes the urine, stops nocturnal emission, treats leukorrhea and dribbling urination.

Aside from these herbal medicines, there are additional medicines collected from flowers, leaves, barks, branches and stems, but they are more difficult to classify than the medicines above that are related to the nutritional and reproductive systems. Leaves have a function similar to the stomach and lungs of animals such as assimilation, dispersing water and breathing. Thus, we can generally observe a lot of action on the Stomach such as the harmonizing the Stomach, clearing the Stomach and dispersing *Qi* from leaves such as agastache, perilla, peppermint and bamboo.

In the function of barks, too, there are properties which are held in common with the leaves of the plants. We can observe a great deal of action occuring on the Lungs and skin. For example, barks such as cinnamon, magnolia and mulberry stop cough, dispel phlegm and promote sweat. I have not yet discovered common functions regarding flowers and branches/stems, but since the season in which flowers blossom is in spring and summer, they can be inferred to act a great deal on the Liver and Heart.

In adolescence, a period in which reproduction is about to begin, the Heart has especially exuberant activity. There is a lot of laughter and the skin is lustrous in order to attract the opposite sex. Similarly, in spring–summer seasons, when pollination begins, brilliant flowers blossom to attract mediators of pollens. The relationship between the Liver and Heart and pregnant women and the function of the Liver, too, was mentioned many times already.

The branches and stems of plants do not have specified organs they act on, but they can be observed to act on the interior of the human body more than the skin. The tip of a branch ascends or reaches four extremities, is active and has intense action (like cinnamon twig). The stem of the plant is passive and stays in the Middle[37] or descends, but its action has a tendency to be slow (like sappan wood). By the way, cases of using the stem of a plant as a medicinal substance are extremely small in number so it is not much of an issue in Oriental medicine.

---

37. Acts on the digestive organs which are in the Middle Burner.

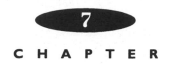

C H A P T E R

THE STUDY OF PRESCRIPTION

I. INTRODUCTION

The purpose of a medicine is in the treatment and the method of treatment is in the prescription. As the symptoms of diseases change continuously and the corresponding treatment methods become varied, it is not feasible to memorize main treatment symptoms nor to recite highly efficacious prescriptions. Even if that were possible, without an understanding of the principles of prescription and pharmacology, memorized facts become dead knowledge and hold little value. In contrast, if one understands the methodology of herbal therapy, assesses herbal properties, observes syndromes and understands the principles of prescription, the etiology will be clearly known even when one is confronted with innumerable disease symptoms. Adapting a prescription to a specific syndrome can then be done easily and effectively.

THE DOCTOR AND THE TAILOR

A doctor creates a prescription much like a tailor weaves a suit. To make a properly fitting suit for one's body, one must go to a skillful tailor and have measurements taken to fit the actual body. After deciding the style and color, basting is done and at last, the complete suit can be made. In order to receive a proper prescription for the individual constitution and disease, one must employ a doctor well–versed in the "Four Methods of Diagnosis" which are looking, listening/smelling, asking and palpating. Then, if the results of ingesting herbs are favorable, it can be considered as an excellent prescription.

In terms of the tailor, since physical constitutions, perceived from the outside, vary from person to person, accurate observation is needed to fit the clothing perfectly. In the case of the doctor, much more accuracy is needed in distinguishing the physiological phenomena and pathological symptoms of a person, which are often much more complex and elusive.

TRADITIONAL FORMULAS AND READY–MADE CLOTHING

The formulas that were prescribed to people in ancient times are comparable to the ready–made clothes crafted by a tailor. Frequently, obtaining ready–made clothes by a skilled tailor are better than ordering custom–made clothes from an unskilled tailor, but what about comparing custom–made clothing from a skilled tailor with ready–made clothing of a skilled tailor? In short, the question really is whether or not one can find a skilled craftsman or an eminent doctor.

The purpose of making a prescription is to treat the patient and in patients with variations of symptoms, it is difficult to find an appropriate prescription among the traditional formulas. Inevitably, formulas that resemble each other closely are all tested haphazardly in order to find the most appropriate formula among them. There are times when the disease gets treated quickly due to luck in picking out the correct formula, but in general, there are many times when one laments over choosing a less applicable or even inappropriate prescription and thus delaying or even impairing the patient's recovery.

II. CLINICAL SYNDROMES
(refer to Chapter 3 on the Syndrome)

DIAGNOSIS AND TREATMENT

The subject for diagnosis in Oriental medicine is not a disease but a living body that displays the disease phenomena – in other words, a diseased body. The goal of the treatment is not in the elimination of a localized disease or each pathological symptom, but in transforming a diseased body in an abnormal physiological state, into a healthy body in a normal physiological state. Therefore, the diagnosis and the treatment of a disease must be holistic.

A disease is always in the whole body. So in a strict sense, such a thing as a purely localized disease cannot exist. Even when the body is damaged due to external stimuli, the activation of substances in areas other than the localized region is needed for the recovery. Accordingly, each organ undergoes individually appropriate changes.

How can one correctly diagnose a disease developed from internal causes by localized observation? There exists an indivisible relationship between every organ within the human body. Consequently, functional impairment of one organ directly influences functional changes in other organs. For example, when the heart valve is damaged, liver enlargement occurs, the quantity of urine is reduced, edema develops, abnormalities in the blood are created and the breathing center is stimulated. The real question is: why did the heart valve get damaged? Although the heart valve damage could be the cause of liver enlargement, one cannot say that the liver enlargement cannot be the cause of the heart valve damage. Abnormalities of the blood can bring about activation of the breathing center and the change in breathing can create a change in the blood. Thus, a change in one organ can be the cause or the result of the changes in other organs. So the true cause of the disease must be found in the physical constitution. For example, when abnormal changes occur in the liver, there is a function which compensates, supports and treats that change inside the body. If that function is sufficiently carried on, then unusual changes in the liver will not be able to bring the body into a diseased state, but when functions such as compensating and healing are incomplete, a disease develops.

All organs of a human body maintain life by going through a cycle of work, fatigue, compensation, recovery and then back to work. When there is no work by the organs, life cannot exist. The result of work is the creation of fatigue in the organs and the fatigue requires compensation and recovery. When there is no compensation and replenishment, the organ's fatigue cannot be recovered and when there is no recovery, the complete work by the organs cannot be maintained, resulting in a disease.

To recover from fatigue, organs mutually compensate and replenish each other within the body, while at the same time, continuously receiving assistance in healing from the outside. However, once the fatigue reaches a pathological state, the possibility of recovering from fatigue and hindrance within the body is small, so the degree of reliance on healing from the outside necessarily becomes greater. This increased demand for assistance in healing and receiving of reinforcement is called the disease symptomatology. Therefore, disease symptoms are very beneficial experiences for us. There are times when we often dislike disease symptoms, but in actuality, this is foolish rather than being humorous. It is equivalent to resenting a warning signal out of fear in dreading a dangerous event. The disease symptoms warn us of the danger and at the same time the symptoms themselves frequently have the direct function of healing. To give a few examples:

1. Sensitivity, pain, itchiness or rash occur in the needed regions of the body surface through the channels to sensitize or strengthen the demand for external treatment stimulation. It is valid to see all changes in the skin that are not caused by external injury as internally related healing phenomena. So not even a single pimple is without significance.
2. Cold sensations demand warmth and warm sensations demand clearing of heat.
3. Thirst is an indication that one is in need of water.
4. Preference for certain foods and sensations of taste are both demands for the appropriate substance necessary for healing.
5. It can be inferred that changes in skin pigment are a response to certain types of chemical actions needed to facilitate the healing process.

Thus, after observing the patient in every direction in order to diagnose holistically, the treatment must be done holistically as well. For example, using sleeping pills when treating insomnia is not a holistic treatment, but a mere symptomatic measure. One might momentarily avoid the suffering of insomnia in this way, but the insomnia itself will not be eliminated. Therefore, in order to treat insomnia, the abnormal physiological state of the diseased body which created insomnia must be corrected.

MANIFESTATION OF SYNDROMES AND THE FORMULAS

Although symptoms are innumerable, the process that is needed in the treatment is distinguishing *Yin–Yang*. To explain in further detail, it is enough to discern the relative balance of Cold–Heat, Deficiency–Excess, Exterior–Interior, pathological changes and the *Zang Fu* organs.

A. Yin–Yang (refer to the detailed discussion in Chapter 1)

B. Cold – Heat

Cold and Heat are manifestations of *Yin–Yang*, so the basic principle is that when *Yin* flourishes, there is Cold and when *Yang* flourishes there is Heat. However, in practice, discerning this becomes a headache for the doctor because the functions of *Yin–Yang* are not expressed simply. There is the addition of the suppressing–promoting relationship between the organs and interference by the complicated order of life force. A doctor will commit an error in treatment if he or she does not properly recognize Cold and Heat. Since warm herbs must be used in Cold disease, mistaking a Cold disease as a Heat disease and using cold herbs would further worsen the disease. Mistaking a Heat disease as a Cold disease and using hot herbs would actually be promoting the disease–causing factors.

1. Cold

(a) Aversion to Cold or Chills

Although "Averson to Cold" or "Chills" implies cold, the actual characteristic is different; it is the feeling of cold even when the outside temperature is not cold. When the whole body feels extremely tense, as in the circumstances of feeling extreme fear, sensing danger or anticipating a violent fight, one feels chills. When listening to a frightening ghost story or to stories of corpses walking around, one feels shivers on the back, one's hair stands on end and the entire body gets goose bumps. When entering an old, empty house at night or hearing a slight rustle when walking the streets at night, one feels chills. Likewise chills occur on the occasion of making a public speech for the first time "on stage" or entering the examination room for a big test, or when an innocent virgin meets the man she adores for the first time, all feel chills. The chill of a disease also has its origin as extreme tension and always results in a strong fever. The chill and fever of lung disease, malaria and typhoid fever are all examples of this. A chill implies the tension or getting "armed" and fever implies the effort and struggle. The chill and fever of a disease in general can be presumed to be caused by an invasion of germs and if not attributed to germs, we can suppose that a chill comes from a sudden stimulus that can endanger one's life. Therefore, one must not perceive all chills as cold and uniformly use hot herbs.

(b) Intolerance to Cold

"Intolerance to Cold" is usually included under a common "chill," but I am distinguishing between them and calling a chill without a fever an "Intolerance to Cold." "Intolerance to Cold" is a physiological demand for an increase in the body temperature, so it disappears when one warms up the room and covers oneself with thick blankets. However, in the case of a "chill" symptom, for a certain period of time, while in the preparation for the effort and struggle, one cannot avoid the shivering chill no matter how thick a blanket is used in a warm room. The body temperature is deficent in the case of an "Intolerance to Cold" because of a *Yang* Deficiency. Thus one can use *Yang* tonics and Heat promoting herbs.

(c) Exterior Cold

When Cold *Qi* exists on the exterior of the body, there is an Intolerance to Cold, cold body, bluish or black facial color, cold hands and feet and sometimes edema.

(d) Interior Cold

When the Cold *Qi* exists in the interior of the body, there is indigestion, nausea, vomiting, epigastric pain, etc. and one likes warm–hot foods and drinks, while disliking cool–cold foods and drinks.

(e) Upper Cold

When the Cold *Qi* is in the upper part of the body, there occurs acid regurgitation, dysphagia, indigestion, etc.

(f) Lower Cold

When the Cold *Qi* is in the lower part of body, there occurs enuresis, loose stool, impotence, cold knees and feet, etc.

2. Heat

Our life maintains itself by consuming energy to create metabolic heat. Hence, in maintaining a healthy body, a certain heat (namely body temperature) must be sustained. When there is a change within the body, the body puts out more effort than usual in order to normalize itself and accordingly, body temperature rises. This is called a fever. Therefore, fever usually accompanies a disease and the severity of the disease can be observed through the degree of the fever. Here is a point that a doctor must pay great attention to, for when there is a disease, there is bodily fever and when there is no disease, the fever drops. Accordingly, the conclusion can be made that it is sufficient to relieve the heat in a disease. The statements are accurate, but to think that cold herbs should be used to relieve heat will have disastrous results. In such a case, without discussing the Cold–Heat principle of the symptoms and herbal properties, the conclusion will be to use cold herbs, since all diseases uniformly have fever. In practice, it does not work that way. Even though all diseases have fever, the methods of relieving the fever are all different.

There are times when the heat is relieved through hot herbs and there are times when heat is relieved through cold herbs. Sometimes, diaphoretics are used to relieve heat and sometimes purgatives are used to relieve heat. The reason for this is that the causes of fever are many and even the types of heat are different. The following is a discussion of the types of Heat.

(a) Fever due to Fatigue

This is a fever resulting from the physiological effort to recover from the strong degree of fatigue caused by mental or physical overstrain. Deficient Heat, False Heat, *Yang* Deficient Heat, *Qi* Deficient Heat and Blood Deficient Heat all belong to this category. Fever due to fatigue requires rest and when the body is rested and nourished, the fever automatically disappears. Thus, it is caused by merely being weak and not from having a particular cause of disease which has been lying dormant, although sometimes this fever combines with the cause of a disease.

(b) Fever due to Stimulation

This fever is due to excitation caused when the activity of the heart becomes exuberant as a result of external stimulation, so that the body temperature suddenly rises. The cause of fever can be psychological as in the case of excessive anger or physical as in the case of ingesting substances such as alcoholic drinks. When such stimulants are taken repeatedly, sometimes the physical constitution changes accordingly and this is called a "Deficiency of *Yin* with Exuberance of Fire," "Stagnated Fire" or "Deficient Fire." The so–called "Night Fever" also belongs to this category.

(c) Fever due to Struggle

When there is an invasion by germs or other unusual changes that can threaten life occur in the body, the effort to eliminate them causes fever. Thus, the fever of diseases generally belongs to this type of fever and is called "Pathogenic Heat" or "Excess Heat." However, there is a "Fever due to Struggle" even in a weak person. This is called "Excess within Deficiency" and is differentiated from the "Fever due to Struggle" of a healthy person. Therefore, all "Fever due to Struggle" should not be regarded in the same light as Excess Heat.

(d) Tidal Fever

This type of fever is the same as "Intermittent Fever" and implies a periodically occuring Fever. It is proper to view this "Tidal Fever" as the "Fever due to Struggle" of generally weak patients, so all effort should be made to increase the power of resistence, namely Original *Qi* in the treatment.

(e) Alternating Chill and Fever

This fever is similar to Tidal Fever, but includes "Intolerance to Cold" or "Aversion to Cold." This fever is a result of the phenomenon of struggle when the body is extremely deficient, having lost the balance of regulating body temperature, or when the stomach is diseased, or when the bacteria–caused disease worsens.

(f) Exterior Heat

When the heat is on the Exterior, there are symptoms such as fever, redness, swelling, rash, etc. In this condition, one will seek to cool his or her body by removing clothing or resting in bed on top of the covers.

(g) Interior Heat

When the heat is in the Interior, there are symptoms such as restlessness, fullness and distention of the chest, irritability, thirst, asthmatic breathing, shouting, mania, constipation, reddish urine, etc.

(h) Upper Heat

When the heat is in the upper region of the body, there are symptoms such as headache, red eyes, flushed feeling, a red face, swelling and pain of the throat, dryness in the nose, a burning sensation on the tongue, a preference for cold things, etc.

(i) Lower Heat

When the heat is in the lower region of the body, there are symptoms such as dry stool, reddish and difficult urination, swelling and pain of the waist and leg, etc.

3. Cold–Heat and the Herbal Formulas

(a) Aversion to Cold (Chills) and Exterior Cold

The diaphoretic method should be used for this condition. With regards to taste and temperature, formulas with pungent, warm, fragrant and dispersing properties should be used. Herbs such as ephedra, cinnamon twig, asarum, fresh ginger and atractylodes are all in this category and they should be used appropriately. In actual practice, however, there are occasions when the "Warming Up the Middle" method or Tonifying *Yang* method is used.

Whether the symptoms are chills or Intolerance to Cold, when there is an External pathogen, the diaphoretic method must be used. When diaphoresis is called for, there are changes in the prescription according to the individual constitution. This is difficult to explain, but one will be able to gradually understand it. When there are chills or Intolerance to Cold without the External Pathogen, the diaphoretic method should not be used.

(b) Interior Cold

For treating this condition, Tonifying *Yang* and "Warming the Middle" herbs such as ginseng, white atractylodes, dried ginger, cinnamon bark, magnolia, evodia, etc. should be used. Chinese angelica, cooked rehmannia and cnidium or eucommia, lycium, aconite, etc. can be combined and used according to the physical constitution.

(c) Upper Cold

When cold is in the upper body, it is enough to use warm or hot herbs. The reason is that many of the *Yang*–natured herbs generally have ascending properties or a combination of ascending–descending properties. Ginseng, white atractylodes, dried ginger, cinnamon bark, licorice, etc. are the herbs to be used and because an herb that supports Original *Yang* like ginseng is complete, it is not necessary to distinguish ascending or descending properties.

(d) Lower Cold

When Cold is in the lower part of the body, warm or hot herbs that descend are used and herbs that combine pungent and bitter taste or warm–hot natured herbs with "Thick taste" can be used. Warm herbs that descend and warm the lower part of the body include magnolia, evodia, fennel, cyperus, lycium, etc. Additionally, herbs from other categories such as ginseng, white atractylodes, dried ginger, cinnamon bark and aconite can also be used to warm the lower part of the body.

(e) Fever due to Fatigue

Qi or Blood tonics such as ginseng, astragalus, Chinese angelica and cooked rehmannia are used for this condition, but depending on the *Yin–Yang* of a person's constitution, warm or cool herbs are added.

(f) Fever due to Stimulation

This condition will automatically resolve itself, but when it affects the physical constitution, *Yin* tonics, *Yang* tonics, *Qi* tonics or Blood tonics can be used according to the symptoms. In addition, herbs that enter the Heart channel, Liver channel, etc. are used according to the organ systems.

(g) Fever due to Struggle

The treatment for this fever is done by finding the cause of a disease. It cannot be simply expressed here, because it will require explanation of the entire method of treating disease.

(h) Tidal Fever and Alternating Chills & Fever

Tonifying the Original *Qi* should be the main focus with this fever and it is good to combine diaphoretics or purgatives according to the symptoms.

(i) Exterior Heat

Since this is like Exterior Cold, warm–dispersing, neutral–dispersing or cool–dispersing formulas are used according to the physical constitutions and symptoms. Ephedra, cinnamon twig, asarum, fresh ginger, atractylodes, schizonepeta, siler, notopterygium, pubescent angelica, bupleurum, cimicifuga, perilla leaf and angelica are all diaphoretic herbs.

(j) Interior Heat

The methods to disperse Interior Heat are different according to the person's constitution and symptoms. The Heat is dispelled through the urine or stool, by clearing Blood or by Tonifying *Yin*.

- **Yin tonics** – cooked rehmannia, dioscorea, cornus, glehnia, scrophularia, ophiopogon, achyranthis, peony
- **Heat–clearing diuretics (herbs that dispel heat by promoting urination)** – poria, alisma, polyporus, akebia, gardenia, plantago seed
- **Purgatives/Laxatives** – rhubarb, mirabilite, immature bitter orange, peach seed, asparagus
- **Clearing and circulating Blood herbs** – rhinocerous horn, raw rehmannia, scutellaria, coptis, peony, rubia

(k) Upper Body Heat

For this condition, cool herbs with fragrant and ascending properties need to be used. The herbs should contain a taste that is bitter and light and *Qi* that is thick and light. The herbs to use are bupleurum, platycodon, rhinocerous horn, cimicifuga, peppermint and scutellaria. Even for Upper Body Heat that is due to an External Pathogen, the treatment principle calls for sweating out the pathogen. When Deficient Fire rises up, *Yin* should be tonified. When there is Upper Heat and Lower Cold, Tonifying *Yang* and "Warming the Middle" method should be used.

(l) Lower Body Heat

For this condition, herbs that tonify *Yin*, or clear heat and promote urination or purge are used.

C. Exterior – Interior

Exterior Syndrome is a disease caused by changes in the weather and consists mainly of Wind–Cold. Since the disease is superficial in Exterior Syndrome, it gets cured by promoting sweating and "Releasing Exterior" with the use of warm or cool diaphoretics. However, when the Exterior Syndrome is prolonged, it combines with an Interior Syndrome. Certain Interior Syndromes resemble Exterior Syndromes, so precise observation is required to differentiate Exterior and Interior Syndromes. In Interior Syndromes, there are many causes of the disease such as digestive disturbance, mental or physical overwork, prolonged strong emotion, overindulgence in alcoholic drinks and excess sexual activity. In the Interior Syndrome, herbs such as *Yang* tonics, Interior Warming, *Yin* tonics, purgatives, diuretics, *Qi* tonics, carminatives, Blood tonics, Breaking up Blood Stagnation, etc. are used according to the physical constitution and the symptoms.

- **Qi tonics** – ginseng, astragalus, white atractylodes
- **Carminatives** – lindera, aquilaria, saussurea, agastache, areca seed, perilla leaf
- **Blood tonics** – cooked rehmannia, Chinese angelica, peony, cnidium
- **Break up Blood Stagnation** – peach seed, carthamus, sappan, sparganium, zedoaria

D. Deficiency – Excess

Distinguishing Deficiency and Excess in treatment is of great importance. Thus, so–called *Yin–Yang*, Deficiency–Excess, Tonifying–Sedating are the critera by which treatment herbs are used. It is sufficient to tonify the Deficient patient and to sedate the Excess patient. If a Deficiency is sedated and Excess tonified, the Deficient patient gets weaker and the Excess patient will get even more excessive, worsening the condition of the disease.

What is meant by Deficiency and Excess? It is reasonable for a weak person to develop a disease, but the concept of disease occuring due to an Excess condition will make a person who looks at the Oriental medical books for the first time suspicious. In actuality, it is not that Original *Qi* is in Excess, instead it is the Pathogenic *Qi* that is in Excess. The statement, "*Zheng Qi* (Upright *Qi*) is deficient in a Deficient patient and Pathogenic *Qi* is excess in an Excess patient" implies just that.

A Deficient Syndrome is obviously due to being weak and deficient, but a disease occurs also in an Excess Syndrome because of being somewhat deficient. So fundamentally, both are deficient and it is only a matter of difference in the degree. If the physiolgical function is carried on completely and the resistive power and recuperative power of the body are vigorous, there will be no reason for the occurrence of the Excess Syndrome. Deficiency and Excess is distinguished by the difference in the proportion of external causes and internal causes of a disease and accordingly, the usage of herbs is different in each treatment. A Deficient Syndrome exists when the internal cause is greater than the external cause and an Excess Syndrome occurs when the external cause is greater than the internal cause. The Excess Syndrome generally includes acute diseases and the Deficient Syndrome generally includes chronic diseases. Even though a person's health is not that weak, when a disease occurs due to a violent change in the weather causing loss of the balance of physiological regulation, then his or her health will instantly recover when that abnormality is eliminated with diaphoretic or diuretic herbs. External causes which are so minor that they would not cause a disease in the average person will cause a disease in an essentially weak patient since he or she cannot endure them. Since a deficiency is the cause, tonics are mainly used and sedating herbs are combined in small amounts, thus this Syndrome is called "Excess within Deficiency." Without any external cause, sometimes the disease symptoms occur when there are abnormalities in the body's physiology or when the body is unable to endure normal amounts of physical activity or work. This is a purely Deficient Syndrome. This degree of Deficiency–Excess is different according to the person and disease and this point must be taken into consideration when selecting appropriate formulas.

1. In case of Exterior Excess, the following diaphoretic herbs should be used: ephedra, cinnamon twig, bupleurum, schizonepeta, siler, asarum, etc.

2. In case of Interior Excess, the following purgatives should be used: rhubarb, mirabilite, peach seed, bitter orange, sparganium, zedoaria, etc.

3. In case of Exterior Deficiency, stop–sweating herbs such as astragalus, zizyphus, peony, etc. are used and *Qi* tonics such as ginseng and white atractylodes can also be used.

4. In case of Interior Deficiency, *Qi* tonics, Blood tonics, *Yin* tonics and *Yang* tonics are used according to the physical constitution.

5. In case of Upper Deficiency, use tonics appropriate for the physical constitution. In some cases, upward–guiding herbs such as astragalus and cimicifuga are combined.

6. In case of Lower Deficiency, tonics that descend or astringents are used.

7. In case of *Qi* Deficiency, *Qi* tonics are used and for Blood Deficiency, Blood tonics are used.

E. Pathological Changes of the Zang Fu Organs

Oriental medical treatments can sufficiently be performed by distinguishing the above stated principles of Cold–Heat, Exterior–Interior and Deficiency–Excess, but in order to give more elaborate treatment, one must diagnose the *Zang Fu* organ with particularly obvious abnormality and apply appropriate treatment to that organ. Thus, by mastering the chapters on the *Zang Fu* organs and herbal properties, one will naturally acquire insights that can make the application of the herbs easier.

The following is a list of the herbs differentiated according to the various syndromes in each *Zang Fu* organ.

1. Heart
- Deficiency – ginseng, cooked rehmannia, Chinese angelica, zizyphus, polygala
- Excess – coptis, gardenia, akebia, red poria
- Heat – raw rehmannia, scutellaria, bamboo leaf, ophiopogon, salvia, gardenia, red poria

2. Lung
- Deficiency – ginseng, astragalus, licorice, dioscorea, lily, ophiopogon
- Excess – mulberry bark, poria, anemarrhena, apricot seed
- Heat – scutellaria, anemarrhena, ophiopogon, platycodon, asparagus
- Cold – white atractylodes, pinellia, ginseng, white mustard seed

3. Spleen
- Deficiency – ginseng, white atractylodes, licorice, astragalus, date
- Excess – peony, scutellaria, rhubarb, anemarrhena, immature bitter orange
- Heat – same as above
- Damp – white atractylodes, atractylodes, tangerine peel, pinellia, magnolia

4. Liver
- Deficiency – Chinese angelica, zizyphus, cornus, Chinese quince
- Excess – bupleurum, gentiana, green tangerine peel, coptis, gardenia

- Heat – red peony, phellodendron, anemarrhena, raw rehmannia, ophiopogon, moutan

5. Kidney
- Deficiency – ginseng, cooked rehmannia, dioscorea, lycium
- Yin Deficiency – cooked rehmannia, dioscorea, cornus, schizandra, scrophularia, raw rehmannia, achyranthis, peony
- Yang Deficiency – ginseng, aconite, dried ginger, cinnamon bark, eucommia
- Excess – alisma, polyporus, poria, plantago seed, lycium bark, phellodendron, anemarrhena
- Heat – use Kidney Excess herbs or *Yin* tonics
- Cold – Kidney *Yang* tonics
- Essence Depletion – rosa, euryale, dioscorea, polygala

6. Stomach
- Deficiency – ginseng, white atractylodes, astragalus
- Excess – immature bitter orange, tangerine peel, rhubarb, gypsum, barley sprout, magnolia, zedoaria, sparganium
- Heat – peony, scutellaria, coptis, ophiopogon, bamboo leaf, gypsum
- Cold – ginseng, white atractylodes, dried ginger, pinellia, cinnamon bark, evodia, nutmeg
- Qi stagnation – saussurea, tangerine peel, hawthorn fruit, agastache, bitter orange, lindera

7. Small Intestine
- Heat – phellodendron, scutellaria, coptis, forsythia, raw rehmannia, moutan, gardenia, akebia
- Cold – white atractylodes, fennel, dried ginger, nutmeg
- Qi stagnation – fennel, nutmeg, clove, saussurea

8. Large Intestine
- Heat – coptis, scutellaria, gypsum, asparagus
- Dryness – Chinese angelica, peony, achyranthis, raw rehmannia, peach seed, cannabis seed, cistanche
- Cold or Damp – dried ginger, nutmeg, aconite, magnolia, white atractylodes, atractylodes, pinellia
- Qi stagnation – bitter orange, tangerine peel, saussurea, areca seed, magnolia, nutmeg

9. Gall Bladder
- Deficiency – Chinese angelica, zizyphus, cooked rehmannia, ginseng
- Excess – gentiana, coptis, bupleurum, gardenia
- Heat – scutellaria, coptis, peony, forsythia

10. Urinary Bladder
- Heat – alisma, polyporus, poria, plantago seed, gardenia

- Bladder Cold – same as Kidney Cold
- Incontinence – cuscuta, black cardamon, psoralea, Chinese leek

THE ESSENTIAL POINTS IN THE OBSERVATION OF SYNDROMES

The intricacies of disease–states and herbal usages are substantially complex. They cannot be explained one by one, but rather only the main principles of syndrome observation can be learned. When the main principles are learned, it is like asking one question, but knowing ten. People often have tedious feelings towards complicated explanations. In acquiring the main principles about syndrome observation as repeatedly explained above, attention should be paid to observing Pulse diagnosis, Color observation, channels, appetite (diet), emotions, etc. Then, if effort is put into differentiating *Yin–Yang*, Cold–Heat, Deficiency–Excess, Exterior–Interior and Above–Below of the symptoms, the main principles will be acquired.

THE NAME OF DISEASE AND THE TREATMENT

A. The Name of a Disease is not related to the Treatment.

In Western medicine, the name of a disease must be determined before treatment can be performed. The goal of diagnosis is determining the name of the disease and once the name of a disease is determined, the treatment for that disease is spelled out within that name. This is because the treatment method has been already determined through experimentation. Therefore, by determining the name of a disease and giving treatment pertinent to that disease, the duty of the doctor is accomplished. In actual practice, determining the name of a disease is not absolutely necessary in the treatment. The disease can be well treated without knowing its name and there are many occasions when the treatment effectiveness is not particularly good even though the name of the disease is known.

The name of a disease is necessary in Western medicine, but in Oriental medicine, there is no hindrance in the treatment even though the name of disease is not known. Oriental medical doctors usually present the names of diseases as Wind, Fire, Phlegm, Damp, Wind–Phlegm, Damp–Phlegm, Phlegm–Fire, Summer Heat, Coolness, Stagnation, Accumulation, *Qi* Deficiency, Blood Deficiency, etc. which are different from the Western medical terminology.

By no means are the so–called "Wind," "Fire," "Coolness" and "Stagnation" inferior as the names of diseases. Rather, the names of diseases are essentially extremely vague.

Why is the name "cranial nerve disease" better than "Wind" as the name of a disease and why is the terminology "metabolic disorders" better than "Dampness?" What is the reason for rheumatism and neuralgia being better terms than "Phlegm?" In fact, in terms of simplicity, Wind, Dampness and Phlegm are more convenient.

The name of a disease is no more than a concept that has descriptive classification as a goal and the treatment cannot be easily determined by that. So the medicine, which cannot give treatment when the name of a disease is not determined, will not be able to treat many diseases which have no specific name. In the medicine that has a fixed treatment method according to the name of disease, there is reason for concern in ignoring the characteristics of individual patients. In other words, no matter how much modern science has developed, it will not be able to say that it is so good and virtuous that it needs no further study or has no margin for further development. There are many diseases that have not yet been studied or discovered as to the name and there is no reason that a disease will not occur just because a name has not been identified. Thus, will there not be a flaw in differentiating an unknown disease with a known disease name and performing treatment based on that known disease?

Since each individual has so–called disease patterns, even though the disease name is the same, the symptoms are all different. That is the reason for treatment not being uniformly based on the name of the disease. Moreover, one can know with the following few examples that the name of a disease does not have much relationship to the treatment according to Oriental medicine. It would be more appropriate to select the treatment method based on the syndromes rather than the name of the disease.

1. The formula is different according to the symptoms of the diseases that have an identical name. To give an example of insomnia – all of the following are formulas for insomnia:

   (a) *Gui Pi Tang* (Restore the Spleen Decoction)[1]
       – insomnia due to Deficiency such as *Qi* Deficiency, indigestion, etc.
   (b) *Bu Zhong Yi Qi Tang* (Tonify the Middle and Augment the *Qi* Decoction)
       – insomnia due to fatigue or with a slight Invasion by External Pathogen
   (c) *Yang Xin Tang* (Nourish the Heart Decoction)
       – insomnia in a deficient person or when the Heart is fatigued with a slight feverish sensation due to overthinking after an illness
   (d) *Ping Wei San* (Calm the Stomach Powder)
       – insomnia due to indigestion or Injury due to improper foods
   (e) *Si Mo Yin* (Four Milled Decoction)
       – insomnia due to intoxication from the gas developed in the digestive organs
   (f) *Li Zhong Tang* (Regulate the Middle Decoction)
       – insomnia due to a *Yang* Deficiency and Excess Cold
   (g) *Wu Ling San* (Five Ingredient Powder with Poria)
       – insomnia due to difficulty in urination
   (h) *Chai Hu Tang* (Bupleurum Decoction)
       – insomnia due to External Invasion of Wind–Cold pathogens

Aside from these, various formulas are used according to a person's constitution and symptoms for insomnia. In beriberi, *Ping Wei San* (Calm the Stomach Powder), *Si Mo Yin* (Four Milled Decoction), *Wu Ling San* (Five Ingredient Powder with Poria), or other formulas can be used. This explains why a treatment method cannot be determined by the name of a disease.

---

1. For the detailed information on the formulas mentioned in this chapter, see appendix II.

2. Diseases that have different names can be effectively treated with an identical formula. For example, the following disorders can be treated with *Bu Zhong Yi Qi Tang* (Tonify the Middle and Augment the *Qi* Decoction):

Lung disease, indigestion, dizziness and vertigo, insomnia, blood in the stools, Hernial disorders, prolapse of anus or uterus, difficult urination, constipation, headache, weak vision, deafness, sinusitis, spermatorrhea, enuresis, cerebrovascular accident, diarrhea, malaria, External Invasion of Wind–Cold pathogen, leukorrhea, diseases occuring after child birth and external diseases.

There are many examples other than these. Looking at the effectiveness of one formula on so many diseases, it would not be wise to determine the treatment method based solely on the name of a disease.

3. The identical disease can have different names, but the same formula. To give an example of appendicitis:

(a) Hernial Disorders – Blood *Shan* (Appendicitis)
     Formula – *Yu Zhu San* (Jade Candle Powder)
               Tao Ren Jian (Decoction of Persica Seed)

"A person with Blood stagnation in the lower abdomen is called Blood *Shan*. In this condition, there is no passing of gas with stagnation of food. The lower abdomen has firmness and mass and there is constipation with a dark stool and scanty urine." *(Zhang Jing Yue)*

(b) Abdominal Pain – Blood Accumulation (Appendicitis)
     Formula – *Yu Zhu San* (Jade Candle Powder)
               Tao Ren Cheng Qi Tang (Order the *Qi* Decoction with Persica Seed)

"When pathogenic *Qi* accumulates in the Lower Burner, body fluid is unable to flow, *Qi* and Blood are unable to circulate, urine is retained or Blood stagnates in the Lower Burner. This produces distention and fullness with firm pain."*(Cheng Wu Ji)*[2]

"There is constipation due to Blood stagnation, where Excess pathogen is not moving or there is constipation due to dryness caused by Blood Deficiency." *(Zhang Jing Yue)*

(c) *Shang Han* – Blood Accumulation (Appendicitis)
     Formula – *Yu Zhu San* (Jade Candle Powder)
               Tao Ren Cheng Qi Tang (Order the *Qi* Decoction with Persica Seed)

"In Injury due to Cold, when there is knotting of Heat in the Interior, it disturbs Blood level and causes stagnation in the Lower Burner which does not move." *(Zhang Jing Yue)*

---

2. Cheng Wu Ji (1062 – 1155 A.D.) is most famous for his commentaries on Zhang Zhong Jing's "Treatise on Febrile Diseases caused by Cold."

(d) External Medicine – Inguinal lymphadenitis or Fecal poisoning (Appendicitis)
Formula – *Yu Zhu San* (Jade Candle Powder)

> *Long Dan Xie Gan Tang* (Gentiana Longdancao Decoction to Drain the Liver)
>
> *Bu Zhong Yi Qi Tang* (Tonify the Middle and Augment the *Qi* Decoction)

"The inguinal lymphadenitis belongs to the Liver channel and is caused by Interior Heat with Exterior Cold or overstrain or excessive sexual activity or Damp–Heat in the Liver channel." (*Bi Li Zi*)[3]

Determining a treatment method only through the name of a disease without knowing the syndrome will not give accurate results.

B. The New Interpretation of Wind, Fire, Phlegm and Damp

Oriental medical doctors often say "Wind" or "Phlegm" or "Fire" or "Damp" when describing a disease. Nevertheless, naming a disease as "Wind" or "Phlegm" is not wrong.

1. Wind

"Wind has image but no shape." *Inner Classic*

That which demonstrates phenomena, but no visible shape is called Wind. The wind of weather implies the phenomenon of air movement and the Wind of the human body implies a change in the nervous system.

(a) Invasion by External Pathogens

So–called "Injury due to Wind," "Contacting Wind," "Wind pathogen" or "Invasion by Pathogenic *Qi*" are diseases which all belong to "*Shang Han*"[4] and are cured by promoting sweat. In the case of "Wind Pathogen" there is a condition called "Middle Wind" or "Windstroke."[5] This is an Internal Injury Syndrome.

(b) Internal Injury

There are diseases of the central nervous system such as Windstroke, childhood convulsion, epilepsy, encephalitis, etc. There are diseases of the peripheral nervous system such as Wind *Bi*, rheumatism, leprosy, etc. In Windstroke, successive generations of doctors have said Windstroke is not due to External Injury. Looking at the herbs they have used, it is generally *Xu Ming Tang* (Extend the Life Decoction). *Xu Ming Tang* is a diaphoretic formula that has ephedra as the king herb, but in the disease due to Internal Injury, diaphoretics are inappropriate. The reason that Windstroke was considered as an incurable disease up to now relates not only to the difficulty of curing cranial nerve

---

3. Bi Li Zi (approx. 1486 – 1558 A.D.) was a physician of the Ming Dynasty. He is the author of "Synopsis of Internal Medicine."

4. See note 15 in Chapter 1, and pages 153 and 154 in Chapter 4.

5. A stroke or cerebrovascular accident in Oriental medicine is called "Middle Wind" or "Windstroke."

disease, but also to the use of inappropriate herbs. It is difficult to cure a disease of the nervous system after it becomes permanently fixed. However, when it is at the beginning stage, it can be restored by eliminating its cause. By using the wrong medicine, the disease becomes permanent and incurable because the proper time frame for treatment has passed. The cause of Windstroke can again be divided into the categories of External Injury and Internal Injury. The cause of epidemic encephalitis is External Injury and the cause of cerebral hemorrhage is Internal Injury. In Windstroke caused by External Injury, the formulas such as *Xu Ming Tang* might be appropriate, but in Windstroke caused by Internal Injury, *Xu Ming Tang* will only worsen the disease and not lessen it. In recent times, diseases with unknown causes are generally attributed to Wind. To give a few examples of disease names related to Wind:

1. *Shang Feng* (Injury due to Wind) – this is Wind pathogen, namely a disease that belongs to *Shang Han*.
2. *Zhong Feng* (Windstroke) – this is a cranial nerve system disease caused by External pathogen (such as epidemic encephalitis).
3. *Fei Feng* (Internal Windstroke) – this is a cranial nervous system disease caused by Internal Injury (cerebral hemorrhage).
4. *Jing Feng* (Fright Wind) – this is a cranial nerve disease of a child.
   • Acute Fright Wind (Externally caused)
   • Chronic Fright Wind (Internally caused)
5 *Feng Chi* (Wind Dementia) – praecox dementia
6. *Xian Feng* (Epileptic Wind) or *Dian Xian Feng* (Psychotic – Epileptic Wind) – epilepsy
7. *Feng Bi* (Wind Bi) or *Tong Feng* (Painful Wind) – neuralgia, rheumatism
8. *Li Jie Feng* (Moving Joint Wind) – rheumatoid arthritis
9. *Da Feng Chuang* (Large Wind Ulcer) – leprosy
10. *E Zhang Feng* (Goose Palm Wind) – skin disease of the palm
11. *Tou Feng* (Head Wind) – skin disease of the head
12. *Shen Feng* (Kidney Wind) – skin disease of the thigh
13. *Po Shang Feng* (Damage by Wind) – tetanus
14. *Dian Feng* – vitiligo or piebald skin
15. *Bai Xue Feng* (White Snow Wind) – dandruff

With these we can see that Wind is a disease generally related to the nervous system. The peripheral nerve spasm such as trembling of the eyelids is also called Wind. The reason for calling the nervous system diseases Wind is because the Wind is said to "have image but no shape." When toxins in the blood invade the central nervous system due to insufficiency of the liver's detoxifying action, abnormality can occur at times in the nervous system.

2. Fire

Even the so–called Fire is extremely vast in its content and cannot be simply explained. Instead I will give the following few examples:

(a) Monarch Fire

It refers to the dynamic force of the Heart, thus the physiological operation of humans depends on the function of this Monarch Fire.

(b) Ministerial Fire

This refers to the endocrine function which regulates the physiological activity of the human so that through Ministerial Fire (the endocrine system) the function of Monarch Fire (the activity of the Heart) is regulated. Fire becomes the source of heat and since physiological activity increases body temperature, the term "Fire" was created. The Monarch and Ministerial Fires are not disease conditions.

(c) Angry Fire

This implies excitement all together. In the state of extreme excitement, the sensation of heat can be consciously felt.

(d) Heart Fire and Liver Fire

These are the acceleration of the physiological function of the Heart or Liver. At this time, emotional excitement accompanies the Fire.

(e) Deficient Fire

This means the same as Deficient Heat and occurs due to an excess effort by the body to make up for a deficiency in the physiological process.

(f) Excess Fire and Pathogenic Fire

These mean the same as Excess Heat and Pathogenic Heat. Since there is an external pathogen, they imply a fever that results from the effort in eliminating that pathogen. (refer to Deficieny – Excess section)

(g) Stomach Fire and Lung Fire

An inflammation or catarrh is called Fire. Stomach catarrh is Stomach Fire and pneumonia is Lung Fire.

(h) Triple Burner Fire:

* Upper Burner Fire refers to pleurisy, inflammation, catarrh or irritable diseases of the lung, apex of the lung, trachea, heart, etc.
* Middle Burner Fire is the general term for inflammation, catarrh or irritable diseases of the stomach, liver, gall bladder, spleen, pancreas, small intestine, etc.
* Lower Burner Fire is the general term for inflammation, catarrh or irritable diseases of the kidney, urinary bladder, uterus, large intestine, small intestine, peritoneum, etc.

(i) Phlegm Fire

This refers to fever due to the stagnation of waste products and other toxins within the body.

■ The method of treating Fire

Diseases such as pleurisy, peritonitis, uteritis, nephritis, cystitis, pulmonary apicitis and large intestine catarrh are all common in recent times and are generally considered difficult to treat. Though all of them manifest signs of Fire such as heat and inflammation, one must not uniformly use cold, Heat–clearing or Fire–sedating herbs. The reason for this is that there are different types of Fire – Deficient Fire and Excess Fire.

When looking at the diseased region, there is always heat. The cause of that heat generally comes from the obstruction of the blood circulation occurring in a certain region as a result of a decline in physiological function and waste products and toxins are stagnated due to insufficient metabolism. At this time, inflammation and catarrh develop. To treat the cause, one should support the Fire or Heat, to strengthen physiological activities in order to invigorate blood circulation to promptly resolve stagnated substances in the diseased region and increase healing force. If that is not done and local symptomatic treatment is used instead, one might see a momentary reduction in symptoms, but the condition of the disease will again return as a consequence of suppressing the activity of the life force in order to eliminate the Fire.

Sometimes, using Fire–sedating diuretics for the nephritis of elders does not necessarily result in recovery. A doctor should not be bound by the name of a disease or symptoms such as inflammation and should properly use *Yin* tonics, *Yang* tonics, warm herbs, cold herbs, *Qi* herbs and Blood herbs according to the person's constitution and symptoms. In basic inflammatory reactions, healing takes place when the blood circulation and eliminating functions are promoted and regulated. It is usually enough to distinguish the *Yin–Yang* and Deficiency–Excess of the physical constitution and match appropriate herbs.

3. Phlegm

When the metabolic products and other substances that are supposed to be excreted to the outside of the body are stagnating inside so that only the disease phenomenon appears, those stagnated substances are called "invisible Phlegm." Mucus, which is the pathological product, that is vomited is also called phlegm. Phlegm is usually thought to be that which is visible to the eye, but in Oriental medicine invisible Phlegm and visible phlegm are identical. There are times when the former is called "Phlegm pain" and is distinguished from the latter and the latter is called "Phlegm–Damp" or "Phlegm–slobber" and is distinguished from the former.

■ Treatment of Phlegm

Phlegm is neither the cause of a disease nor the disease itself, rather, it is the result of a disease. The Phlegm that is mentioned in the *Inner Classic* was not originally a pathological name, but a trend for calling Phlegm a disease seems to have started at the time of *Zhang Zhong Jing*. At present, Oriental Doctors frequently speak about the names of disease with Phlegm. Some of them say, "Nine out of ten diseases are Phlegm" or "Phlegm is the mother of all disease" and they often consider the disease as Phlegm and concentrate on the treatment to eliminate Phlegm. However, this is a big mistake for they have mistaken the means for the end. It is not that the disease has occurred due to the Phlegm, but rather Phlegm has occurred because of the disease. If Phlegm–dissolving and Phlegm–eliminating herbs are used, the Phlegm that has already developed might be eliminated, but these herbs cannot prevent new Phlegm from forming and the Original *Qi* gets even weaker due to the herbs. Thus, other than eliminating small amounts of excess Phlegm, Phlegm treating formulas have many disadvantages in treating diseases. When the Phlegm is left as it is and proper treatment is given through distinguishing Cold–Heat, Exterior–Interior and Deficiency–Excess, the Phlegm will automatically disappear.

(a) Deficient Phlegm

This is Phlegm due to a Deficient Syndrome so a person's constitution should be properly tonified and when it combines with Invasion by External Pathogen, use diaphoretics properly.

(b) Excess Phlegm

This is Phlegm occuring in the Excess Syndrome, so sedate properly.

(c) Wind–Phlegm

Since this is Phlegm related to the abnormality in the nervous system, its cause must be eliminated.

(d) Phlegm–Fire or Heat–Phlegm

This implies a Phlegm related to fever and is called Phlegm–Fire when Phlegm is considered the cause of the heat.

(e) Damp–Phlegm

This implies Phlegm related to the decline of metabolic function, especially an abnormality of the eliminating system.

(f) Spleen/Stomach Phlegm

This is Phlegm related to indigestion.

(g) Kidney Phlegm

The Phlegm related to an abnormality in the urinary system and phlegm secreted from the respiratory system are generally considered to be related to the Kidneys. Phlegm in the cough of elders is due to *Yang* Deficiency of the Kidneys and the phlegm in lung disease is due to *Yin* Deficiency of the Kidneys.

(h) Phlegm of Wind–Cold

This phlegm occurs due to Invasion by External pathogens.

(i) Phlegm in the channels

When there is "Phlegm pain," it is called "Phlegm in the channels." Neuralgia, rheumatism and arthritis all belong to Phlegm pain and hemiplegia can be considered as Wind–Phlegm in the channels. Aside from these, there are Phlegm in Exterior, Phlegm in Interior, Phlegm above the diaphragm, Phlegm between the stomach and intestines, Phlegm in the extremities, Phlegm in the Middle Burner, Phlegm below the hypochondrium, subcutaneous Phlegm, Phlegm that moves around, Phlegm due to alcohol, and Phlegm due to food stagnation. However, it is enough to just understand the Phlegm itself.

4. Dampness

The general term for the diseases caused by obstruction in metabolic function is called "Dampness." The Damp Syndrome is a disease generally related to the heart and kidneys and it specifically implies symptoms caused by functional impairment of the kidneys. There is a relationship between the Damp Syndrome and dampness in nature, so one develops Damp Syndrome easily when dwelling in damp regions. As a proof, consider that a person who lives on a tatami mat in the city frequently develops beriberi during the rainy season each year. When wearing sweat–laden clothes and living in a back room of a shop that does not have sunshine or heat, one's health cannot help but be harmed by the dampness. Beriberi is a clear manifestation of this. Dampness implies moisture and Damp

Syndrome is a disease related to moisture.

In Damp Syndrome, abnormality first develops in urination and bowel movements. In the Cold–Damp Syndrome, one has frequent diarrhea. In the Damp–Heat Syndrome, there is constipation. In either case, there is difficulty in urination. Edema occurs due to stagnation of water within the tissue and is typical of Damp Syndrome.

■ **Treatment method for Dampness**

The key in treating Dampness lies in regulating urination and bowel movements, but that regulation is difficult. Since there is no certain treatment method, one must give proper treatment based on *Yin–Yang*, Cold–Heat, Deficiency–Excess and Exterior–Interior of a person's physical constitution and symptoms.

(a) Damp–Heat: This is a Damp Syndrome combined with Heat and since there are symptoms such as irritability, thirst, reddish and difficult urination, constipation, and flooding + slippery + full + rapid pulse (increase in blood pressure), the Heat–clearing diuretics are used.

(b) Cold–Damp: This is a Damp Syndrome combined with Cold which occurs most frequently. Aside from these, there are names such as Wind–Damp, Damp–Phlegm, Damp *Bi* Syndrome, Damp–rash (eczema), etc. The variations in Damp Syndrome are endless, but all are related to blood circulation and metabolism.

With the above explanations, I hope readers will roughly understand what Wind, Fire, Phlegm and Dampness are. I have given a brief summary of the treatment methods, but it is difficult to express the treatment methods more clearly. It is the characteristic of Oriental medicine that a "principal treatment medicine" cannot be spoken of. When looking from the viewpoint of Wind, all diseases are Wind Syndrome and when looking from the viewpoint of Phlegm, all diseases are Phlegm Syndrome. It is the same whether looking from the viewpoint of Fire, Damp, *Qi* or Blood. That is why the name of the disease cannot be roughly estimated. It is nothing but a representation of one aspect of the disease phenomenon.

III. PRESCRIPTIONS

A prescription is the preparation of different herbs to fit the syndrome. If one already has sufficient understanding of the study of syndromes and has correctly learned the study of herbal properties, a prescription should automatically evolve from it. Since the prescription in Oriental medicine is like the tactics of a military strategist or the negotiation of a diplomat where proper decisions according to circumstances are needed rather than mechanical operation, appropriate herbs that correspond to the syndromes are needed. Hence, it is possible for doctors to display personal technique when making a prescription. One thing to pay attention to is to avoid doing unreasonable acts. Needless to say, the utmost sincerity or responsibility is needed in diplomacy or military affairs which are related to the benefit and rise and fall of a country. Prescriptions, which are related to the health and life of human beings, are analogous to that. The fight against disease, on no account should be carelessly handled, just like defending a country. I am going to provide the following summary of prescriptions for reference.

OUTLINE OF THE PRESCRIPTIONS

A. The Theory of King, Minister, Assistant and Conductant

Since King, Minister, Assistant and Conductant are mentioned often in prescriptions, I must comment on this. The theory of King, Minister, Assistant and Conductant compares the combination of herbs in a prescription to the political system to facilitate understanding. There are two meanings to this theory.

1. It is a theory that looks through the properties of herbs. The herbs that increase the vital force of a person, namely top quality herbs in *Shen Nung's Herbal* are selected as the Kings. Manifestation or symptom–treating herbs which directly expel diseases, namely middle and inferior quality herbs, are selected as the Ministers, Assistants and Conductants.

Dao Hong Jing[6] said: "Herbs that nourish life are mostly Kings, herbs that nourish one's nature are mostly Ministers and herbs that treat diseases are mostly Assistants."

The way to distinguish "Life nourishing herbs" and "Nature nourishing herbs" cannot be known here and it is difficult to guess the distinctions of high, middle and low quality herbs mentioned in *Shen Nung's Herbal*. Chinese angelica, peony and antler horn are good enough to be in the category of high quality, but were put into middle quality. Platycodon and bean sprout are commonly used as food, but were nevertheless put into the category of low quality. Mirabilite, ephedra and gentiana cannot be ingested in great amounts but were put into the category of high quality.

Li Shi Zhen has said, "Since the three classifications lead to confusion, there is no need to follow the traditional method of classification." So one can know that the basis for classification of three qualities is weak and accordingly, defining King, Minister, Assistant and Conductant by three qualities is inappropriate. Also, there are plenty of herbs that were added after *Shen Nung's Herbal* and it is not shown to which quality among the three those herbs belong to. Since deciding King, Minister, Assistant and Conductant through these qualities is not especially needed in making a prescription, the information given thus far will be sufficient as a general knowledge in Oriental medicine.

2. It is a theory which appoints an herb that has the main force in treatment as the King and classifies herbs that have the supporting role as Minister, Assistant and Conductant.

If one takes the trouble to discuss the King–Minister–Assistant–Conductant theory, selecting this "Main force herb as King theory" seems proper. In actuality, it is not

---

6. Dao Hong Jing (452 – 536 A.D.) is a famous Taoist–medical doctor who compiled "Shen Nung's Herbal" even though it is often times attributed to have been written by legendary emperor Shen Nung.

necessary to distinguish the King, Minister, Assistant and Conductant because there are times when each herb has an equal footing without distinctions of the King, Minister, Assistant or Conductant. When making a prescription, do not hold onto the notion of King–Minister–Assistant–Conductant. Only try to observe the manifestation of the syndrome accurately and combine herbs properly for that manifestation. Then it will automatically become matched with the principle of King–Minister–Assistant–Conductant. Putting the name of an herb on the name of a prescription is done by generally selecting the King herb and that King herb can be sometimes a high quality herb or an herb that has the most effect or it can indicate both types. Also at certain times, it is represented by the high priced herb or commonly used herb. The following examples demonstrate this. The King herb is in brackets.

- **Bai Zhu San (White Atractylodes Powder)**
  pueraria (8 grams), ginseng, [**white atractylodes**], poria, saussurea, agastache, licorice (4 grams each)
- **Ren Shen Yang Wei Tang (Ginseng Nourish the Stomach Decoction)**
  Atractylodes (6 grams), tangerine peel, magnolia, pinellia (5 grams each), red poria, agastache (4 grams each), [**ginseng**], tsaoko, licorice (2 grams each)
- **Lu Rong Da Bu Tang (Antler Horn Great Tonifying Decoction)**
  cistanche, eucommia (4 grams each), peony, white atractylodes, aconite, ginseng, cinnamon bark, pinellia, dendrobium, schizandra (3 grams each), [**Antler horn**], astragalus, Chinese angelica, poria, cooked rehmannia (2 grams each), licorice (1 gram)
- **Mai Men Dong Tang (Ophiopogon Decoction):**
  licorice (11 grams), [**ophiopogon**] (8 grams), rice (180 grams)
- **Ma Huang Tang (Ephedra Decoction)**
  [**ephedra**], cinnamon twig (113 grams each), licorice (38 grams), apricot seed (70 pieces)
- **Ge Gen Tang (Pueraria Decoction)**
  [**pueraria**] (150 grams), ephedra, fresh ginger (113 grams each), cinnamon twig, peony, licorice (75 grams each), date (12 pieces)
- **Zheng Chai Hu Yin (Upright Bupleurum Decoction)**
  [**bupleurum**] (11 grams), peony (8 grams), tangerine peel (6 grams), siler, licorice (4 grams each)
- **Ren Shen Bai He Tang (Ginseng and Lily Decoction)**
  white atractylodes, poria, [**lily**], donkey–hide gelatin, asparagus (4 grams each), peony, [**ginseng**], schizandra, pinellia, apricot seed (3 grams each), asarum, carthamus, cinnamon twig, licorice (1 grams each)
- **He Zi Ren Shen Tang (Chebula and Ginseng Decoction)**
  [**chebula**], [**ginseng**], poria, white atractylodes, licorice, lotus seed, cimicifuga, bupleurum (in equal amounts)
- **Zhu Sha Liang Ge Wan (Cinnabar Cooling the Diaphragm Pill)**
  coptis, gardenia (38 grams each), ginseng, poria (19 grams each), [**cinnabar**] (11 grams), borneol (2 grams)
- **Niu Huang Wan (Cow Gallstone Pill)**
  siler, scutellaria, anemarrhena, gentiana, acorus, peony, scorpion, mercury, licorice (19

grams each), asparagus, ophiopogon, ginseng, poria (15 grams each), rhinocerous horn, amber, dragon teeth (8 grams each), [**cow gallstone**], musk (2 grams each), wasp's nest (3 pieces), gold sheet, silver sheet (70 pieces each)

B. Seven Prescriptions

There are seven types of prescriptions known as: Large prescription, Small prescription, Moderate prescription, Urgent prescription, Odd prescription, Even prescription and Complex prescription. Like the King–Minister–Assistant–Conductant classification, this should also be understood for reference purpose only and is not necessary for making a prescription in actual practice. Thus, it is not a matter of fitting a prescription into a certain pattern, rather it is enough to have simplicity as the main guide in the herbal usage.

1. **Large prescription** – There are two types of Large prescription: Large prescription in the total number and Large prescription in the total volume. In the Large prescription of number, the number of herbs that are combined are many types and in the Large prescription of volume, the dosage of herbs are made greater and are ingested in greater amounts at one time. It is said that a Large prescription is used in "distal disease" and a Small prescription is used in "local disease." To make an interpretation, the place where herbs go quickly is referred to as "local" and less quickly is "distal." Thus, the difference is in the time of delivery of herbs. This type of prescription is used for serious illness, with two or more syndromes occuring together, that requires immediate attention. *Wang Bing*[7] has said, "Heart and Lungs are local and Liver and Kidneys are distal" and *Liu He Gan* has said, "Exterior of body is distal and Interior of body is local."

2. **Small prescription** – This is opposite to the Large prescription.

   "There are two types of Small prescription. There is a Small prescription with one King and two Ministers which is used for the disease without multiple syndromes. Since there is only one pathogenic *Qi*, the disease can be treated with just a few herbs. Another is a Small prescription with a small quantity and is taken frequently and is appropriate for the disease of the Heart, Lung and the upper region." *(Zhang Cong Zheng)*[8]

3. **Moderating prescription** – This is a prescription that slows and relaxes the effects of herbs and makes treatment come about naturally and spontaneously. It is for long term use such as for a patient with Deficient Fever.

4. **Urgent prescription** – This is a prescription that gives immediate effect in the symptomatic treatment of an acute disease.

---

7. A Tang dynasty physician who wrote the "Commentary on the Inner Classic" in 762 A.D.

8. Also known as Zhang Zi He (1156 – 1228 A.D.). He is the founder of the "Purging" school of thought. He said that all diseases arise from the accumulation of Pathogenic Qi. By eliminating this pathogen, the body can be returned to a harmonious state. Thus, he used formulas that promote perspiration and bowel movement.

"In treating the Host, the moderate way is proper. This is treating the root of the disease. In treating the Guest, the urgent way is proper. This is treating the manifestation of the disease. Exterior, Interior, sweating and purging of the disease all have proper moderateness and urgency." *(Wang Hao Gu)*

"Host" is Original *Qi* and "Guest" is Pathogenic *Qi*, thus treat the Host in the Deficient Syndrome and the Guest in the Excess Syndrome. Treating the "root" is treating the cause of a disease and treating the manifestation is treating the symptoms of a disease.

5. **Odd prescription** – It is a single herb prescription or combining the herbs in odd numbers. This prescription is used for diseases that have a simple cause that can be cured with only few herbs.

"The Odd prescription that uses a single herb is appropriate for diseases in the upper region and for local diseases. The Odd prescription that combines herbs in *Yang* numbers such as one, three, five, seven and nine are appropriate for purging but not for sweating." *(Zhang Cong Zheng)*

6. **Even prescription** – indicates a two herb combination or a combination of herbs in an even number. This prescription is used for more complicated diseases.
Zhang Cong Zheng considered the prescription that combined two traditional prescriptions as an Even prescription and the prescription that combined three or more traditional prescriptions as a Complex prescription. It is appropriate, however, to see a prescription that combines two prescriptions as the Complex prescription like the theory of *Wang Bing*.

"There is an Even formula that combines two types of herbs and that which combines two traditional formulas are appropriate for all diseases that are in the lower region and are distal. There is an Even formula that combines herbs in *Yin* numbers such as two, four, six, eight and ten which are appropriate for sweating but not for purging." *(Zhang Cong Zheng)*

7. **Complex prescription** – indicates mutual combination of traditional prescriptions or indicates a complicated prescription.

I know that with the preceding description, readers will roughly guess what the seven prescriptions are. In fact, the seven prescriptions can be omitted since it can sometimes cause confusion in the beginners of Oriental medical study. Since they are usually recorded in the medical texts without mention of whether or not to follow those rules, I have purposely described them here for critical examination.

C. Ten Formulas
This is classified by *Xu Zhi Cai*[9] and I am introducing them here for certain points that can serve as a reference in using the herbs.

---

9. A sixth century physician.

1. **Disseminating formulas**
   These are the formulas to disperse obstruction, thus aromatic fragrant herbs in general such as ginger, tangerine peel and agastache are commonly used.

2. **Unblocking formulas**
   These circulate the stagnation and consist of diuretics such as akebia, stephania, poria and polyporus.

3. **Tonifying formulas**
   These formulas make a weak person stronger. On the whole, they regulate and invigorate physiological functions and provide nourishment. The herbs in these formulas include ginseng, cooked rehmannia, Chinese angelica and astragalus.

4. **Purging formulas**
   These formulas purge stagnation and consist of herbs that are bitter–cold and sinking–descending such as rhubarb, mirabilite and descurainia seed.

5. **Light formulas**
   This implies diaphoretic formulas. The herbs in these formulas include ephedra, pueraria, peppermint and cinnamon twig.

6. **Heavy formulas**
   This implies calming formulas and generally contains mineral types of herbs such as magnetite, cinnabar, calcite, minium, pearl and hematite. A heavy formula is sometimes used as the nickname for metal and stone formulas, namely formulas with minerals.

7. **Slippery formulas**
   These formulas make things that are stagnated and rough slippery and generally consist of diuretics and laxatives. They have something in common with the unblocking, purging and lubricating formulas. The herbs in these formulas include abutilon seed, cannabis seed, bush–cherry seed, talc and plantago seed.

8. **Astringent formulas**
   These contain herbs that prevent leakage and dispersion, thus for symptoms such as diarrhea, incontinence, enuresis, spermatorrhea, nocturnal emission, profuse sweating and loss of blood, the astringent formula is needed. The herbs in these formulas include cornus, oyster shell, dragon bone, mantis egg–case, schizandra, Chinese gall, mume, pomegranate rind, opium poppy capsule and ephedra root.

9. **Drying formula**
   These contain herbs that are used when there is a surplus of water in the body. Herbs that are pungent and warm or diuretic are used – morus bark, aduki bean, aconite, black pepper, white atractylodes, tangerine peel, saussurea and atractylodes.

10. **Lubricating formula**

These formulas moisten dryness due to Deficiency of Water in the body. The herbs in these formulas include cannabis seed, donkey–hide gelatin, Chinese angelica, cooked rehmannia, ophiopogon, trichosanthes root, cistanche and lycium.

D. Herbs that treat All Symptoms

I have already said repeatedly that Oriental herbs, by nature, are difficult to specify as the "main treatment medicine" due to the nature of Oriental medicine. Since there are probably some feelings of ambiguity regarding this for a novice and for the purpose of enabling one to have an initial reference in making a prescription in actual practice, I am going to briefly write about the suitable herbs for the various symptoms.

Herbs that are enumerated as suitable herbs have properties necessary for strongly eliminating the symptoms, but one must keep in mind that those herbs contain many other properties as well. This point must be well understood. Also, it is not that those herbs must suit the symptoms, instead one must keep in mind that when the cause of illness is fundamentally eliminated, the disease can be cured easily without using symptomatic herbs. Moreover, it is wiser to treat without using symptomatic herbs.

Compendium of Materia Medica Chapter 3: Herbs to treat various diseases

1. **Hot and Warm Herbs**
   – aconite, cinnamon bark, dried ginger, white atractylodes, ginseng

2. **Cold and Cool Herbs**
   – rhubarb, coptis, scutellaria, raw rehmannia, red peony, achyranthis, ophiopogon, asparagus, phellodendron, anemarrhena

3. **Yang Tonics**
   – ginseng, aconite, eucommia, lycium

4. **Yin Tonics**
   – cooked rehmannia, dioscorea, glehnia, achyranthis, ophiopogon

5. **Qi Tonics**
   – ginseng, white atractylodes, astragalus

6. **Blood Tonics**
   warm – cooked rehmannia, Chinese angelica, cnidium, antler horn
   cool – peony, achyranthis, raw rehmannia

7. **Diaphoretics**
   warm – ephedra, cinnamon twig, atractylodes, fresh ginger, schizonepeta, siler, asarum, angelica, notopterygium
   cool – bupleurum, peucedanum, cimicifuga, peppermint

8. **Detoxifying Herbs** (herbs ingested internally for external disorders)

warm – angelica, schizonepeta, siler, tangerine peel, frankincense, myrrh, gleditsia, cnidium

neutral – astragalus, anteater shell

cool – forsythia, rhinocerous horn, lonicera, peony, trichosanthes root, bupleurum, prunella, trichosanthes seed

9. **Hemostatic** (hematemesis, hemoptysis, epistaxis, hemafecia, hematuria, metrorrhagia)

slightly warm – donkey–hide gelatin, black ink

cool – bamboo shavings, rubia, imperata, biota tops, astragalus, coptis, anemarrhena, sanguisorba

10. **Alternating Chills and Fever**

– bupleurum, scutellaria

For root treatment, refer to (The Syndromes and corresponding formulas).

11. **Discharge Gas, Spread Qi and Harmonize Middle Burner**

warm – tangerine peel, saussurea, agastache, cyperus, magnolia, and other fragrant warm herbs

cool – bitter orange, green tangerine peel

12. **Heat Pain of the Upper Region** (pain and swelling in the throat, etc.)

– bupleurum, cimicifuga, platycodon, scutellaria, peppermint

These are cool herbs that ascend but they do not need to be used when treating the original cause.

13. **Cold Pain in the Lower Region** (lower abdominal pain, Hernial disorders, etc.)

warm herbs that descend – evodia, magnolia, fennel, dried ginger, cinnamon bark

14. **Cough**

warm – white atractylodes, pinellia, white mustard seed, tangerine peel, honey

cool – apricot seed, morus bark, scutellaria, platycodon, asparagus, ophiopogon, fritillary

neutral – schizandra, lily, donkey–hide gelatin

15. **Vomiting**

warm herbs for Stomach Cold – ginseng, white atractylodes, dried ginger, pinellia, black pepper

cool herbs for Stomach Heat – peony, immature bitter orange, coptis, ophiopogon

16. Indigestion

warm – white atractylodes, pinellia, dried ginger, cardamon, nutmeg, magnolia, tsaoko, tangerine peel, radish seed

cool – immature bitter orange, peony, scutellaria, coptis

neutral – hawthorn fruit, barley sprout, medicated leaven

17. Constipation

- Moisten dry

  warm – Chinese angelica, cooked rehmannia

  cool – peony, achyranthis, scutellaria

  neutral – cistanche, cannabis seed
- Support Heat – ginseng, pinellia, magnolia
- Tonify *Qi* – ginseng, astragalus, white atractylodes, licorice
- Discharge Gas – bitter orange, immature bitter orange, areca, tangerine peel, magnolia
- Purgatives and Cathartics

  cold – rhubarb, mirabilite, belamcanda, kansui root

  warm – croton, ricini, genkwa

It is better not to use the purgatives and cathartics.

18. Diarrhea

- Support Heat – ginseng, dried ginger, cinnamon bark, pinellia, aconite, white atractylodes, atractylodes, magnolia, evodia
- Diuretic – poria, polyporus, alisma, plantago seed, akebia, gardenia
- Tonify *Qi* – ginseng, astragalus, white atractylodes, licorice
- Discharge gas – nutmeg, katsumadai, saussurea, magnolia, clove
- Astringe – dioscorea, mume, schizandra, opium poppy capsule

19. Difficult urination

– poria, polyporus, alisma, akebia, plantago seed, gardenia

20. Incontinence or enuresis

– black cardamon, cuscuta, lindera, Chinese leek

21. Spermatorrhea, nocturnal emission or leukorrhea.

– cuscuta, dioscorea, rosa fruit, euryale, donkey–hide gelatin, dragon bone, oyster shell

22. Blood stagnation

– peach seed, carthamus, sappan wood, sparganium, zedoaria

23. Prolapse of anus or prolapse of uterus

– astragalus, cimicifuga, ginseng

24. Profuse sweating
 – astragalus, ginseng, peony, zizyphus, biota seed

25. Restlessness of Heart (insomnia, forgetfulness, palpitations, fright palpitations, etc.)
 – spirit of poria, zizyphus, polygala, biota seed

E. Contrary Theory

Treating Heat Syndrome with cold herbs and Cold Syndrome with hot herbs is called "normal treatment;" treating Cold Syndrome with cold herbs and Heat Syndrome with hot herbs is called "contrary treatment." Normal treatment goes against the disease and contrary treatment follows the disease.

In a Heat disease, cold herbs should be used, but when a patient cannot take cold herbs, adding hot herbs to the cold herbs or warming up and ingesting cold herbs is what is called contrary treatment. It is also the same when hot herbs cannot be taken in the Cold disease.

F. Yin Deficiency Theory and Yang Deficiency Theory

The theory that *Yang* is always in surplus, but *Yin* is always in deficiency is the "Theory of Surplus *Yang* and Deficient *Yin*." Contrary to that theory is "Theory of Surplus *Yin* and Deficient *Yang*." The person who advocated the *Yin* Deficiency Theory is *Zhu Dan Xi* and the person who refuted that theory and advocated the *Yang* Deficiency Theory is *Zhang Jing Yue*.

Since the theory in dispute is not contemporary, I do not feel the need to introduce the two sides here, but to presume the basis for the development of the differences in the opinions of these two persons is that, in the *Yin* Deficiency Theory of *Zhu Dan Xi*, the diseases of humans always include a fever. The heat being the function of *Yang*, it seems to have stemmed from the feeling that *Yin* is always in deficiency and *Yang* is always in surplus in clinical practice. In the *Yang* Deficiency Theory of *Zhang Jing Yue*, since *Yang* is the life energy and *Yin* is death energy, the life of a human always ends when *Yang* is cut off and *Yin* is flourishing at the height of prosperity. So he felt that *Yang* is always in deficiency. In actuality, the *Yang* Deficiency Theory of *Zhang Jing Yue* is a reactionary statement to refute the *Yin* Deficiency Theory of *Zhu Dan Xi* since *Zhang Jing Yue* himself admitted that "*Yang* always being deficient is but a biased opinion."

Since both theories represent somewhat biased opinions, in actual practice one must discern each individual's constitution to distinguish whether *Yang* or *Yin* is in deficiency. In addition, I am going to add as a remark that the medical sect of *Zhu Dan Xi* is called the Tonifying *Yin* Sect and there is a tendency to use cold herbs excessively. The Tonifying *Yin* Theory of *Zhu Dan Xi* for the most part was learned from *Liu He Gan*.

G. A Theory of "Not Tonifying Kidney in Children"

This is the theory of *Wang Ju Jie*[10] which says that it is not necessary to use Kidney tonics for children. In actual practice, Kidney tonics are often required for children and

---

10. Wang Ju Jie (approximately middle of 15th century to beginning of 16th century) was a government official and a physician of the Ming Dynasty. He is the author of "Essential Collection of Materia Medica."

Liu Wei Di Huang Tang (Six Rehmannia Decoction) is the Kidney tonic that supports *Yin* within the Kidneys. This formula is the most appropriate for children. Lung disease can be prevented with this formula and this is the reason for commonly giving Six Rehmannia Decoction to children. For the infant's green stool, *Wei Guan Jin* (Stomach Gate Decoction) is most efficacious. It is a Kidney tonic that supports *Yang* within the Kidneys.

H. Theory of "Warm–Hot Herbs are Contraindicated in the Summer Time."

This is a theory that says warm–hot natured herbs should not be used during the summer season; this too is the theory of *Zhu Dan Xi*. I am just going to say that in practice, warm–hot herbs are needed plentifully in the summer season.[11]

I. "All Forms of Dysentery are Damp–Heat" Theory

This is the theory of *Liu He Gan* and *Zhu Dan Xi* that says regardless of red, white or other dysentery, they are all diseases caused by Damp–Heat, so the treatment must use the bitter–cold formula with coptis and phellodendron as the main herbs.

Although some dysenteries are due to Heat, all cannot be considered to be due to Heat, so using bitter–cold herbs uniformly is incorrect practice. Therefore, the cold–heat and tonifying–sedating properties of the herbs must be selected by holistically observing the constitution and symptoms of an individual.

ANALYSIS OF THE FAMOUS TRADITIONAL FORMULAS

A. Si Wu Tang (Four Substance Decoction)

Four Substance Decoction is a Blood tonic and is exemplary of women's herbs. Let us look at the ingredients of that formula now:

1. The taste and temperature of cooked rehmannia is pure, having warm properties without stimulating properties to smoothly increase body temperature. Its sweet taste assists the Spleen and nutrition, the slightly bitter taste recuperates the fatigue of the Heart, the slightly sour taste tonifies the Liver and the black color constituents tonify the Kidneys.[12]
2. Chinese angelica is a Blood tonic that smooths out the Blood circulation and softens stools. It has slight disinfecting powers due to its fragrant property and also opens up breathing.
3. Cnidium invigorates the Blood circulation, assists the function of sweating to lighten the whole body and it is presumed to have fairly strong disinfecting power.
4. Since peony is a Blood tonic with cool properties, it assists the Blood Level without increasing the body temperature. It relieves fatigue of the Liver through its sour taste, restrains excessive activity of the Heart, maintains physiological regulation by

---

11. In the summer time, we lose a lot of Yang energy through sweating and overactivity. That is why the author mentions that we need to use plenty of warm–hot herbs to replenish our Yang energy.

12. The color of rehmannia is black and it is said to affect the Kidneys. The color black belongs to the Water Element and so does the Kidneys.

controlling the dispersing properties of cnidium, prevents excessive sweating through its astringent function, clears up stagnated Blood of the digestive organs to increase appetite, clears Blood and relieves Heat.

A combination of the above four herbs is called the Four Substance Decoction and there is no further need to extol its benefit. Since women in particular lose blood each month, it supplements blood production. Also, much blood is required to nourish a fetus, thus it is a self–evident truth that the Four Substance Decoction can become a miraculous medicine. The ratio of the combination is usually divided into equal parts, but it can be freely added or subtracted according to the physical constitution.

B. Si Jun Zi Tang (Four Gentlemen Decoction)
The Four Gentlemen Decoction is typical of the *Qi* tonics.

1. Ginseng fundamentally assists Original *Yang* and Original *Qi* to invigorate the physiological function.
2. White atractylodes increases digestive power and makes the function of the Lung healthy to invigorate Original *Qi*.
3. Licorice increases nutrition, harmonizes and moderates the function of all organs to prevent overstrain and has the function of softening and moderating all toxins and violent substances in the body.
4. *Qi* and *Yang* tonics in general have warm–hot properties and consolidating–ascending properties, so in order to eliminate side effects of the functions of ginseng, white atractylodes, licorice and poria are used. Since poria has descending and diuretic properties, it functions to promote urination and to eliminate excessive Heat.

Due to the harmonizing action of the above four herbs, a *Qi* deficient person can be effectively tonified naturally without strain.

C. Ba Wu Tang or Ba Zhen Tang (Eight Substance Decoction or Eight Precious Decoction)
This is a combination of the Four Substance Decoction and Four Gentlemen Decoction. It is a formula that equally tonifies *Qi* and Blood.

D. Shi Quan Da Bu Tang (All Inclusive Great Tonifying Decoction)
It is the Eight Substance Decoction with the addition of astragalus and cinnamon bark and is an effective formula for tonifying *Qi* and the Blood especially in a person with a stronger degree of *Qi* and *Yang* Deficiency. Astragalus tonifies *Qi* and cinnamon bark assists Heat.

E. Liu Wei Di Huang Tang (Six Rehmannia Decoction)
This is superior as a Kidney *Yin* tonifying and Water strengthening formula. It is effective for Deficient Water with Exuberant Fire due to *Yin* Deficiency within the Kidneys. The superiority of the Six Rehmannia Decoction lies in tonifying *Yin* without injuring *Yang*.

1. Cooked rehmannia which is purely a *Yin*, Blood and Kidney tonic, assists Water (*Yin*) while having warm properties. This cooked rehmannia is regarded as the King herb. (16 grams)
2. Dioscorea has a sweet and bland taste with a neutral temperature, thus it most properly supports nutrition and Kidney Water. (8 grams)
3. Cornus, similar to cooked rehmannia and dioscorea, nourishes Kidney Water, but it too has a neutral temperature. Due to a sour taste, it assists *Yin* of the Liver channel and has an astringing action. (8 grams)
4. Moutan has a slightly cool property to reduce Heat and has the function of cooling Blood. (6 grams)
5. Poria has a neutral temperature and bland taste to assist the Kidneys and it smoothly eliminates water to lower sudden increases in the body temperature. (6 grams)
6. Alisma has a slightly cool temperature and sweet, bland taste and has the function of promoting urination and eliminating Dampness. (6 grams)

The ratio of the herbs is:

rehmannia (slightly warm)	8
dioscorea (neutral)	4
cornus (neutral)	4
poria (neutral)	3
moutan (slightly cool)	3
alisma (slightly cool)	3

The ratio of slightly warm property is eight, neutral eleven and slightly cool six, thus in all, the temperature is neutral. However, because the properties of all the herbs support Water and *Yin*, a slight reduction of cold herbs is needed for the *Yang* Deficient constitution. The wisdom of the person who made this formula can be known on one hand by Water being made to increase without stagnating within the body and on the other hand, by making the diuretic function active. This will become an excellent formula for a child prone to high fever or an adolescent with a constitution tending toward a *Yin* Deficiency.

F. Bu Zhong Yi Qi Tang (Tonify Middle and Support Qi Decoction)

The characteristic of this formula is its efficacy for both Invasion by External Pathogen and Internal Injury. It is effective for indigestion, Wind pathogen, Cold pathogen, malaria, lung disease, leukorrhea and diarrhea and is the best formula for the prolapse of the anus and prolapse of the uterus. This is truly an excellent formula.

astragalus	4 to 6 grams
ginseng	4 to 6 grams
white atractylodes	4 to 6 grams
licorice	4 to 6 grams
Chinese angelica	2 to 4 grams

tangerine peel	2 grams
bupleurum	1 grams
cimicifuga	1 grams

Astragalus, ginseng and white atractylodes assist Original *Qi*; ginseng and Chinese angelica tonify the Blood; ginseng and licorice provide nutrition; ginseng, white atractylodes and tangerine peel assist digestion; ginseng and astragalus stops Deficient sweating; bupleurum and cimicifuga disperse and release Invasion due to External Pathogen; tangerine peel eliminates toxic gas in the digestive organs; Chinese angelica and tangerine peel lubricate the stool; cimicifuga clears the Stomach channel and bupleurum clears the Liver channel.

Thus, Tonify Middle and Support *Qi* Decoction is just about the cure–all medicine, but it is inappropriate when the Fire rises upward due to the Deficiency of *Yin* and Water.

THE PRACTICAL APPLICATION OF THE PRESCRIPTIONS

A. Lung Disease

[Example: 1]
1. The complexion has a tinge of redness, showing excitement.
2. The pulse is flooding and rapid.
3. Emotionally, easily angered and impatient
4. In breathing, there is weak inhalation and strong exhalation.
5. The person has good digestion or has fullness in the stomach with no appetite (there is a tongue coating).
6. Thirsty and likes cold drinks
7. The chest region feels distended, full and irritable as if being pressed upward.
8. Constipation with dark and difficult urination
9. Fever in the afternoon which decreases at night
10. Occasional cough

For such a patient, the degree of *Yin* Deficiency is fairly high so Tonifying *Yin* and Clearing Fire methods are combined for the treatment.

■ **Jia Wei Di Huang Tang** (Rehmannia Decoction with additions)

cooked rehmannia	19 grams
peony, ophiopogon, dioscorea	8 grams each
cornus, poria, alisma, moutan	4 grams each
platycodon, schizandra	2 grams each

[Example: 2]
1. Complexion is pale
2. Pulse is empty and rapid
3. The person has indigestion and likes heat, but dislikes cold.

4. There is a low grade fever
5. Has cough

For such a patient, one must gently tonify and moisten the Lungs.

- **Jia Wei Bu Fei Tang** (Tonify Lung Decoction with additions and subtractions):
  cooked rehmannia, cornus, lycium   8 grams each
  ophiopogon, tangerine peel, donkey–hide gelatin 4 grams each
  moutan, platycodon   3 grams each
  ginseng, Chinese Angelica, schizandra, licorice 2 grams each

B. Neurasthenia

[Example: 1]
1. Sexually weak with symptoms such as spermatorrhea, nocturnal emission, premature ejaculation, impotence, etc.
2. Always tired and has no endurance
3. Has several other deficient symptoms

- **Bi Yuan Jian** (Conserving the Source Decoction)
  dioscorea, euryale, zizyphus, rosa fruit 8 grams each
  white atractylodes, poria   6 grams each
  ginseng, astragalus, licorice   4 grams each
  polygala   3 grams

[Example: 2]
1. Heart is weak, so with slight exertion, there is extreme fatigue and Deficient Fever
2. Overly sensitive and gets frightened easily over small matters
3. Occasionally, the heart palpitates as if scared
4. Has insomnia and always feels frightened, getting scared without reason (seems like ghosts are coming out and the faces of dead people appear before the eyes, etc.)

- **Yang Xin Tang** (Nourish the Heart Decoction)
  Chinese angelica, cooked rehmannia, spirit of poria 8 grams each
  ginseng, ophiopogon   6 grams each
  zizyphus, biota seed   4 grams each
  schizandra, licorice   2 grams each

[Example: 3]
1. Has severe indigestion and no appetite
2. Frequently has Deficient sweating
3. Has much rumination so there is idle dreaming and worry
4. Has insomnia
5. Head always feels unclear and has dizziness and headache

- **Jia Wei Gui Pi Tang** (Restore the Spleen Decoction with additions)

ginseng, astragalus, white atractylodes	8 grams each
zizyphus, Chinese angelica, tangerine peel, spirit of poria	4 grams each
polygala, licorice	2 grams each

C. Indigestion

[Example: 1]
1. *Yang* is deficient.
2. Likes warm–hot foods

- **Wen Wei Yin** (Warm the Stomach Decoction)

white atractylodes, ginseng	8 grams each
tangerine peel, dried ginger, licorice	4 grams each

[Example: 2]
1. Likes cool or cold types of food and feels comfortable after eating those foods
2. Has thirst and constipation
3. Develops abnormal sensation in the Stomach channel and especially feels pain at ST–8 and the pain is most severe between two to three hours after eating

- **Qing Wei Yin** (Clear the Stomach Decoction)

peony, immature bitter orange	8 grams each
tangerine peel, barley sprout, hawthorn fruit	4 grams each

[Example: 3]
1. Develops gas in the stomach so that the abdomen always feels full and at times has abdominal pain and joint pain and always feels tired
2. Always belches, but has an appetite. There is no problem during eating, but shortly after eating, the abdomen gradually feels distended and full, becoming uncomfortable.

- **Xu Qi Yin** (Spread the Qi Decoction) – *Wen Wei Yin* can be substituted.

tangerine peel, bitter orange, hawthorn fruit	6 grams each
magnolia, saussurea, lindera	3 grams each

A NOTE ON
APPENDIX I & II

$\mathcal{T}$he following appendices are on the herbs and formulas that are mentioned in this book. They were gathered from several texts, including the original author's text. For reference purposes, the texts that were used in compiling these charts are listed in the bibliography section of this book. As you will see in the charts, a single herb or a single formula can be used for a wide range of disorders. In contrast to Western medicine, the names of diseases or individual symptoms are not as important in Oriental medicine. It is the syndrome differentiation, as mentioned in the text, that is the most important aspect in applying herbs or formulas. Upon further inspection, it should be noticed that one indication can be treated by several herbs or formulas, but the auxiliary functions should be considered carefully in order to pick the most appropriate medicine to administer. This reflects the simplistic elegance of Oriental medicine in which one etiopathology can cause several complaints. A good practitioner will be able to correctly identify the underlying cause and by judiciously choosing the correct herbs or formulas, one will have great success in treating the complaints.

As for the names of the formulas that are in appendix II, I have used some of the translations from Dan Bensky's *Formulas and Strategies* whenever possible.

The following abbreviations were used in appendix I: Bk = bark, Ca = Caulis, Fl = flower, Fr = fruit, Hb = herb, Mn = mineral, Rt = root, Rz = rhizome and Sd = seed.

APPENDIX I: A TABLE OF HERBS

HERB	TASTE & TEMP.	CHANNELS	ACTIONS	INDICATIONS
Abutilon Sd. *Dong Kui Zi* 6 - 12grams	sweet, cold	large and small intestine	1. Promote urination and bowel movement 2. Promote secretion of mother's milk	edema, hot, painful and difficult urination, urinary tract stone, breast swelling, breast abscess, constipation • Cautioned during pregnancy
Achyranthes Rt. *Huai Niu Xi* 9 - 15g	bitter, sour, neutral	liver, kidney	1. Circulate Blood 2. Tonify Liver and Kidney 3. Strengthen bones and tendons 4. Descend Blood and Fire	amenorrhea, dysmenorrhea, abdominal mass, retention of lochia, pain and weakness in low back and knees, urinary tract infection, vaginal discharge, bleeding (urine, vomit, nose, gum, etc.), hypertension • Contraindicated during pregnancy
Aconite Rt. *Fu Zi* 1.5 - 9g	pungent, sweet, very hot, toxic	heart, spleen, kidney	1. Warm up Middle Burner 2. Restore Heart and Kidney Yang 3. Dispel Wind, Cold and Damp	abdominal pain, chills, cold extremities, shock, collapse, edema, diarrhea, arthritis, chronic diseases with cold symptoms, skin disorders • Contraindicated during pregnancy
Acorus Rz. *Shi Chang Pu* 3 - 9g	pungent, bitter, warm	heart, stomach, liver	1. Open orifice, calm Spirit and dispel Phlegm 2. Harmonize Stomach and dispel Damp	epilepsy, insanity, melancholy, deafness, dizziness, forgetfulness, impaired consciousness, chest and abdominal distention, abdominal pain, abscesses, trauma
Aduki Bean *Chi Xiao Dou* 9 - 30g	sweet, sour, neutral	spleen, heart, small intestine	1. Promote urination 2. Clear Heat and detoxify 3. Dispel pus	edema, difficult urination, sores, carbuncles, furuncles, jaundice
Agastache Hb. *Huo Xiang* 3 - 9g	pungent, slightly warm	lung, spleen, stomach	1. Clear Summer heat and Damp 2. Dispel Exterior Cold and Damp 3. Stop vomiting	chest fullness, poor appetite, indigestion, malaise, nausea, vomiting, abdominal pain and distention, morning sickness, common cold, edema, bad breath, alcohol intoxication
Akebia Ca. *Mu Tong* 3 - 9g	bitter, cold	heart, small intestine, bladder	1. Clear Heat and promote urination 2. Promote menstruation and lactation	edema, scanty urine, acute urinary tract infection, amenorrhea, scanty lactation, breast abscesses, jaundice • Contraindicated during pregnancy

Herb	Taste/Temp	Channels	Functions	Indications
Alisma Rz. *Ze Xie* 6 - 15g	sweet, cold	kidney, bladder	1. Promote urination and dispel Damp 2. Clear Damp-Heat in Lower Burner	edema, difficult urination, diarrhea, nephritis, night sweating, dizziness, tinnitus, fatty liver, high cholesterol
Allium Bulb *Cong Bai* 2 - 5 bulbs	pungent, warm	lung, stomach	1. Release Exterior and promote sweating 2. Invigorate Yang Qi to dispel Cold	common cold, abdominal pain, coldness and fullness, nasal congestion ● Used externally for sores and abscesses
Amber Resin *Hu Po* 1 - 3g	sweet, neutral	heart, liver, bladder	1. Calm the Spirit and stop spasm 2. Promote urination 3. Circulate Blood and remove stasis	insomnia, excess dreams, palpitations, epilepsy, infantile convulsion, acute urinary tract infection, urinary tract stone, amenorrhea, tumors, sores, carbuncles, ulceration
American Ginseng Rt. *Xi Yang Shen* 3 - 9g	sweet, slightly bitter, cool	lung, kidney, heart	1. Nourish Yin 2. Tonify Qi 3. Promote body fluid	chronic cough, low grade fever, fatigue, weakness, dryness, coughing up blood, loss of voice
Anemarrhena Rz. *Zhi Mu* 6 - 12g	bitter, cold	lung, stomach, kidney	1. Clear Heat in Lung and Stomach 2. Nourish Yin and promote body fluids	high and low fever, thirst, irritability, fidgeting, chronic bronchitis, tuberculosis, oral ulcers, bleeding (gums, cough, nose, etc.), low back pain, diabetes
Angelica Rt. *Bai Zhi* 3 - 9g	pungent, warm	lung, stomach	1. Dispel Wind and Cold 2. Dispel pus and reduce swelling 3. Stop pain 4. Open sinus passage	common cold, headache, rhinitis, sinusitis, toothache, boils, lung and intestinal carbuncle, skin diseases, vaginal discharge
Anteater Scales *Chuan Shan Jia* 3 - 9g	salty, slightly cold	liver, stomach	1. Circulate Blood 2. Reduce swelling and dispel pus 3. Promote menstruation and lactation	amenorrhea, dysmenorrhea, scanty lactation, boils, tumors, abscesses, scrofula, rheumatic arthritis, external trauma ● Contraindicated during pregnancy
Antler Horn *Lu Rong* 1 - 4.5g	sweet, salty, warm	liver, kidney	1. Tonify Kidney Yang 2. Nourish Blood, Yin, and Essence 3. Strengthen bones and tendons	weakness, fatigue, intolerance to cold, weakness of libido, impotence, spermatorrhea, infertility, vaginal discharge, uterine bleeding, delayed growth in children ● One of the best known aphrodisiacs

HERB	TASTE & TEMP.	CHANNELS	ACTIONS	INDICATIONS
Apricot Sd. *Xing Ren* 3 - 9g	bitter, slightly warm, slightly toxic	lung, large intestine	1. Stop cough and asthma 2. Lubricate Intestine	cough, asthma, acute or chronic bronchitis, constipation, dog bites
Aquilaria Wood *Chen Xiang* 1.5 - 3g	pungent, bitter, warm, aromatic	spleen, stomach, kidney, lung	1. Circulate Qi and stop pain 2. Dispel Cold 3. Descend Qi	chest and abdominal pain and distention, abdominal mass, hiccough, vomiting, belching, diarrhea, asthma, rheumatic pain, pulmonary emphysema
Areca Peel *Da Fu Pi* 6 - 9g	pungent, slightly warm	spleen, stomach, large and small intestines	1. Circulate Qi and remove food stagnation 2. Promote urination and dispel Damp	food stagnation, acid regurgitation, belching, abdominal distention, constipation, edema
Areca Sd. *Bing Lang* 6 -12g	pungent, bitter, warm	stomach, large intestine	1. Circulate Qi and remove food stagnation 2. Promote urination and dispel Damp 3. Kill parasites	abdominal pain and distention, constipation, edema, tenesmus, pinworm, roundworm, tapeworm, blood flukes, malaria, beriberi, alcohol intoxication
Asafoetida Resin *E Wei* 1 - 2g	pungent, bitter, warm	liver, spleen, stomach	1. Kill parasites 2. Detoxify 3. Promote digestion	parasites, dysentery, tumors, food stagnation ● Contraindicated during pregnancy
Asarum Hb. *Xi Xin* 1 - 3g	pungent, warm	lung, kidney	1. Dispel Wind-Cold and stop pain 2. Warm up Lung and resolve phlegm 3. Open nasal passages	common cold, internal cold, headache, severe toothache, rheumatic pain, chronic bronchitis, nasal and sinus congestion, spasm in joints, bad breath
Asparagus Rt. *Tian Men Dong* 6 - 15g	sweet, bitter, very cold	lung, kidney	1. Nourish Yin and body fluids 2. Resolve phlegm	tidal fever, night sweat, seminal emission, muscular atrophy, irritability, extreme thirst, dry throat, cough with sticky or bloody phlegm, asthma, constipation, diabetes

Herb	Properties	Channels	Functions	Indications
Aster Rt. *Zi Wan* 3 - 9g	sweet, bitter, slightly warm	lung	1. Stop cough and resolve phlegm	cough with thick phlegm, chronic cough, chronic bronchitis, tuberculosis
Astragalus Rt. *Huang Qi* 9 - 30g	sweet, slightly warm	spleen, lung	1. Tonify and raise Qi 2. Stop sweating 3. Dispel pus and promote healing 4. Promote urination	fatigue, weakness, spontaneous or night sweat, prolapse of organs (uterus, anus, stomach, etc.), abscesses, chronic ulcers, uterine bleeding, vaginal discharge, edema
Atractylodes Rz. *Cang Zhu* 4.5 - 9g	pungent, bitter, warm	spleen, stomach	1. Tonify Spleen and dry Damp 2. Dispel Wind, Cold and Damp	poor appetite, indigestion, nausea, vomiting, abdominal distention, diarrhea, rheumatic arthritis, night blindness • Similar to white atractylodes but has stronger dispersing/diaphoretic action
Atractylodes Rz. (White) *Bai Zhu* 4.5 - 9g	bitter, sweet, warm	spleen, stomach	1. Tonify Spleen and dry Damp 2. Calm fetus	poor appetite, indigestion, fatigue, weakness, abdominal pain and distention, diarrhea or loose stool, vomiting, copious clear sputum, edema, restless fetus, threatened miscarriage
Bamboo Lf. *Zhu Ye* 6 - 12g	sweet, bland, cold	heart, lung, stomach, gall bladder	1. Clear Heat 2. Promote body fluids 3. Promote urination	irritability, thirst, infantile convulsion, poor appetite, vomiting, bleeding (nose, vomit, etc.) • Cautioned during pregnancy
Bamboo Sap *Zhu Li* 30 - 60g	sweet, very cold	heart, lung, stomach	1. Clear Heat-Phlegm in Heart, Lung and Stomach	irritability, thirst, cough with yellow phlegm, convulsion, epilepsy, unconsciousness, post stroke complications
Bamboo Shavings *Zhu Ru* 4.5 - 9g	sweet, slightly cold	lung, stomach, gall bladder	1. Clear Heat-Phlegm in Lung 2. Clear Stomach Heat 3. Calm fetus 4. Stop bleeding	cough with yellow phlegm, vomiting, chronic gastritis, threatened miscarriage, bleeding (nose, vomit, cough, urine, etc.)
Barley Sprout *Mai Ya* 6 - 15g	sweet, neutral	spleen, stomach	1. Promote digestion 2. Stop lactation 3. Circulate Qi	indigestion, poor appetite, belching, vomiting, regurgitation of milk, breast distention

HERB	TASTE & TEMP.	CHANNELS	ACTIONS	INDICATIONS
Bean Sprout (Soybean) *Dou Juan* 9 - 15g	sweet, neutral	spleen, stomach	1. Clear Summer heat and Damp-Heat	early stage of Summer heat, warm-febrile disease (with joint pain, heavy sensation, little sweating), diarrhea, edema
Belamcanda Rt. *She Gan* 1.5 - 9g	bitter, cold	lung	1. Clear Heat and detoxify 2. Resolve phlegm and reduce swelling	acute tonsillitis, acute laryngitis, edema of glottis, cough with yellow phlegm ● Contraindicated during pregnancy
Biota Sd. *Bai Zi Ren* 6 - 18g	sweet, neutral	heart, liver, spleen, kidney, large intestine	1. Nourish Heart and calm Spirit 2. Lubricate Intestine 3. Stop sweating	palpitation, insomnia, anxiety, irritability, forgetfulness, constipation (elderly, debilitated, post partum, etc.), night sweating
Biota Tops *Ce Bai Ye* 6 - 15g	bitter, astringent, slightly cold	lung, heart, liver, large intestine	1. Cool Blood and stop bleeding 2. Resolve phlegm 3. Detoxify	bleeding (cough, vomit, urine, stool, gum, uterine, etc.), chronic bronchitis, cough with sticky phlegm, erysipelas, epidemic parotitis, bacterial dysentery, hair loss, arthritic pain, burns
Bitter Orange Fr. *Zhi Ke* 3 - 9g	sour, bitter, slightly cold	spleen, stomach	1. Circulate Qi and harmonize Stomach 2. Dispel hardening and food stagnation	indigestion, chest, hypochondriac and abdominal distention and fullness, constipation, prolapse of organs (uterus, rectum, stomach, etc.)
Bitter Orange Fr. (Immature) *Zhi Shi* 3 - 9g	sour, bitter, slightly cold	spleen, stomach	1. Circulate Qi and harmonize Stomach 2. Resolve hardening and food stagnation	same as above but is stronger in removing food stagnation and constipation ● Cautioned during pregnancy
Black Cardamon Fr. *Yi Zhi Ren* 3 - 9g	pungent, warm	spleen, kidney	1. Warm up and astringe Kidney 2. Warm up Spleen and stop diarrhea	enuresis, incontinence, frequent urination, spermatorrhea, seminal emission, abdominal pain, diarrhea, excessive salivation, vaginal discharge

Herb	Properties	Channels	Actions	Indications
Black Pepper *Hu Jiao* 2 - 4g	pungent, warm	stomach, large intestine	1. Warm up Spleen and Stomach 2. Promote digestion	poor appetite, indigestion, vomiting, diarrhea, abdominal pain and distention, dysentery, cholera, food poisoning
Borneol Resin *Bing Pian* 0.3 - 0.9g	pungent, bitter, slightly cold	heart, lung	1. Resuscitate 2. Clear Heat and stop pain	high fever, loss of consciousness, convulsion, stomatitis, tonsillitis, pharyngitis, laryngitis, sores, scabies, photophobia, excessive tearing ● Cautioned during pregnancy
Bugleweed Hb. *Ze Lan* 3 - 9g	pungent, slightly warm, aromatic	liver, bladder	1. Circulate Blood and promote menstruation 2. Promote urination	menstrual irregularities, dysmenorrhea, postpartum abdominal pain, abdominal mass, edema, incontinence, ulcers, furuncles, bleeding (vomit, urine, etc.), traumatic injury, joint pain ● Cautioned during pregnancy
Bupleurum Rt. *Chai Hu* 3 - 12g	bitter, slightly cold	liver, gall bladder, pericardium, triple burner	1. Clear Wind-Heat 2. Circulate Liver Qi 3. Raise Yang Qi	common cold, malaria, chest and hypochondriac pain and distention, prolapse of organs (uterus, rectum, anus, etc.)
Bush-cherry Sd. *Yu Li Ren* 3 - 9g	pungent, sweet, bitter, neutral	spleen, small and large intestine	1. Lubricate Intestine 2. Promote urination	constipation, edema ● Cautioned during pregnancy
Calcite Mn. *Han Shui Shi* 9 -30g	pungent, salty, cold	heart, stomach, kidney	1. Clear Heat and Fire	fever, thirst and vomiting in febrile disease, sore throat, oral ulcers, burns, scalds, erysipelas
Cannabis Sd. *Huo Ma Ren* 9 - 15g	sweet, neutral	spleen, stomach, large intestine	1. Lubricate Intestine 2. Nourish Yin	constipation (elderly, debilitated, post partum, etc.), diabetes, scanty lactation
Capillaris Hb. *Yin Chen Hao* 9 - 15g	bitter, slightly cold	spleen, stomach, liver, gall bladder, bladder	1. Dispel Damp-Heat 2. Treat jaundice 3. Release Exterior	jaundice, hepatitis, cholecystitis, intermittent chills and fever, difficult urination, rheumatic pain

HERB	TASTE & TEMP.	CHANNELS	ACTIONS	INDICATIONS
Cardamon Fr. *Sha Ren* 1.5 - 6g	pungent, warm, aromatic	spleen, stomach, kidney	1. Dispel Cold and Damp 2. Warm up Spleen 3. Calm fetus	poor appetite, indigestion, nausea, vomiting, abdominal pain, fullness and distention, diarrhea, threatened miscarriage
Carthamus Fl./ Safflower *Hong Hua* 3 - 9g	pungent, slightly sweet, warm	liver, heart	1. Circulate Blood and remove Blood stagnation 2. Stop pain	amenorrhea, dysmenorrhea, abdominal pain, abdominal mass, traumatic injury, enlargement of liver and spleen ● Contraindicated during pregnancy ● Excellent herb for post partum recovery
Celosia Sd. *Qing Xiang Zi* 3 - 15g	bitter, slightly cold	liver	1. Sedate Liver Fire 2. Clear Wind-Heat 3. Brighten eyes	red, painful and swollen eyes, blurred vision, cataract, tinnitus, hypertension ● Contraindicated for glaucoma patients
Chebula Fr. *He Zi* 3 - 9g	bitter, sour, astringent, neutral	lung, stomach, large intestine	1. Astringe Lung and Intestine	chronic diarrhea and dysentery, chronic cough, wheezing, hoarseness of voice
Chinese Angelica Rt. *Dang Gui* 3 - 15g	sweet, pungent, warm	liver, heart, spleen	1. Tonify Blood and regulate menstruation 2. Circulate Blood 3. Lubricate Intestine	amenorrhea, dysmenorrhea, anemia, abdominal pain, traumatic injury, arthritis, coronary heart disease, angina pectoris, constipation, sores, abscesses ● Best known for treating a variety of women's disorders
Chinese Gall *Wu Bei Zi* 1.5 - 6g	sour, salty, astringent, cold	lung, kidney, large intestine	1. Astringe Lung and Intestine 2. Stop bleeding	chronic cough, chronic diarrhea or dysentery, rectal prolapse, spontaneous or night sweats, profuse urination, bleeding (cough, stool, sputum, etc.), sores, ringworm
Chinese Leek Sd. *Jiu Zi* 3 - 9g	pungent, salty, warm	kidney, liver	1. Tonify Liver and Kidney 2. Tonify Yang and consolidate Essence	incontinence, frequent urination, impotence, spermatorrhea, vaginal discharge, pain and weakness in low back and knees

Herb	Taste/Nature	Channels	Functions	Indications
Chinese Quince Fr. *Mu Gua* 4.5 - 12g	sour, warm	liver, spleen	1. Relax tendons and activate channels 2. Harmonize Stomach and dispel Damp	rheumatic pain, spasm, vomiting, diarrhea, indigestion, weakness in low back and knees, beriberi
Cicada Moulting *Chan Tui* 3 - 9g	slightly sweet, salty, cool	lung, liver	1. Dispel Wind-Heat 2. Eliminate rash 3. Clear eyes 4. Extinguish Internal Wind	common cold, sore throat, rash, measles (early stage), red, swollen and painful eyes, convulsions, spasms
Cimicifuga Rz. *Sheng Ma* 1.5 - 9g	pungent, sweet, slightly bitter, cool	lung, spleen, stomach, large intestine	1. Dispel Wind-Heat 2. Clear Heat and detoxify 3. Raise Yang Qi	common cold, sore throat, measles, rash, carbuncles, furuncles, headache, inflammation of gums and mouth, prolapse of organs (uterus, rectum, anus, etc.)
Cinnabar Mn. *Zhu Sha* 0.3 - 2.7g	sweet, slightly cold, toxic	heart	1. Calm Spirit 2. Stop convulsion 3. Clear Heat and detoxify	palpitations, restlessness, insomnia, epilepsy, convulsion, boils, furuncles, carbuncles, sore throat, snake bite ● Highly toxic/ contraindicated during pregnancy
Cinnamon Bk. *Rou Gui* 1.5 - 4.5g	pungent, sweet, very hot	spleen, kidney, liver, heart,	1. Warm up Spleen 2. Tonify Kidney Yang 3. Warm up channels and stop pain	chronic diarrhea, aversion to cold, cold hands and feet, scanty urination, edema, impotence, abdominal, hypochondriac and low back pain, amenorrhea, dysmenorrhea, boils, abscesses ● Cautioned during pregnancy
Cinnamon Twig *Gui Zhi* 3 - 9g	pungent, sweet, warm	heart, lung, bladder	1. Dispel Wind-Cold 2. Adjust Ying and Wei 3. Circulate Yang Qi in chest 4. Warm up channels and circulate Blood	common cold, chest and abdominal pain, palpitation, angina pectoris, abdominal fullness, arthritic pain, amenorrhea, dysmenorrhea, uterine tumors
Cistanche Hb. *Rou Cong Rong* 9 - 21g	sweet, salty, warm	kidney, large intestine	1. Tonify Kidney Yang 2. Lubricate Intestine 3. Warm up womb	impotence, premature ejaculation, spermatorrhea, genital pain, frequent urination, incontinence, low back and knee pain and weakness, chronic constipation in elderly and debilitated, infertility, uterine bleeding, vaginal discharge

HERB	TASTE & TEMP.	CHANNELS	ACTIONS	INDICATIONS
Clematis Rt. *Wei Ling Xian* 6 - 12g	pungent, salty, warm	bladder	1. Dispel Wind-Damp 2. Circulate Qi and stop pain	rheumatic pain, fish bone stuck in throat, abdominal distention, tumors
Clove Fl. *Ding Xiang* 1.5 - 4.5g	pungent, warm	spleen, stomach, kidney	1. Warm up Spleen and Stomach and descend Qi 2. Warm up Kidney Yang	hiccup, poor appetite, vomiting, diarrhea, abdominal pain and distention, impotence, vaginal discharge, alcohol intoxication
Cluster Fr. *Bai Dou Kou* 3 - 6g	pungent, warm	spleen, stomach, lung	1. Dispel Damp and circulate Qi 2. Descend Qi	abdominal pain and fullness, indigestion, nausea, vomiting
Cnidium Fr. *She Chuang Zi* 3 - 9g	pungent, slightly, warm	spleen, kidney	1. Tonify Kidney Yang 2. Dry Damp and kill parasites	impotence, frequent urination, low back and knee pain and weakness, colic, vaginal discharge, eczema, pruritis, trichomonas vaginitis, scabies, ringworm
Cnidium Rz. *Chuang Xiong* 3 - 6g	pungent, warm	liver, pericardium, gall bladder	1. Circulate Qi and Blood 2. Stop pain	headache, bodyache, amenorrhea, dysmenorrhea, irregular menstruation, difficult labor, retention of lochia, cerebral embolism, coronary heart disease ● Cautioned during pregnancy
Coix Sd./ Job's Tear *Yi Yi Ren* 9 - 30g	sweet, slightly cold	spleen, stomach, lung, large intestine, kidney	1. Promote urination 2. Tonify Spleen 3. Expel Wind-Damp 4. Clear Heat or Damp-Heat	edema, ascites, scanty urination, tinea of the foot, lung and intestinal abscess, warts, diarrhea, rheumatic arthritis, beriberi ● Cautioned during pregnancy
Coptis Rz. *Huang Lian* 1.5 - 9g	bitter, cold	heart, liver, stomach, large intestine	1. Clear Heat and Damp 2. Calm Spirit 3. Detoxify 4. Cool Blood	irritability, thirst, insomnia, delirium due to high fever, diarrhea, acute enteritis and dysentery, bleeding (nose, vomit, urine, stool, etc.), inflammation of the mouth and tongue, bad breath, hemorrhoids, leukemia, conjunctivitis, otitis media, carbuncles

Herb	Properties	Channels	Functions	Indications
Cornus Fr. *Shan Zhu Yu* 3 - 12g	sour, slightly warm	liver, kidney	1. Tonify Liver and Kidney 2. Astringe	low back and knee pain and weakness, dizziness, vertigo, impotence, frequent urination, spermatorrhea, nocturnal emission, incontinence, spontaneous or night sweat, uterine bleeding, vaginal discharge
Corydalis Rz. *Yan Hu Suo* 4.5 - 12g	pungent, bitter, warm	heart, liver, spleen, stomach	1. Circulate Blood and Qi and remove stagnation 2. Stop pain 3. Calm Spirit	low back pain, dysmenorrhea, irregular menstruation, hernia, chest and abdominal pain, traumatic injury, insomnia ● One of the best herbs for stopping various types of pain/contraindicated during pregnancy
Croton Sd. *Ba Dou* 0.1 - 0.3g	pungent, hot, toxic	stomach, large intestine, lung	1. Purge water 2. Dispel Cold, accumulation and food stagnation 3. Kill parasites	constipation, abdominal distention and pain, wheezing, diarrhea, dysentery, edema, ascites, warts, furuncles, ulcers, dermatitis ● Contraindicated during pregnancy
Curculigo Rz. *Xian Mao* 3 - 9g	pungent, warm, slightly toxic	kidney, spleen, liver	1. Warm up Kidney Yang 2. Strengthen bones and tendons 3. Dispel Cold and Damp	impotence, premature ejaculation, nocturnal emission, frequent urination, incontinence, intolerance to cold, low back and knee pain, abdominal pain and coldness, diarrhea, pain and spasm of limbs, climacteric hypertension
Cuscuta Sd. *Tu Si Zi* 9 - 15g	pungent, sweet, neutral	liver, kidney	1. Tonify Spleen and Kidney Yang 2. Tonify Liver and brighten eyes 3. Calm the fetus	impotence, premature ejaculation, spermatorrhea, vertigo, frequent urination, incontinence, low back and knee pain and weakness, decreased eyesight, threatened miscarriage, chronic diarrhea, vaginal discharge
Cyperus Rz. *Xiang Fu* 4.5 - 12g	pungent, slightly bitter, neutral	liver, stomach, triple burner	1. Circulate Liver Qi and stop pain 2. Harmonize Stomach 3. Regulate menstruation	abdominal and hypochondriac pain, indigestion, diarrhea, chest and abdominal fullness and distention, hernia, uterine bleeding, dysmenorrhea, irregular menstruation
Date Fr. (Red) *Da Zao* 3 - 12 pieces	sweet, warm	spleen, stomach	1. Tonify Spleen and Stomach Qi 2. Nourish Blood 3. Calm the Spirit 4. Harmonize other herbs	fatigue, weakness, lack of appetite, diarrhea or loose stool, shortness of breath, anemia, palpitation, irritability, hysteria

HERB	TASTE & TEMP.	CHANNELS	ACTIONS	INDICATIONS
Dendrobium Hb. *Shi Hu* 9 - 20g	sweet, bland, slightly cold	lung, stomach, kidney	1. Tonify Lung and Stomach Yin 2. Clear Heat	thirst, dry mouth, dry cough, vomiting, abdominal pain, chronic tidal fever
Descurainia Sd. *Ting Li Zi* 3 - 9g	pungent, bitter, very cold	lung, bladder	1. Stop cough and asthma 2. Purge water	cough, asthma, edema, scanty urination, pleurisy ● Contraindicated during pregnancy
Dioscorea Rt. *Shan Yao* 9 - 30g	sweet, neutral	lung, spleen, kidney	1. Tonify Spleen, Lung and Kidney Qi 2. Astringe Essence	poor appetite, chronic diarrhea, enuresis, frequent urination, dry cough, asthma, spermatorrhea, nocturnal emission, vaginal discharge, diabetes, carbuncles, boils, abscesses ● Very good herb for all weaknesses and deficiencies
Dipsacus Rt. *Xu Duan* 6 - 21g	bitter, pungent, slightly warm	liver, kidney	1. Tonify Liver and Kidney 2. Strengthen bones and tendons 3. Stop bleeding and calm fetus 4. Circulate Blood and stop pain	low back, joint and rheumatic pain, bone fracture, external trauma or injury, frequent urination, spermatorrhea, bleeding (nose, vomit, urine, stool, etc.), vaginal discharge, threatened miscarriage, hemorrhoids
Dittany Bark *Bai Xian Pi* 6 - 9g	bitter, cold	spleen, stomach	1. Clear Heat and detoxify 2. Dispel Wind and Damp	sores, scabies, rubella, jaundice, arthritic pain, urinary difficulty, vaginal pain and swelling
Dolichos Sd. *Bai Bian Dou* 9 - 21g	sweet, neutral	spleen, stomach	1. Clear Summer heat 2. Tonify Spleen and Stomach	sunstroke, fever, thirst, poor appetite, vomiting, diarrhea, vaginal discharge, infantile malnutrition
Donkey-hide Gelatin *E Jiao* 3 - 15g	sweet, neutral	lung, liver, kidney	1. Tonify Blood and Yin 2. Stop bleeding 3. Calm fetus	palpitations, bleeding (nose, cough, urine, uterine, etc.), irritability, paralysis, dry cough with bloody sputum, lung abscess, tuberculosis, anemia, threatened miscarriage

Herb	Properties	Channels	Functions	Indications
Dragon Bone *Long Gu* 15 - 30g	sweet, astringent, cool	heart, liver, kidney	1. Calm Spirit 2. Descend Liver Yang 3. Astringe	palpitations, insomnia, restlessness, excess dreaming, headache, dizziness, spontaneous sweating, vaginal discharge, uterine bleeding, seminal emission, hypertension, seizures, chronic sores and ulcerations
Dragon Teeth *Long Chi* 9 - 15g	astringent, cool	heart, liver	1. Calm Spirit	palpitations, insomnia, excess dreaming, neurasthenia, epilepsy
Elsholtzia Hb. *Xiang Ru* 3 - 9g	pungent, slightly warm, aromatic	lung, stomach	1. Release Exterior and Clear Summer heat 2. Promote urination	common cold, summer heat, irritability, edema, scanty urination, vomiting, abdominal pain, bad breath
Ephedra Hb. *Ma Huang* 1.5 - 9g	pungent, bitter, warm	lung, bladder	1. Dispel Wind-Cold 2. Descend Lung Qi 3. Promote urination	common cold, cough, asthma, edema
Ephedra Rt. *Ma Huang Gen* 9 - 15g	sweet, bitter, neutral	lung	1. Stop sweating	spontaneous sweating, night sweating, post partum sweating
Epimedium Hb. *Yin Yang Huo* 6 - 15g	pungent, sweet, warm	liver, kidney, triple burner	1. Tonify Kidney Yang 2. Dispel Wind-Damp 3. Stop cough and asthma	impotence, spermatorrhea, frequent urination, genital pain, low back pain, fatigue, arthritis, low back and leg numbness and weakness, hypertension, chronic bronchitis
Eucommia Bk. *Du Zhong* 6 - 15g	sweet, slightly pungent, warm	liver, kidney	1. Tonify Liver and Kidney 2. Strengthen bones and tendons 3. Calm fetus 4. Lower blood pressure	impotence, spermatorrhea, frequent urination, incontinence, low back and knee pain and weakness, threatened miscarriage, hypertension
Euryale Sd. *Qian Shi* 9 - 15g	sweet, astringent, neutral	spleen, kidney	1. Tonify Spleen 2. Astringe Kidney	chronic diarrhea, seminal emission, premature ejaculation, vaginal discharge, copious and frequent urination, enuresis

HERB	TASTE & TEMP.	CHANNELS	ACTIONS	INDICATIONS
Evodia Fr. *Wu Zhu Yu* 3 - 9g	pungent, bitter, hot, slightly toxic	spleen, stomach, liver, kidney	1. Warm up Spleen and dispel Cold and stop pain 2. Descend Qi 3. Kill parasites	headache, cold sensation in stomach, abdominal pain and distention, vomiting, acid regurgitation, early morning diarrhea, mouth and tongue sores, edema
Fennel Sd. *Xiao Hui Xiang* 3 - 9g	pungent, warm	spleen, stomach, liver, kidney	1. Regulate Qi and harmonize Stomach 2. Warm up Kidney, dispel Cold and stop pain	abdominal pain, coldness and distention in abdomen, hernia, poor appetite, indigestion, vomiting, pain in testis, beriberi, toothache
Fleeceflower Rt. *He Shou Wu* 9 - 30g	sweet, bitter, astringent, slightly warm	liver, kidney	1. Tonify Blood 2. Tonify Liver and Kidney 3. Lubricate Intestine 4. Calm Spirit 5. Detoxify	dizziness, blurred vision, early greying of hair, low back and knee pain and weakness, neurasthenia, insomnia, palpitation, spermatorrhea, nocturnal emission, vaginal discharge, constipation in elderly, boils, abscesses, goiter, scrofula, rash, high cholesterol level, anemia
Forsythia Fr. *Lian Qiao* 6 - 15g	bitter, slightly cold	lung, heart, liver, gall bladder	1. Clear Heat and detoxify 2. Dispel Wind-Heat 3. Dispel lumps and hardening	common cold, flu, high fever, thirst, delirium, urinary tract infection, scrofula, sores, abscesses ● Superior herb for skin disorders
Frankincense Resin *Ru Xiang* 3 - 9g	pungent, bitter, warm	heart, liver, spleen	1. Circulate Blood and stop pain 2. Promote healing	amenorrhea, dysmenorrhea, abdominal pain, rheumatic pain, traumatic injury and wounds, ulcers, carbuncles, furuncles ● Contraindicated during pregnancy
Fritillary Bulb *Chuan Bei Mu* 3 - 12g	bitter, sweet, slightly cold	lung, heart	1. Clear Heat-Phlegm 2. Moisten Lung and stop cough 3. Dispel lumps and hardening	dry cough or cough with scanty sputum, chronic bronchitis, tuberculosis, lung or breast abscess, goiter, scrofula, jaundice, sores, nodules ● Milder in action than Zhe Bei Mu, this herb is used more for chronic condition
Fritillary Bulb *Zhe Bei Mu* 3 - 9g	bitter, cold	lung, heart	1. Clear Heat-Phlegm 2. Dispel lumps and hardening	cough with thick sputum, acute bronchitis, pneumonia, subcutaneous swelling, lung abscess, scrofula, goiter, jaundice

Herb	Properties	Organs	Functions	Indications
Galanga Rz. *Gao Liang Jiang* 1.5 - 9g	pungent, hot	spleen, stomach	1. Warm up Stomach and stop pain	abdominal pain and coldness, indigestion, nausea, vomiting, hiccough, diarrhea, chronic enteritis, alcohol intoxication
Gardenia Fr. *Zhi Zi* 3 - 12g	bitter, cold	heart, lung, liver, gall bladder, stomach, triple burner	1. Clear Heat, sedate Fire and cool Blood 2. Clear Damp-Heat 3. Reduce swelling and detoxify	high fever, thirst, fidgeting, insomnia, red eyes, acute hepatitis, jaundice, bleeding (nose, vomit, urine, etc.), external injury, swelling, difficult urination
Gastrodia Rz. *Tian Ma* 3 - 9g	sweet, neutral	liver	1. Extinguish Liver Wind 2. Dispel Wind-Damp	headache, dizziness, vertigo, spasm, convulsion, hypertension, post stroke complications, epilepsy, tetany
Genkwa Fl. *Yuan Hua* 1.5 - 3g	bitter, pungent, warm, toxic	lung, kidney, large intestine	1. Purge water 2. Stop cough and dispel phlegm 3. Kill parasites	severe edema, ascites, chronic bronchitis, scabies, ringworm, constipation ● Contraindicated during pregnancy
Gentiana Rt. *Long Dan Cao* 3 - 9g	bitter, cold	liver, gall bladder, stomach	1. Clear Damp-Heat 2. Sedate Liver Fire	jaundice, headache, red eyes, conjunctivitis, sore throat, bitter taste in mouth, dizziness, tinnitus, ear pain, sudden deafness, acute urinary tract infection, swollen testicles, vaginal discharge, spasm, convulsion, mania, diarrhea, eczema, hypertension
Ginger (dried) Rz. *Gan Jiang* 3 - 12g	pungent, hot	heart, lung, spleen, stomach	1. Warm up Spleen and Stomach 2. Restore Yang 3. Warm up Lung and resolve phlegm	coldness in extremities and abdomen (shock), nausea, vomiting, diarrhea, abdominal pain and distention, chronic bronchitis, uterine bleeding ● Cautioned during pregnancy
Ginger (fresh) Rz. *Sheng Jiang* 3 - 9g	pungent, warm	lung, spleen, stomach	1. Dispel Wind-Cold 2. Harmonize Stomach and stop vomiting 3. Resolve phlegm 4. Harmonize Ying and Wei	common cold, cough with thin white sputum, vomiting, diarrhea, abdominal fullness and pain ● Best known herb for stopping vomiting

HERB	TASTE & TEMP.	CHANNELS	ACTIONS	INDICATIONS
Ginseng Rt. *Ren Shen* 1 - 9g	sweet, slightly bitter, slightly warm	spleen, lung, heart	1. Tonify Qi and promote body fluids 2. Tonify Spleen and Lung 3. Calm Spirit	fatigue, extreme weakness, shortness of breath, feeble breathing, poor appetite, chronic diarrhea, palpitation, insomnia, forgetfulness, dehydration ● The most well known herb in the world
Gleditsia Spine *Zao Jiao Ci* 0.6 - 1.5g	pungent, warm	liver, stomach	1. Dispel lumps and swellings and discharge pus 2. Circulate Blood 3. Dispel Wind and kill parasites	sores, inflammation, tonsillitis, ringworm, leprosy ● Contraindicated during pregnancy
Glehnia Rt. *Bei Sha Shen* 9 - 15g	sweet, slightly cold	lung, stomach	1. Tonify Lung and Stomach Yin 2. Promote body fluids	dry cough with thin, sticky sputum or bloody sputum, thirst, dry throat, hoarseness, constipation, dry and itchy skin
Gypsum Mn. *Shi Gao* 9 - 30g	pungent, sweet, very cold	lung, stomach	1. Clear Heat and sedate Fire 2. Promote body fluids	high fever, tidal fever, fidgeting, thirst, asthma, headache, inflammation of gums, toothache, burns, abscesses, eczema, constipation, diabetes
Hawthorn Fr. *Shan Zha* 9 - 15g	sour, sweet, slightly warm	spleen, stomach, liver	1. Dispel food stagnation 2. Circulate Blood and remove stagnation	indigestion (especially due to meat and fats), acid regurgitation, abdominal fullness and distention, abdominal tumor, retention of lochia, amenorrhea, postpartum abdominal pain, hypertension, coronary heart disease, elevated cholesterol
Hematite Mn. *Dai Zhe Shi* 9 - 30g	bitter, cold	heart, liver	1. Descend Liver Yang 2. Descend Qi 3. Cool Blood and stop bleeding	hypertension, headache, vertigo, tinnitus, redness and pressure in eyes, belching, vomiting, nausea, hiccough, asthma, bleeding (nose, vomit, uterine, etc.) ● Cautioned during pregnancy
Honey *Feng Mi* 15 - 30g	sweet, neutral	lung, spleen, large intestine	1. Nourish Lung and stop cough 2. Nourish Spleen and Stomach 3. Lubricate Intestine 4. Moderate and detoxify	dry cough, chronic cough, sore throat, dry stool, constipation in elderly, ulcer, chronic hepatitis

Herb	Taste/Nature	Channels	Functions	Indications
Imperata Rz. *Bai Mao Gen* 9 - 18g	sweet, cold	lung, stomach, small intestine	1. Cool Blood and stop bleeding 2. Clear Heat and promote urination	various bleeding (cough, vomit, nose, urine, etc.), edema, difficult urination, jaundice, abdominal distention, thirst, wheezing, nausea
Inula Fl. *Xuan Fu Hua* 3 - 12g	salty, warm	lung, spleen, stomach, liver	1. Resolve Cold-Phlegm 2. Descend Lung and Stomach Qi	cough, asthma, copious phlegm, belching, vomiting, hiccough
Kansui Rt. *Gan Sui* 1.5 - 3g	bitter, cold, toxic	lung, spleen, kidney	1. Purge water 2. Clear Heat and reduce swelling and lumps	severe edema, ascites, pleurisy, painful urination, constipation, liver cirrhosis, inflammation ● Contraindicated during pregnancy
Katsumadai Sd. *Cao Dou Kou* 1.5 - 6g	pungent, warm, aromatic	spleen, stomach	1. Tonify and warm Spleen and Stomach 2. Dry Damp	poor appetite, abdominal pain, fullness and distention, vomiting, diarrhea
Large-leaf Gentian Rt. *Qin Jiao* 4.5 - 12g	pungent, bitter, slightly cold	stomach, liver, gall bladder	1. Dispel Wind-Damp 2. Clear Deficient Heat 3. Lubricate Intestine	rheumatic pain, mouth and tooth pain, mouth ulcers, low-grade fever, steaming heat sensation in bones, constipation, allergic inflammation, jaundice, hepatitis
Leonurus Hb. *Yi Mu Cao* 9 - 60g	pungent, bitter, slightly cold	liver, heart, kidney, bladder	1. Circulate Blood and remove stagnation 2. Promote urination 3. Cool Blood and detoxify	irregular menstruation, dysmenorrhea, retention of lochia, postpartum abdominal pain, abdominal tumors, bleeding (uterine, stool, etc.), edema, nephritic edema, eczema, abscesses ● Contraindicated during pregnancy ● Frequently given after childbirth for speedy recovery
Licorice Rt. *Gan Cao* 2 - 12g	sweet, neutral	all 12 channels (mainly heart, lung, spleen, stomach)	1. Tonify Spleen and Stomach Qi 2. Clear Heat and detoxify 3. Stop spasm and pain 4. Moisten Lung, stop cough and resolve phlegm 5. Harmonize other herbs	palpitation, shortness of breath, weakness, fatigue, loose stool, sore throat, boils, carbuncles, cough, asthma, spasm in abdomen or legs, peptic ulcer, Addison's disease ● Raw - clears heat and detoxify ● Baked - more tonifying

HERB	TASTE & TEMP.	CHANNELS	ACTIONS	INDICATIONS
Lily Bulb *Bai He* 9 - 30g	sweet, slightly bitter, slightly cold	heart, lung	1. Tonify Lung Yin 2. Stop cough and resolve phlegm 3. Calm Spirit	cough, hemoptysis, sore throat, low grade fever, insomnia, fidgeting, palpitation, fright, breast abscess, constipation
Lindera Rt. *Wu Yao* 3 - 9g	pungent, warm	lung, spleen, stomach, kidney, bladder	1. Circulate Qi 2. Dispel Cold and stop pain 3. Warm up Kidney	abdominal pain and distention, indigestion, menstrual pain, enuresis, incontinence, frequent urination, diarrhea, hernial disorders
Long Pepper Fr. *Bi Ba* 1.5 - 4.5g	pungent, hot	spleen, stomach, large intestine	1. Warm up Interior and dispel Cold 2. Descend Qi 3. Stop pain	abdominal pain and coldness, nausea, vomiting, belching, borborygmus, acid regurgitation, diarrhea, headache, toothache, rhinitis
Longan Fr. *Long Yan Rou* 6 - 15g	sweet, warm	heart, spleen	1. Tonify Blood 2. Calm Spirit 3. Tonify Heart and Spleen	insomnia, palpitation, irritability, dizziness, forgetfulness, postpartum weakness
Lonicera Fl. *Jin Yin Hua* 9 - 15g	sweet, bitter, cold	lung, stomach, large intestine	1. Clear Heat and detoxify 2. Clear Wind-Heat and Damp-Heat	common cold, febrile disease with high fever, thirst, upper respiratory infection, sore throat, boils, carbuncles, furuncles, scrofula, enteritis, dysentery, syphilis
Lotus Sd. *Lian Zi* 6 - 15g	sweet, astringent, neutral	heart, spleen, kidney	1. Tonify Spleen 2. Tonify Kidney 3. Calm Spirit	chronic diarrhea, poor appetite, seminal emission, vaginal discharge, insomnia, palpitation, anxiety, insomnia, premature ejaculation, spermatorrhea, uterine bleeding
Lycium Bk. *Di Gu Pi* 6 - 15g	sweet, cold	lung, kidney	1. Clear Yin Deficiency Heat 2. Clear Lung Heat 3. Clear Heat and Cool Blood	chronic low grade fever, irritability, thirst, night sweat, steaming heat sensation in bones, cough, asthma, bleeding (nose, vomit, urine, etc.), toothache, tuberculosis, hypertension, diabetes

Herb	Properties	Channels	Functions	Indications
Lycium Fr. *Gou Qi Zi* 6 - 18g	sweet, neutral	liver, lung, kidney	1. Tonify Yin, Blood and Essence 2. Tonify Liver and Kidney 3. Brighten eyes	impotence, nocturnal emission, low back and knee pain, chronic cough, dizziness, vertigo, blurred vision, diabetes ● A tonic that increases overall vitality
Magnetite Mn. *Ci Shi* 9 - 30g	pungent, salty, cold	heart, lung, liver, kidney	1. Calm Spirit 2. Descend Liver Yang 3. Tonify Kidney and stop asthma	insomnia, palpitation, restlessness, dizziness, epilepsy, convulsion, mania, tinnitus, deafness, blurred vision, chronic asthma, anemia
Magnolia Bk. *Hou Po* 3 - 9g	pungent, bitter, warm, aromatic	spleen, stomach, lung, large intestine	1. Circulate Qi and dry Damp 2. Tonify Spleen and Stomach 3. Descend Lung and Stomach Qi	poor appetite, indigestion, chest and abdominal pain and distention, vomiting, acid regurgitation, diarrhea, cough, asthma, profuse phlegm, constipation ● Cautioned during pregnancy
Mantis Egg-case *Sang Piao Xiao* 3 - 9g	sweet, salty, astringent, neutral	liver, kidney	1. Tonify Kidney and astringe Essence	frequent and profuse urination, enuresis, seminal emission, impotence, vaginal discharge
Medicated Leaven *Shen Qu* 6 - 15g	sweet, warm	spleen, stomach	1. Harmonize Stomach and remove food stagnation	indigestion, poor appetite, abdominal fullness and distention, vomiting, borborygmus, tumors ● Cautioned during pregnancy
Minium Mn. *Qian Dan* 0.3 - 0.6g	pungent, salty, cold, toxic	heart, spleen, liver	1. Detoxify 2. Promote healing 3. Eliminate Phlegm and calms fright	carbuncles, furuncles, ulcers, sores, epilepsy, delirium, palpitation, irritability, insomnia, malaria
Mirabilite Mn. *Mang Xiao* 3 - 9g	bitter, salty, very cold	stomach, large intestine	1. Promote bowel movement 2. Clear Heat and reduce swelling	constipation, mastitis, appendicitis, conjunctivitis, ulcerated mouth and throat ● Contraindicated during pregnancy
Morinda Rt. *Ba Ji Tian* 6 - 15g	pungent, sweet, warm	liver, kidney	1. Tonify Kidney Yang 2. Strengthen bones and tendons 3. Dispel Wind-Damp	impotence, spermatorrhea, infertility, irregular menstruation, frequent urination, incontinence, low back and knee pain and weakness, arthritis, muscular atrophy

HERB	TASTE & TEMP.	CHANNELS	ACTIONS	INDICATIONS
Morus Bk. *Sang Bai Pi* 6 - 15g	sweet, cold	lung, spleen	1. Stop cough and asthma 2. Resolve phlegm 3. Promote urination	cough, asthma, thirst, coughing up blood, difficult urination, edema, hypertension, parasites
Morus Fr. *Sang Shen* 6 - 15g	sweet, slightly cold	heart, liver, kidney	1. Tonify Blood and Yin 2. Lubricate Intestine	anemia, insomnia, dizziness, tinnitus, neurasthenia, premature graying of hair, hypertension, thirst, diabetes, constipation
Morus Lf. *Sang Ye* 4.5 - 15g	sweet, bitter, cold	lung, liver	1. Dispel Wind-Heat 2. Clear Liver Heat and eyes 3. Clear pathogenic Heat and stop bleeding	common cold with fever, headache, sore throat, red, swollen and painful eyes, vomiting of blood
Morus Twig *Sang Zhi* 3 - 15g	bitter, sweet, neutral	liver	1. Dispel Wind-Damp 2. Promote urination	rheumatic pain and spasms, edema, high blood pressure ● Especially treats pain in upper extremities
Moutan Bk. *Mu Dan Pi* 6 - 12g	pungent, bitter, slightly cold	heart, liver, kidney	1. Clear Heat and cool Blood 2. Circulate Blood and remove stagnation	high fever, bleeding (nose, vomit, uterine, subcutaneous, etc.), abdominal tumors, amenorrhea, dysmenorrhea, appendicitis, boils, sores, carbuncles, traumatic injury ● Contraindicated during pregnancy
Mugwort Lf. *Ai Ye* 3 - 9g	pungent, bitter, warm	lung, liver, spleen, kidney	1. Warm up channel and stop bleeding 2. Dispel Cold and stop pain 3. Calm fetus	abdominal pain, vaginal discharge, bleeding (uterine, vomit, stool, etc.), threatened miscarriage, infertility, dysmenorrhea, malaria ● Best known for treating women's disorder due to cold ● Used as sole or main ingredient in moxibustion
Mulberry Mistletoe Stem *Sang Ji Sheng* 9 - 30g	bitter, neutral	liver, kidney	1. Tonify Liver and Kidney 2. Tonify Blood and calm fetus 3. Strengthen bones and tendons 4. Dispel Wind-Damp	low back and leg pain, numbness, weakness and atrophy of bones and tendons, arthritis, threatened miscarriage, uterine bleeding, dry and scaly skin, hypertension, coronary heart diseases

Herb	Properties	Channels	Functions	Indications
Mume /Black Plum *Wu Wei* 3 - 9g	sour, astringent, warm	liver, spleen, lung, large intestine	1. Astringe Lung and Intestine 2. Promote body fluids 3. Kill parasites	chronic cough, chronic diarrhea, extreme thirst, lung abscess, pulmonary tuberculosis, diabetes, alcohol intoxication, tinea, intestinal parasites, corns, warts
Mung Bean *Lu Dou* 15 - 30g	sweet, bland, cool	stomach	1. Clear Summer heat 2. Clear Heat and eliminate phlegm 3. Stop thirst 4. Calm Spirit	thirst, vomiting, bleeding (vomit, stool, urine, etc.), diarrhea, abdominal distention, constipation, erysipelas, urticaria, dry skin, carbuncle, smallpox, measles, diabetes
Musk *She Xiang* 0.06 - 0.15g	pungent, warm	heart, spleen, liver	1. Aromatically open up orifices 2. Circulate Blood and remove stagnation	loss of consciousness in acute infectious disease, convulsion, delirium, apoplexy, abdominal tumors, boils, furuncles, carbuncles, Buerger's disease, retention of lochia, alcohol intoxication ● Contraindicated during pregnancy
Myrrh Resin *Mo Yao* 3 - 12g	bitter, neutral	heart, liver, spleen	1. Circulate Blood and remove stagnation 2. Stop pain and promote healing	traumatic pain and swelling, amenorrhea, abdominal tumors, chest and abdominal pain, sores, carbuncles, hemorrhoids ● Contraindicated during pregnancy
Notopterygium Rt. *Qiang Huo* 6 - 15g	pungent, bitter, warm, aromatic	kidney, bladder	1. Dispel Wind, Cold and Damp 2. Stop pain	common cold, headache, heavy sensation over the body, rheumatic pain (especially upper body), carbuncles, furuncles
Nutmeg Sd. *Rou Dou Kou* 1.5 - 9g	pungent, warm	spleen, stomach, large intestine	1. Warm up Spleen and Stomach 2. Astringe Intestine 3. Circulate Qi	chronic diarrhea (early morning), vomiting, poor appetite, indigestion, abdominal pain and distention, flatulence, undigested food in stool, alcohol intoxication
Ophiopogon Rz. *Mai Men Dong* 6 - 15g	sweet, slightly bitter, slightly cold	heart, lung, stomach	1. Tonify Lung and Stomach Yin 2. Calm Spirit 3. Lubricate Intestine	extreme thirst, dry mouth and throat, vomiting, nosebleed, dry cough, thin or bloody sputum, dry stool, palpitations, insomnia, fearfulness, scanty lactation

HERB	TASTE & TEMP.	CHANNELS	ACTIONS	INDICATIONS
Opium Poppy Capsule *Ying Su Ke* 1.5 - 6g	sour, astringent, neutral, toxic	lung, kidney, large intestine	1. Astringe Lung and Intestine 2. Stop pain	chronic diarrhea and dysentery, abdominal pain, stomach pain, chronic cough and asthma, lung abscess, tuberculosis, copious urination, spermatorrhea, vaginal discharge ● Treats all types of pain
Ox Gallstone/ Bezoar *Niu Huang* 0.15 - 1g	bitter, sweet, cool, slightly toxic	heart, liver	1. Extinguish Liver Wind 2. Clear Heat and aromatically open orifices 3. Clear Heat, reduce swelling and detoxify	loss of consciousness, delirium, convulsions, stroke, epilepsy, lock-jaw, tetany, pharyngitis, laryngitis, inflammation of mouth and skin, sores, carbuncles, ulcerated throat ● Contraindicated during pregnancy
Oyster *Hao* 10 - 25 pieces	sweet, bland, salty, cool	lung, liver, heart, spleen, kidney	1. Tonify Blood 2. Tonify Kidney 3. Clear mind	thirst, insomnia, palpitations, stress, nervousness, goiter, tuberculosis of lymph node, excess perspiration, premature ejaculation ● Strengthens whole body and beautifies complexion
Oyster Shell *Mu Li* 15 - 30g	salty, astringent, slightly cold	liver, kidney	1. Calm Spirit 2. Astringe 3. Soften and dispel lumps and hardening	headache, dizziness, palpitation, insomnia, neurasthenia, night or spontaneous sweat, vaginal discharge, uterine bleeding, enuresis, spermatorrhea, nocturnal emission, scrofula, goiter, enlarged spleen, peptic ulcer, hypertension
Peach Sd. *Tao Ren* 4.5 - 9g	sweet, bitter, neutral	lung, liver, heart, large intestine	1. Circulate Blood and remove stagnation 2. Lubricate Intestine 3. Stop cough and asthma	amenorrhea, dysmenorrhea, abdominal pain, lung and intestinal abscess, traumatic pain, constipation, cough, asthma, parasites ● Contraindicated during pregnancy
Pear *Li* 1 - 2 pieces	sweet, slightly sour, cool	lung	1. Moisten Lung 2. Promote urination and bowel movement 3. Cool Heart	thirst, irritability, cough, asthma, edema, constipation, alcohol intoxication

Herb	Properties	Channels	Functions	Indications
Pearl *Zhen Zhu* 0.3 - 0.9g	sweet, salty, cold	heart, liver	1. Sedate Heart 2. Clear Liver 3. Promote healing	palpitations, seizures, childhood convulsions, pterygium, ulcers
Peony Rt. (white) *Bai Shao Yao* 6 - 15g	sour, bitter, slightly cold	liver, spleen	1. Tonify Blood and Yin 2. Soften Liver 3. Regulate Qi and stop pain 4. Harmonize Ying and Wei	headache, eye pain, tinnitus, dizziness, irritability, irregular menstruation, dysmenorrhea, uterine bleeding, spontaneous and night sweats, vaginal discharge, chest, flank and abdominal pain, spasms, hypertension
Peony Rt. (red) *Chi Shao Yao* 4.5 - 9g	sour, bitter, slightly cold	liver, spleen	1. Clear Heat and cool Blood 2. Circulate Blood and stop pain 3. Sedate Liver Fire	fever, red, swollen and painful eyes, amenorrhea, dysmenorrhea, menorrhagia, traumatic injury, bleeding (nose, uterine, vomit, etc.), rash, boil, abscesses
Peppermint Lf. *Bo He* 1.5 - 6g	pungent, cool, aromatic	lung, liver	1. Dispel Wind-Heat, clear head and eyes 2. Promote measle eruption 3. Regulate Liver Qi	common cold, headache, pharyngitis, conjunctivitis, chest and hypochondriac pain, distention and fullness, scrofula, ulcers, rash, scabies, measles (early stage)
Perilla Lf. *Zi Su Ye* 3 - 9g	pungent, warm, fragrant	lung, spleen	1. Dispel Wind-Cold 2. Circulate Spleen and Stomach Qi 3. Detoxify fish poisoning	common cold, chest fullness, vomiting, abdominal pain and distention, cough, asthma, fish and crab poisoning, snake and dog bites, beriberi, threatened miscarriage ● Very good for vomiting during pregnancy
Perilla Sd. *Zi Su Zi* 3 - 9g	pungent, warm	lung, large intestine	1. Stop cough and resolve phlegm 2. Lubricate Intestine	cough with thin white sputum, asthma, chest fullness, constipation, chronic bronchitis
Peucedanum Rt. *Qian Hu* 4.5 - 9g	pungent, bitter, slightly cold	lung, spleen	1. Descend Lung Qi 2. Dispel Wind-Heat 3. Resolve phlegm	cough, thick sputum, asthma, irritability, headache, common cold, upper respiratory tract infection
Phellodendron Rt. *Huang Bai* 3 - 12g	bitter, cold	kidney, bladder, large intestine	1. Clear Heat and dry Damp 2. Clear Yin Deficient Heat 3. Detoxify	thirst, diarrhea, dysentery, jaundice, vaginal discharge, acute urinary tract infection, abscesses, eczema, boils, furuncles, tidal fever, night sweat, spermatorrhea, nocturnal emission

HERB	TASTE & TEMP.	CHANNELS	ACTIONS	INDICATIONS
Pinellia Rz. *Ban Xia* 4.5 - 12g	pungent, warm, toxic	lung, spleen, stomach	1. Resolve Cold-Phlegm 2. Warm up Stomach and descend Qi 3. Dispel lumps	cough, copious thin clear sputum, nausea, vomiting, morning sickness, chest and hypochondriac pain and fullness, vaginal discharge, scrofula, goiter, carbuncles, furuncles, ulcer ● Contraindicated during pregnancy (in raw form)
Plantago Sd. *Che Qian Zi* 4.5 - 9g	sweet, slightly cold	lung, liver, kidney, bladder, small intestine	1. Clear Heat and promote urination 2. Stop cough and resolve phlegm	edema, scanty urination, diarrhea, urinary tract infection, cough with profuse phlegm, irritability, red, dry and swollen eyes, cataracts, vertigo ● Contraindicated during pregnancy
Platycodon *Jie Geng* 3 - 9g	pungent, bitter, neutral	lung	1. Resolve Cold or Heat-Phlegm 2. Circulate Lung Qi and eliminate pus	cough, profuse sputum, sore throat, lung or throat abscess, loss of voice ● One of the best herbs for throat disorders
Polygala Rt. *Yuan Zhi* 3 - 9g	pungent, bitter, slightly warm	lung, heart, kidney	1. Calm Spirit 2. Resolve Phlegm 3. Reduce abscess	insomnia, palpitation, irritability, forgetfulness, neurasthenia, disorientation, seizures, nocturnal emission, ulcer, boils, furuncles, carbuncles, acute or chronic bronchitis, cloudy urination, vaginal discharge
Polygonatum Rz *Yu Zhu* 9 - 15g	sweet, slightly cold	lung, stomach	1. Tonify Lung and Stomach Yin 2. Promote body fluids	thirst, irritability, dry throat, dry cough, constipation, spasm of tendons, diabetes, lung disease, coronary heart disease
Polyporus Fungus *Zhu Ling* 6 - 15g	sweet, bland, neutral	spleen, kidney, bladder	1. Promote urination and eliminate Damp	edema, scanty urination, vaginal discharge, cloudy urination, diarrhea, jaundice
Pomegranate Rind *Shi Liu Pi* 3 - 9g	sour, astringent, warm, toxic	kidney, large intestine, stomach	1. Astringe Intestine and Kidneys 2. Kill parasites	chronic diarrhea and dysentery, intestinal parasites, rectal prolapse, uterine bleeding, vaginal discharge, spermatorrhea, premature ejaculation

Herb	Properties	Channels	Actions	Indications
Poria Fungus *Fu Ling* 9 - 15g	sweet, bland, neutral	lung, spleen, heart, bladder	1. Promote urination 2. Tonify Spleen and eliminate Damp 3. Calm Spirit	edema, scanty urination, poor appetite, diarrhea, abdominal distention, insomnia, palpitation, forgetfulness
Poria (Red) *Chi Fu Ling* 6 - 12g	sweet, bland, neutral	spleen, bladder	1. Clear Damp-Heat 2. Promote urination	scanty and/or turbid urination, diarrhea, dysentery, gonorrhea
Poria (Spirit of) *Fu Shen* 9 - 15g	sweet, bland, neutral	heart, spleen	1. Calm Spirit 2. Promote urination	palpitation, insomnia, forgetfulness, difficulty in urination ● Similar to Fu Ling but more for calming the mind
Prunella Spike *Xia Ku Cao* 9 - 15g	bitter, pungent, cold	liver, gall bladder	1. Clear Liver Heat and brighten eyes 2. Dispel nodules	redness, swelling and pain of eyes, headache, vertigo, acute mastitis, breast abscess, mumps, lymphoid tuberculosis, goiter, scrofula, hypertension
Psoralea Sd. *Bu Gu Zhi* 3 - 9g	pungent, bitter, very warm	kidney, spleen	1. Tonify Spleen and Kidney Yang 2. Astringe Intestine 3. Aid Kidney grasp Qi	impotence, spermatorrhea, nocturnal emission, frequent, copious urination, incontinence, borborygmus, abdominal pain, chronic diarrhea, vaginal discharge, rheumatic pain, low back pain and weakness, asthma
Pubescent Angelica Rt. *Du Huo* 3 - 9g	pungent, bitter, slightly sweet, slightly warm	kidney, bladder	1. Dispel Wind-Damp 2. Stop pain	common cold, headache, body ache, rheumatic pain (especially lower body), toothache
Pueraria Rt *Ge Gen* 6 - 12g	sweet, pungent, cool	spleen, stomach	1. Dispel Wind-Cold or Wind-Heat 2. Stop pain 3. Promote body fluids 4. Promote measle eruption	common cold, stiff neck, febrile diseases, measles, diabetes, hypertension, alcohol intoxication

HERB	TASTE & TEMP.	CHANNELS	ACTIONS	INDICATIONS
Quisqualis Fr. *Shi Jun Zi* 4.5 - 12g	sweet, warm	spleen, stomach	1. Kill parasites 2. Promote digestion	ascariasis, enterobiasis, poor appetite, abdominal distention, malnutrition and indigestion in children, weak constitution ● Commonly used for children
Radish Sd. *Lai Fu Zi* 6 - 12g	pungent, sweet, neutral	lung, spleen, stomach	1. Promote digestion 2. Circulate and descend Qi 3. Resolve phlegm	indigestion, poor appetite, abdominal fullness and distention, acid regurgitation, tenesmus, cough, wheezing, chronic bronchitis
Rehmannia Rt. (Cooked) *Shu Di Huang* 9 - 30g	sweet, slightly warm	heart, liver, kidney	1. Tonify Blood and Essence 2. Tonify Kidney Yin	pale face, palpitations, insomnia, dizziness, tinnitus, menstrual disorders, chronic low grade fever, night sweats, dry mouth, low back pain, nocturnal emission, anemia, diabetes
Rehmannia Rt. (Raw) *Sheng Di Huang* 9 - 30g	sweet, bitter, cold	heart, liver, kidney	1. Clear Heat and cool Blood 2. Nourish Yin, Blood and Fluids 3. Stop bleeding	high or low grade fever, thirst, dry mouth, irritability, bleeding (nose, vomit, urine, uterine, etc), constipation, mouth and tongue sores, diabetes ● Dried Rehmannia (*Gan Di Huang*) is used more for tonifying essence and to stop bleeding due to blood deficiency
Rhinoceros Horn *Xi Jiao* 1 - 2g	salty, cold	heart, liver, stomach	1. Clear Heat and cool Blood 2. Calm Spirit 3. Detoxify	high fever, bleeding (nose, vomit, cough, etc.), thirst, delirium, convulsion, mania, loss of consciousness, skin disorders (maculation, erysipelas, etc.) ● Contraindicated during pregnancy
Rhubarb Rz. *Da Huang* 3 - 12g	bitter, cold	liver, heart, spleen, stomach, large intestine	1. Clear Heat and promote bowel movement 2. Circulate Blood and remove stagnation 3. Detoxify	fever, constipation, abdominal fullness, bleeding (vomit, nose, stool, etc.), dysmenorrhea, amenorrhea, abdominal mass, jaundice, dysentery, acute urinary tract infection, appendicitis, burns, carbuncles, furuncles, suppurative skin disease, burns, traumatic injury ● Cautioned during pregnancy/ contraindicated for nursing mothers

Herb	Properties	Channels	Functions	Indications
Ricini Sd. *Bi Ma Zi* 1.5 - 4.5g	sweet, pungent, neutral, slightly toxic	large intestine, lung	1. Purge water and promote bowel movement 2. Detoxify and eliminate pus	edema, constipation, abdominal distention, difficult urination, scrofula, carbuncles, furuncles • Contraindicated during pregnancy
Rosa Fr. *Jin Ying Zi* 4.5 - 9g	sour, sweet, astringent, neutral	kidney, bladder, large intestine	1. Astringe Kidney 2. Astringe Intestine	excessive and frequent urination, incontinence, spermatorrhea, nocturnal emission, vaginal discharge, chronic diarrhea, bleeding (nose, vomit, etc.)
Rubia Rt. *Qian Cao Gen* 6 - 9g	bitter, cold	heart, liver, lung	1. Clear Heat and stop bleeding 2. Circulate Blood and remove stagnation 3. Stop cough and resolve phlegm	external injury or trauma, bleeding (nose, cough, vomit, stool, uterine, etc.), chronic bronchitis, breast abscess, enlargement of spleen and liver, retention of lochia
Rubus Fr. *Fu Pen Zi* 3 - 15g	sweet, sour, slightly warm	liver, kidney	1. Tonify Liver and Kidney 2. Astringe Essence and urine 2. Brighten eyes	frequent urination, enuresis, impotence, spermatorrhea, premature ejaculation, nocturnal emission, poor eyesight, soreness in the low back and knees
Rush Pith *Deng Xin Cao* 1.5 - 4.5g	sweet, cold	lung, heart, small intestine	1. Clear Heat 2. Promote urination	thirst, restlessness, insomnia, sore throat, edema, acute urinary tract infection, morbid crying of babies, jaundice
Salvia Rt. *Dan Shen* 6 - 15g	slightly bitter, slightly cold	heart, pericardium, liver	1. Circulate Blood and remove stagnation 2. Clear Heat and calm Spirit 3. Tonify Yin and Blood	dysmenorrhea, amenorrhea, retention of lochia, angina pectoris, coronary heart disease, ulcers, carbuncles, insomnia, palpitation, irritability, restlessness, chest, abdominal and hypochondriac pain
Sanguisorba Rt. *Di Yu* 6 - 15g	bitter, slightly sour, slightly cold	liver, stomach, large intestine	1. Clear Heat and stop bleeding 2. Astringe Intestine 3. Promote healing	peptic ulcer, bleeding (nose, vomit, urine, stool, uterine, etc.), diarrhea, dysentery, hemorrhoids, sores, ulcers, burns
Sappan Wood *Su Mu* 3 - 9g	pungent, slightly salty, neutral	liver, heart, spleen	1. Circulate Blood and remove stagnation 2. Eliminate pus and stop pain	amenorrhea, dysmenorrhea, irregular menstruation, postpartum abdominal pain, traumatic injury • Contraindicated during pregnancy

HERB	TASTE & TEMP.	CHANNELS	ACTIONS	INDICATIONS
Saussurea Rt. *Mu Xiang* 1.5 - 9g	pungent, bitter, warm	spleen, stomach, liver, gall bladder, large intestine	1. Circulate Qi 2. Tonify Spleen and Stomach 3. Stop pain	chest, hypochondriac and abdominal pain, indigestion, hiccough, vomiting, diarrhea, flatulence, jaundice, gall bladder pain
Schizandra Fr. *Wu Wei Zi* 1.5 - 9g	sour, warm	lung, heart, kidney	1. Tonify Heart, Lung and Kidney 2. Promote body fluids 3. Astringe 4. Calm Spirit	palpitations, insomnia, forgetfulness, neurasthenia, chronic dry cough, asthma, spontaneous and night sweating, chronic diarrhea, spermatorrhea, nocturnal emission, vaginal discharge, diabetes
Schizonepeta Hb. *Jing Jie* 3 - 9g	pungent, warm, aromatic	lung, liver	1. Release Exterior 2. Stop bleeding 3. Promote measle eruption	common cold, bleeding (nose, stool, uterine, etc.), measles, urticaria, abscesses, swellings, ulcers, scrofula, scabies
Scorpion *Quan Xie* 2.4 - 4.5g	salty, pungent, neutral, toxic	liver	1. Extinguish Internal Wind 2. Detoxify 3. Open collaterals and stop pain	spasm, tics, convulsion, stroke, tetanus, deviations of eyes and mouth, hemiplegia, swellings, abscesses, goiter, headache, rheumatic pain, malaria ● Contraindicated during pregnancy
Scrophularia Rt. *Xuan Shen* 9 - 30g	bitter, sweet, salty, cold	lung, stomach, kidney	1. Clear Heat and cool Blood 2. Tonify Yin and Fluids 3. Soften hard and detoxify	extreme thirst, dry mouth, irritability, restlessness, insomnia, dizziness, dry cough, coughing blood, tuberculosis, sore and swollen throat, boils, carbuncles, scrofula, goiter, constipation
Scutellaria Rt. *Huang Qin* 6 - 15g	bitter, cold	lung, heart, stomach, gall bladder, large intestine	1. Clear Heat and dry Damp 2. Detoxify 3. Stop bleeding 4. Calm fetus	high fever, thirst, diarrhea, dysentery, jaundice, red eyes, acute urinary tract infection, cough, bleeding (cough, stool, uterine, etc.), lung and breast abscess, hypertension, threatened miscarriage, ulcers, rash
Shave Grass Hb. *Mu Zei* 3 - 9g	sweet, bitter, neutral	lung, liver	1. Dispel Wind-Heat 2. Clear eyes 3. Clear Heat and stop bleeding	headache, redness, pain and swelling of eyes, excessive tearing, blurred vision, cataracts, conjunctivitis, pterygium, hemorrhoids, blood in stool, anal prolapse ● Cautioned during pregnancy

Herb	Properties	Channels	Functions	Indications
Siler Rt. *Fang Feng* 3 - 9g	pungent, sweet, slightly warm	lung, liver, spleen, bladder	1. Dispel Wind, Cold and Damp 2. Stop pain and spasm	common cold, migraine, rheumatic pain, tetanus, blood in stool
Sophora Rt. *Ku Shen* 3 - 15g	bitter, cold	liver, kidney, bladder, heart, large and small intestines	1. Clear Heat and dry Damp 2. Dispel Wind and stop itching 3. Clear Heat and promote urination 4. Kills parasites	dysentery, jaundice, vaginal discharge, sores, scabies, genital itching, painful urination, edema
Sparganium Rt. *San Leng* 3 - 9g	pungent, bitter, neutral	liver, spleen	1. Circulate Blood and remove stagnation 2. Circulate Qi and stop pain	amenorrhea, dysmenorrhea, postpartum abdominal pain, tumors, abdominal pain and distention, indigestion ● Contraindicated during pregnancy
Stephania Rt. *Fang Ji* 3 - 15g	pungent, bitter, cold	lung, spleen, bladder, kidney	1. Dispel Wind-Damp and stop pain 2. Promote urination	rheumatic arthritis, edema, scanty urination, wheezing, beriberi
Sweet Wormwood Hb. *Qing Hao* 3 - 9g	bitter, cold	liver, gall bladder, kidney	1. Clear Summer heat 2. Clear malaria 3. Clear Yin Deficiency Heat	malaria, low grade fever, tidal fever, purpuric rash, nosebleed
Talc Mn. *Hua Shi* 9 - 18g	sweet, bland, cold	stomach, bladder	1. Promote urination 2. Clear Damp-Heat 3. Clear Summer heat	thirst, irritability, acute enteritis, acute urinary tract infection, scanty urination, diarrhea, eczema ● Contraindicated during pregnancy
Tangerine Peel *Chen Pi* 3 - 9g	pungent, bitter, warm, aromatic	lung, spleen, stomach	1. Circulate and descend Qi 2. Tonify Spleen 3. Resolve Damp and Phlegm	poor appetite, indigestion, abdominal distention, loose stool, fatigue, cough, profuse phlegm, hiccough, nausea, vomiting, acid regurgitation, alcohol intoxication
Tangerine Peel (Green) *Qing Pi* 3 - 9g	pungent, bitter, warm	liver, gall bladder, stomach	1. Circulate Liver Qi 2. Remove food stagnation 3. Resolve Damp and Phlegm	chest and hypochondriac pain, abdominal pain and distention, enlargement of liver and spleen, liver cirrhosis, low blood pressure

HERB	TASTE & TEMP.	CHANNELS	ACTIONS	INDICATIONS
Torreya Sd. *Fei Zi* 9 - 15g	sweet, astringent, neutral	large intestine, lung, stomach	1. Kill parasites 2. Moisten lung and stop cough	hookworm, pinworms, tapeworms, roundworms, mild cough
Tortoise Plastron or Turtle Shell *Gui Ban* 9 - 30g	salty, sweet, cold	heart, liver, kidney	1. Descend Yang 2. Tonify Kidney and strengthen bones 3. Cool Blood and stop bleeding	chronic tidal fever, night sweats, dry mouth and throat, anxiety, insomnia, palpitations, low back and knee pain and weakness, vertigo, tinnitus, osteomalacia, rickets, uterine bleeding, sores, ulceration, spasms, tremors ● Contraindicated during pregnancy
Tortoise Shell *Bie Jia* 9 - 30g	salty, slightly cold	liver, spleen, kidney	1. Tonify Yin and descend Yang 2. Circulate Blood and resolve lumps	night sweats, chronic tidal fever, abdominal mass, enlargement of liver and spleen, amenorrhea, excessive menstruation, malaria ● Contraindicated during pregnancy
Tribulus Fr. *Ci Ji Li* 6 - 12g	pungent, bitter, neutral	liver, lung	1. Extinguish Internal Wind 2. Dispel Wind-Heat and brighten eyes 3. Stop itching	headache, dizziness, vertigo, mastitis, insufficient lactation, lung abscess, acute conjunctivitis, hives, vitiligo, scabies, hemorrhoids, hypertension ● Cautioned during pregnancy
Tricho-santhes Rt. *Tian Hua Fen* 9 - 15g	slightly sweet, bitter, sour, cold	lung, stomach	1. Clear Heat-Phlegm 2. Promote body fluids 3. Reduce swelling	thirst, dry cough or cough with thick phlegm, coughing blood, sores, abscesses, carbuncles, diabetes, hemorrhoids ● Contraindicated during pregnancy
Tricho-santhes Sd. *Gua Lou Ren* 9 - 12g	sweet, cold	lung, stomach, large intestine	1. Clear Heat-Phlegm 2. Moisten Lung and Intestine	cough, asthma, dry mouth, thirst, irritability, chest pain and fullness, breast abscess and swelling, sores, constipation, dry stool, pulmonary infection
Tsaoko Fr. *Cao Guo* 1.5 - 6g	pungent, warm	spleen, stomach	1. Warm up and circulate Stomach Qi 2. Clear malaria	nausea, vomiting, indigestion, acid regurgitation, diarrhea, abdominal pain, fullness and distention, malaria, alcohol intoxication, seafood poisoning

Turmeric Rz. *Jiang Huang* 3 - 9g	pungent, bitter, warm	liver, spleen, stomach	1. Activate Blood and remove stagnation 2. Circulate Qi and stop pain	traumatic injury, chest and abdominal pain, amenorrhea, dysmenorrhea, arthritic pain, tumors, carbuncles
Wasp's Nest *Lu Feng Fang* 6 - 12g	sweet, neutral, toxic	lung, liver, stomach	1. Dispel Wind and stop pain 2. Detoxify 3. Kill parasites	convulsions, tumors, chronic cough, gum pain and swelling, rash, itching of skin, suppuration, sores, carbuncle, scabies, ringworm
Watermelon *Xi Gua* 6 - 15g	sweet, cold	heart, stomach, bladder	1. Clear Summer heat 2. Stop thirst 3. Promote urination	irritability, scanty and difficult urination, edema, mouth ulcers, dry heaves, jaundice, icteric hepatitis
White Mustard Sd. *Bai Jie Zi* 3 - 9g	pungent, warm	lung, stomach	1. Clear Cold-Phlegm 2. Circulate Qi and resolve lump	cough, profuse sputum, pleurisy, joint pain and numbness, vomiting, abdominal pain, fullness and distention
Xanthium Fr. *Cang Er Zi* 3 - 9g	sweet, pungent, bitter, warm, toxic	lung	1. Dispel Wind-Damp 2. Open nose and sinus 3. Stop pain and itching	allergic or chronic rhinitis, sinusitis, headache, rheumatic arthritis, chronic low back or knee pain, leprosy, itching of skin, scrofula
Zedoaria Rz. *E Zhu* 3 - 9g	pungent, bitter, warm	liver, spleen	1. Circulate Blood and remove stagnation 2. Circulate Qi and stop pain	chest and abdominal pain and mass, amenorrhea, traumatic injury, indigestion, acid regurgitation, vomiting, cervical cancer, childhood nutritional impairment • Contraindicated during pregnancy
Zizyphus Sd. *Suan Zao Ren* 9 - 18g	sweet, sour, neutral	liver, heart	1. Calm Spirit 2. Stop sweating 3. Nourish Blood	palpitations, insomnia or excessive sleeping, irritability, restlessness, forgetfulness, night or spontaneous sweat • Use charred for insomnia/ raw for excessive sleeping

APPENDIX II: A TABLE OF FORMULAS

FORMULA	INGREDIENTS	ACTIONS	INDICATIONS	APPLICATIONS
Ba Wu Tang/ Ba Zhen Tang (Eight Precious Decoction)	ginseng, white atractylodes, poria 4g each, baked licorice 2g, cooked rehmannia, Chinese angelica, cnidium, peony 4g each	1. Tonify Qi and Blood	**Qi and Blood Deficiency** - pale or sallow face, fatigue, weak extremities, poor appetite, abdominal distention, dizziness, shortness of breath, thirst, palpitations, dry and rough skin, a pale tongue with thin white coating, thready and weak or large and weak pulse ● One of the best known formulas for women's disorders	anemia, irregular menstruation, uterine bleeding, circulatory ailments, chronic abscess, chronic hepatitis, chronic nephritis, weakness during convalescence
Bai Zhu San (White Atractylodes Powder)	pueraria 8g, ginseng, white atractylodes, poria, saussurea, agastache, licorice 4g each	1. Tonify Spleen and Stomach 2. Resolve Dampness 3. Stop vomiting and diarrhea	**Spleen and Stomach Deficiency** - poor appetite, fatigue, abdominal pain and distention, diarrhea, nausea, vomiting, irritability, thirst with desire to drink warm water, a pale tongue with greasy white coat, slow and weak pulse ● Especially effective in treating children's digestive disorders	infantile diarrhea, infantile malnutrition, gastric ulcer, chronic gastroenteritis, diabetes
Bi Yuan Jian (Conserve the Source Decoction)	dioscorea, euryale, zizyphus, rosa fruit 8g each, white atractylodes, poria 6g each, ginseng, astragalus, licorice 4g each, polygala 3g	1. Tonify Kidney and Spleen 2. Astringe 3. Calm Spirit	**Heart, Kidney and Spleen Deficiency** - pale face, palpitations, insomnia, frightened easily, fatigue, poor appetite, diarrhea or loose stools, dizziness, cold extremities, pain and soreness in low back and legs, a pale tongue with white coating, and thready, weak, deep and slow pulse	neurasthenia, spermatorrhea, nocturnal emission, leukorrhea, infertility, anemia, gastric ulcer, chronic gastroenteritis, ulcerative colitis, Crohn's disease, infantile diarrhea, malnutrition
Bu Zhong Yi Qi Tang (Tonify the Middle	astragalus, ginseng, white atractylodes, licorice 4g each,	1. Tonify Qi of Spleen and Stomach	**Spleen and Stomach Qi Deficiency with prolapse of organs** - poor appetite, fatigue, loose stool, chronic diarrhea, spontaneous	neurasthenia, anemia, common cold, chronic bronchitis, anorexia, chronic

Formula	Ingredients	Actions	Symptoms	Indications
and Augment the Qi Decoction)	Chinese angelica, tangerine peel 2g each, bupleurum, cimicifuga 1g each	2. Raise the Yang Qi	sweating, shortness of breath, mild fever, headache, thirst, irritability, prolapse of organs (anus, rectum, uterus, etc.), a pale tongue with thin white coating, weak or empty pulse • Most well known for treating prolapse of various organs due to weakness of Spleen	gastroenteritis, chronic hepatitis, hernia, myasthenia gravis, gastroptosis, hypotension, hemorrhoids, cerebral arteriosclerosis, monoplegia, impotence, uterine bleeding, leukorrhea, recurrent miscarriage, chronic gonorrhea, leukopenia, persistent malaria, corneal ulcers
Chai Hu Tang or Zheng Chai Hu Yin (Bupleurum Decoction or Upright Bupleurum Decoction)	bupleurum 11g, peony 8g, tangerine peel 6g, siler, licorice 4g each, fresh ginger 3 pieces	1. Release Exterior (diaphoretic)	**Wind-Cold** - fever, chills, headache, bodyache, nasal obstruction, sweating, superficial pulse	common cold, influenza, malaria
Da Fen Qing Yin (Major Separate the Pure Decoction)	red poria, alisma, akebia, polyporus, gardenia, bitter orange, plantago seed 4g each	1. Clear Heat and promote urination	**Urinary Difficulty due to Heat Accumulation** - frequent, urgent and painful urination, bloody urine, turbid urine, red tongue with yellow coat, wiry or tight pulse • Commonly used for gonorrhea or acute urinary tract infection	acute urinary tract infection, urethritis, cystitis, acute prostatitis, urolithiasis, acute nephritis, acute pyelonephritis, jaundice
Ge Gen Tang (Pueraria Decoction)	pueraria 12g, ephedra, cinnamon twig, peony 8g each, fresh ginger, licorice 4g each, date 5 pieces	1. Release Exterior 2. Release muscle 3. Promote body fluids	**Wind-Cold Attack with Stiff Neck** - chills, fever, nasal obstruction, absence of sweating, neck and upper back pain and stiffness, diarrhea, a pink tongue with white coating, superficial and tight pulse • Frequently used for treating common cold	common cold, influenza, stomach flu, pneumonia, bronchitis, allergic rhinitis, otitis media, acute cervical myositis, tendonitis or bursitis of the shoulder, eczema, urticaria, early-stage polio or encephalitis, meningitis

FORMULA	INGREDIENTS	ACTIONS	INDICATIONS	APPLICATIONS
Gui Pi Tang (**Restore the Spleen Decoction**)	ginseng, astragalus, longan, white atractylodes, poria, zizyphus, polygala 4g each, saussurea 2g, licorice 1g	1. Tonify Qi and Blood 2. Tonify Heart and Spleen	**Heart and Spleen Deficiency** - pale or sallow face, fatigue, palpitations, insomnia, dream disturbed sleep, forgetfulness, phobias, poor appetite, abdominal distention, loose stools, chronic bleeding, a pale and swollen tongue with white coat, thready and weak or empty pulse ● Commonly used as a tonic for women. This formula treats a wide variety of women's problems. It is also used for weakness due to mental and physical over-strain.	neurasthenia, myasthenia gravis, congestive heart disease, neurotic palpitations, gastric and duodenal ulcers, thrombocytopenic or allergic purpura, aplastic anemia, general anemia, amenorrhea, functional uterine bleeding, menorrhagia, irregular menstruation, cervicitis, endometritis, impotence, nocturnal emission, chronic gonorrhea
He Zi Ren Shen Tang (**Chebula and Ginseng Decoction**)	chebula, ginseng, poria, white atractylodes, licorice, lotus seed, cimicifuga, bupleurum 6g each	1. Tonify Spleen 2. Astringe	**Spleen Deficiency with Chronic Diarrhea** - pale face, fatigue, poor appetite, indigestion, abdominal distention, loose stools or diarrhea, a pale tongue with white coat, weak or empty pulse	chronic gastroenteritis, gastric ulcer, gastroptosis, infantile diarrhea, anemia, leukorrhea
Jia Wei Bu Fei Tang (**Tonify Lung Decoction with Modifications**)	cooked rehmannia, cornus, lycium 8g each, ophiopogon, tangerine peel, donkey hide gelatin 4g each, moutan, platycodon 3g each, ginseng, Chinese angelica, schizandra, licorice 2g each	1. Tonify Qi and Blood 2. Tonify Lung and Kidney Yin	**Lung and Kidney Deficiency** - pale face, shortness of breath, dry cough, little sputum sometimes with tinge of blood, wheezing, low back and knee soreness and weakness, low grade fever, heat sensation in palms and soles, night sweats, a red tongue with scanty coating, thready and rapid or empty and rapid pulse	cough, hemoptysis, bronchial asthma, chronic bronchitis, asthmatic bronchitis, emphysema, pulmonary tuberculosis, diabetes mellitus, chronic nephritis, spermatorrhea ● Commonly used to strengthen respiratory system
Jia Wei Di Huang Tang (**Rehmannia Decoction with Modifications**)	cooked rehmannia19g, peony, ophiopogon, dioscorea 8g each, cornus, poria, alisma, moutan 4g each,	1.Tonify Lung and Kidney Yin	**Lung and Kidney Yin Deficiency** - cough with blood, asthma, thirst, irritability, restlessness, malar flush, tidal fever, night sweats, nocturnal emission, spermatorrhea, constipation, dark, difficult urination, a red	cough, asthma, hoarseness, chronic pharyngitis, hemoptysis, pulmonary tuberculosis, spermatorrhea, chronic nephritis, diabetes

Formula	Ingredients	Actions	Pattern / Symptoms	Western Conditions
	platycodon, schizandra 2g each		tongue with little coating, thready and rapid or flooding and rapid pulse	mellitus
Jia Wei Gui Pi Tang (Restore the Spleen Decoction with Modifications)	ginseng, astragalus, white atractylodes 8g each, zizyphus, Chinese angelica, tangerine peel, spirit of poria 4g each, polygala, licorice 2g each	Same as Gui Pi Tang	Same as Gui Pi Tang	Same as Gui Pi Tang
Li Zhong Tang (Regulate the Middle Decoction)	ginseng, white atractylodes, dried ginger 8g each, licorice 4g	1. Warm up and tonify Spleen and Stomach 2. Dispel Cold	**Deficiency and Coldness in Spleen and Stomach** - poor appetite, fullness in the epigastrium and stomach, pale face, fatigue, no thirst, vomiting, diarrhea or loose stool, a pale tongue with white coating, deep, slow and weak pulse • A general tonic for the digestive system especially when there is coldness	acute and chronic gastro-enteritis, gastroduodenal ulcer, gastroptosis, gastrectasis, chronic colitis, irritable bowel syndrome, diabetes, cholera, anemia, excessive salivation, fright in children with vomiting, chronic bronchitis, leukorrhea, oral herpes
Liu Wei Di Huang Tang (Six Rehmannia Decoction)	cooked rehmannia 16g, cornus, dioscorea 8g each, alisma, moutan, poria 6g each	1. Tonify Liver and Kidney Yin	**Liver and Kidney Yin Deficiency** - dry mouth, dizziness, vertigo, tinnitus, deafness, chronic dry and sore throat, tidal fever, night sweats, heat sensation in the palms and soles, weakness of low back and knees, chronic toothache, spontaneous or nocturnal emission, a red tongue with little or no coating, thready and rapid pulse • The best known Yin tonic in Oriental medicine. It is commonly used as a tonic for children, elderly or weak and debilitated persons.	neurasthenia, impotence, delayed growth in children, deafness, tinnitus, senility, lumbago, optic neuritis, central retinitis, optic nerve atrophy, pulmonary tuberculosis, hypertension, hyperthyroidism, Addison's disease, functional anovular uterine bleeding, chronic nephritis, chronic glomerulo-nephritis, chronic urinary tract infection, diabetes

FORMULA	INGREDIENTS	ACTIONS	INDICATIONS	APPLICATIONS
Long Dan Xie Gan Tang (Gentiana Longdancao Decoction to Drain the Liver)	gentiana, akebia, alisma, bupleurum 4g each, scutellaria, gardenia, plantago seed, raw rehmannia, Chinese angelica, licorice 2g each	1. Purge Liver and Gall Bladder Fire 2. Clear Damp-Heat in the Lower Burner	**Liver Fire or Damp-Heat in the Lower Burner** - irritability, short temper, severe splitting headaches, red and painful eyes, thirst with desire to drink cold water, red face, bitter taste in the mouth, chest and hypochondriac pain, dizziness, swollen ears, deafness, tinnitus, dark urine, constipation, difficult and painful urination, short menstrual cycle with reddish purple blood, a red tongue with yellow coat, wiry and rapid or slippery and rapid pulse ● Best known clinically for treating acute urinary tract infection and a variety of herpes	urethritis, acute icteric hepatitis, acute cholecystitis, herpes zoster, herpes simplex, acute pyelitis, acute cystitis, acute pelvic inflammation, urethritis, acute prostatitis, scrotal eczema, orchitis, epididymitis, leukorrhea, genital itching, acute conjunctivitis, central retinitis, acute otitis media, boils and carbuncles of the vestibular and external auditory canal, hypertension, hyperthyroidism
Lu Rong Da Bu Tang (Antler Horn Great Tonifying Decoction)	cistanches, eucommia 4g each, peony, white atractylodes, aconite, ginseng, cinnamon bark, pinellia, dendrobium, schizandra 3g each, antler horn, astragalus, Chinese angelica, poria, cooked rehmannia 2g each, licorice 1g	1. Tonify Qi, Blood, Yin and Yang	**Qi, Blood and Yang Deficiency** - pale or sallow face, dizziness, listlessness, intolerance to cold, cold and weak extremities, low back pain and weakness, poor appetite, fatigue, shortness of breath, cough, palpitations, a pale tongue with thin white coat, thready, weak and slow pulse ● This formula is especially good for general Yang Deficiency. It is one of the most commonly used tonic formulas in Korea.	anemia, emaciation, debility after sickness, surgery or childbirth, decreased eyesight and hearing, cardiac failure, spermatorrhea, infertility, menopause, leukemia, chronic sores and abscess, poliomyelitis, nephrophthisis
Ma Huang Tang (Ephedra Decoction)	ephedra, cinnamon twig, apricot seed 9g each, baked licorice 6g	1. Release Exterior 2. Stop cough and asthma	**Wind-Cold Invasion** - chills, fever, headache, body ache, nasal congestion, absence of sweating, cough, asthma, a pink tongue with thin white coating, superficial and tight pulse	common cold, influenza, bronchial asthma, acute bronchitis, bronchial asthma, lobar pneumonia, rhinitis, rheumatoid arthritis

Mai Men Dong Tang (Ophiopogon Decoction)	licorice 11g, ophiopogon 8g, rice 180g	1. Promote fluids in Stomach 2. Descend Qi	**Lung and Stomach Yin Deficiency** - cough with thin sputum, shortness of breath, wheezing, dry throat and mouth, thirst, nausea, vomiting, belching, hiccup, hoarseness of voice, a dry red tongue with scanty coating, a weak and rapid pulse	gastritis, peptic ulcer, esophageal reflux, tuberculosis of pharynx, chronic bronchitis, bronchial asthma, pertussis, acute or chronic laryngitis, pulmonary tuberculosis, pulmonary atelectasis, diabetes, hypertension
Niu Huang Wan (Cow Gallstone Pill)	siler, scutellaria, anemarrhena, gentiana, acorus, peony, scorpion, mercury, licorice 19g each, asparagus, ophiopogon, ginseng, poria 15g each, cinnabar, rhinoceros horn, amber, dragon teeth 8g each, cow gallstone, musk 2g each, wasp's nest 3 pieces, gold sheet, silver sheet 70 pieces each	1. Clear Heat and detoxify 2. Dispel Phlegm and open Orifice 3. Calm Spirit	**Heat attacking Pericardium** - high fever, thirst, delirium, irritability, restlessness, loss of consciousness, a red or deep red tongue, rapid pulse **Windstroke or Convulsion** - loss of consciousness, stiff tongue, deviation of eyes and mouth, very cold and frigid extremities ● This formula is commonly taken in Korea by many people to calm and settle the mind, including students before a big exam.	cerebrovascular accident, infantile convulsion, acute encephalitis, acute meningitis, acute hepatitis, hepatic coma, arteriosclerosis, pneumonia, dysentery, uremia, neurasthenia, hysteria, schizophrenia ● Contraindicated during pregnancy
Ping Wei San (Calm the Stomach Powder)	atractylodes 8g, tangerine peel 5g, magnolia 4g, licorice 2g, fresh ginger 3 pieces, date 2 pieces	1. Dry Dampness 2. Circulate Spleen and Stomach Qi	**Cold-Damp in the Spleen and Stomach** - loss of taste, poor appetite, nausea, vomiting, belching, abdominal fullness and distention, acid regurgitation, loose stool or diarrhea, easily fatigued, heavy sensation in extremities, a pale and swollen tongue with greasy white coat, moderate or slippery pulse ● Commonly used formula in Korea for digestive disturbances	acute and chronic gastritis, functional gastric neurosis, gastric ulcer, obesity ● Cautioned during pregnancy

FORMULA	INGREDIENTS	ACTIONS	INDICATIONS	APPLICATIONS
Qing Wei Yin (Clear the Stomach Decoction)	peony, immature bitter orange 8g each, tangerine peel, barley sprout, hawthorn fruit 4g each	1. Circulate Qi in Spleen and Stomach	**Qi Stagnation in Spleen and Stomach** - poor appetite, indigestion, abdominal pain, distention and fullness, flatulence, belching, headache, thirst, constipation	chronic gastritis, peptic ulcer, functional gastrointestinal disorders, hepatitis, acute or chronic cholecystitis
Ren Shen Bai He Tang (Ginseng and Lily Decoction)	white attractylodes, poria, lily, donkey hide gelatin, asparagus 4g each, peony, ginseng, schizandra, pinellia, apricot seed 3g each, asarum, carthamus, cinnamon twig, licorice 1g each	1. Tonify Qi and Blood 2. Nourish Lung Yin 3. Descend Qi and Resolve phlegm	**Lung Qi and Yin Deficiency with Phlegm** - dry cough, coughing up blood, thirst, shortness of breath, fatigue, weakness	cough, hemoptysis, pharyngitis, chronic bronchitis, bronchial asthma, pulmonary emphysema
Ren Shen Yang Wei Tang (Ginseng to Nourish the Stomach Decoction)	atractylodes 6g, tangerine peel, magnolia, pinellia 5g each, red poria, agastache 4g each, ginseng, tsaoko, licorice 2g each	1. Eliminate Cold-Damp 2. Release Exterior 3. Circulate and tonify Spleen and Stomach Qi	**Cold-Damp in Spleen and Stomach with External Wind-Cold** - poor appetite, indigestion, vomiting, abdominal fullness, acid regurgitation, belching, chills, mild fever ● This is a variation of Ping Wei San (Calm the Stomach Powder) with a stronger effect in tonifying and circulating Qi.	acute and chronic gastritis, functional gastric disorder, gastric ulcer, malaria, obesity
Shi Quan Da Bu Tang (All Inclusive Great Tonifying Decoction)	ginseng, white atractylodes, poria, baked licorice, cooked rehmannia, Chinese angelica, peony, cnidium, astragalus, cinnamon bark 5g each	1. Tonify Qi and Blood 2. Tonify Yang	**Qi, Blood and Yang Deficiency** - pale or sallow face, dizziness, listlessness, intolerance to cold, cold and weak extremities, poor appetite, fatigue, shortness of breath, cough, palpitations, a pale tongue with thin white coat, thready, weak and slow pulse ● The most famous tonic formula in Oriental medicine	anemia, emaciation, debility after sickness, surgery or childbirth, decreased eyesight and hearing, cardiac failure, spermatorrhea, uterine bleeding, menopause, bloody dysentery, hemorrhoidal bleeding, leukemia, chronic sores and abscesses, malaria, poliomyelitis, nephrophthisis

Formula	Ingredients	Actions	Indications / Pattern	Diseases
Si Jun Zi Tang (Four Gentlemen Decoction)	ginseng, white atractylodes, poria, baked licorice 5g each	1. Tonify Qi 2. Strengthen Spleen and Stomach	**Spleen and Stomach Qi Deficiency** - fatigue, pale face, low and weak voice, poor appetite, abdominal distention, vomiting, borborygmus, diarrhea or loose stool, weakness in the extremities, a pale tongue, weak or empty pulse • One of the most well known Qi tonics in Oriental medicine	gastritis, gastric and duodenal ulcers, irritable bowel syndrome, anemia, bleeding, monoplegia, enuresis, uterine fibroid, diabetes, neurasthenia
Si Ling San (Four Ingredient Powder with Poria)	alisma 9g, poria, polyporus, white atractylodes 6g each	1. Tonify Spleen and eliminate Dampness	Same as Wu Ling San but without complications. This formula is used more for digestive disturbances with loose stools and urinary difficulty.	Same as Wu Ling San.
Si Mo Yin (Four Milled Decoction)	areca, aquilaria, saussurea, lindera 6g each	1. Circulate and descend Qi 2. Eliminate stagnation	**Constipation due to Qi Stagnation** - poor appetite, indigestion, belching, flatulence, epigastric and abdominal pain, distention and fullness	chronic gastritis, gastrectasis, peptic ulcer, functional gastrointestinal disorders, intercostal neuralgia
Si Wu Tang (Four Substance Decoction)	cooked rehmannia, Chinese angelica, cnidium, peony 5g each	1. Tonify and nourish Blood 2. Regulate Blood circulation	**General Blood Deficiency** - pale or sallow face, pale lips and nails, dry skin, dizziness, vertigo, blurred vision, irregular, menstruation, amenorrhea, abdominal pain during pregnancy, intestinal or anal bleeding, generalized muscle tension, a pale tongue, thready/weak or thready/choppy pulse • One of the most famous formulas for treating women's disorders	anemia, dysmenorrhea, irregular menstruation, menorrhagia, threatened miscarriage, lochioschesis, insufficient lactation, post-partum anemia, urticaria, neurogenic headache
Tao Ren Cheng Qi Tang (Peach Pit Decoction to Order the Qi)	persica, cinnamon twig, rhubarb, mirabilitum 6g each, baked licorice 3g	1. Clear Heat 2. Activate Blood and remove stagnation	**Heat and Blood Stagnation in the Lower Burner** - acute, sharp lower abdominal pain, incontinence, restlessness, irritability, thirst, night fever, delirium, mania, deep, full, or choppy pulse • Contraindicated during pregnancy	habitual constipation, intestinal obstruction, irregular menstruation, dysmenorrhea, amenorrhea, endometritis, pelvic inflammatory disease, lochioschesis, gallstones

FORMULA	INGREDIENTS	ACTIONS	INDICATIONS	APPLICATIONS
Tao Ren Jian (Decoction of Persica Seed)	Chinese angelica, red peony, raw rehmannia, cyperus, moutan, carthamus, corydalis, peach seed 4g each	1. Activate Blood and remove stagnation 2. Circulate Qi and stop pain	**Blood Stagnation** - fixed stabbing pain, resists pressure, abdominal mass, purple or purplish red tongue, choppy or wiry, tight pulse ● Contraindicated during pregnancy	coronary artery disease, rheumatic valvular heart disease, dysmenorrhea, traumatic injury
Wei Guan Jian (Stomach Gate Decoction)	cooked rehmannia 12g, dioscorea, dolichoris, white atractylodes, dried ginger 8g each, licorice 4g, evodia 3g	1. Tonify and warm Spleen, Stomach and Kidneys 2. Stop diarrhea	**Diarrhea due to Spleen, Stomach and Kidney Deficiency** - poor appetite, fatigue, abdominal pain and fullness, diarrhea or loose stool, cold extremities, aversion to cold, a pale tongue with moist white coat, deep and weak pulse	infantile diarrhea, infantile malnutrition, chronic gastroenteritis, gastric ulcer
Wei Ling Tang (Calm the Stomach and Poria Decoction)	alisma, poria, polyporus, white atractylodes, atractylodes, magonia, tangerine peel 4g each, cinnamon twig, licorice 2g each, fresh ginger 3 pieces, date 2 pieces	1. Eliminate Dampness 2. Regulate Qi in Spleen and Stomach	**Dampness in the Spleen and Stomach** - poor appetite, indigestion, abdominal fullness, distention and pain, nausea, vomiting, heaviness of head and body, edema of face and eyes, diarrhea or loose stool, scanty urine, a pale tongue with greasy white coat, slippery pulse	acute and chronic gastritis, gastric neurosis, acute enteritis, colitis, ascites, nephritic and cardiac edema, urinary retention, acute nephritis, chronic renal failure, scrotal hydrocele, neuralgia
Wen Wei Yin (Warm the Stomach Decoction)	white atractylodes, ginseng 8g each, tangerine peel, dried ginger, licorice 4g each	1. Tonify and warm Spleen and Stomach 2. Circulate Qi	**Spleen and Stomach Cold and Deficiency** - poor appetite, abdominal pain, no thirst, diarrhea or loose stool, nausea, vomiting, vomiting clear sputum	acute and chronic gastroenteritis, gastroduodenal ulcer, gastrectasis, gastroptosis, chronic colitis, cholera, fright in children with vomiting, anemia
Wu Ling San (Five Ingredient Powder with Poria)	alisma 9g, poria, polyporus 6g each, white atractylodes 6g, cinnamon 2g	1. Tonify Spleen and eliminate Dampness (diuretic) 2. Release	**1. Water Stagnation with Exogenous Invasion of Wind-Cold** - fever, headache, irritability, thirst, vomiting immediately after drinking water, difficult urination, superficial pulse	acute gastroenteritis, gastroptosis, cardiac edema, gastrectasis, Meniere's disease, cholera, diabetes, indigestion, ascites due to

				liver cirrhosis, infectious hepatitis, genito-urinary tract infection, acute or chronic nephritis, chronic renal failure, urinary retention, uremia, scrotal hydrocele, toxemia during pregnancy
		Exterior (diaphoretic)		
Xiao Fen Qing Yin (Minor Separate the Pure Decoction)	red poria, alisma, polyporus, gardenia, coix, magnolia 4g each	1. Clear Heat and promote urination	**2. Spleen Deficiency with Dampness and Water Retention** - diarrhea, edema, vomiting, difficult and painful urination, abdominal pain **3. Water Stagnation in Lower Burner** - vomiting frothy saliva, vertigo, cough, shortness of breath, palpitations below umbilicus ● One of the most frequently used diuretic formulas. It is used for milder cases of edema.	acute urinary tract infection, urethritis, cystitis, urolithiasis, acute prostatitis, acute nephritis, acute pyelonephritis, jaundice
Xu Ming Tang (Prolong Life Decoction)	apricot seed, cinnamon bark, ginseng, cnidium, ephedra, gypsum, Chinese angelica, licorice 4g each, dried ginger 3 pieces	1. Clear Heat and dispel Wind 2. Tonify Zheng Qi	**Damp-Heat in the Lower Burner** - frequent, urgent and painful urination, spermatorrhea, difficult urination, turbid urine, red tongue with yellow greasy coat, wiry or tight pulse ● Similar in action to Da Fen Qing Yin but milder with more Dampness **Windstroke or Invasion of Exogenous Wind with Qi and Blood Deficiency** - paralysis, convulsions, loss of consciousness (in extreme cases), deviation of eyes and mouth, stiff or deviated tongue with slow and slurred speech, generalized pain and stiffness, low-grade fever, cough, edema, dry stool, a thin yellow coating or greasy yellow coating on the tongue, wiry and full or slippery and rapid pulse	cerebrovascular accident, cerebromalacia, aphasia, central and peripheral facial paralysis, monoplegia, hemiplegia, neuralgia, rheumatoid arthritis, urticaria, edema, hypertension, bronchitis
Xu Qi Yin (Spread the Qi Decoction)	tangerine peel, bitter orange, hawthorn fruit 6g each, magnolia, saussurea, lindera 3g each	1. Regulate Qi and stop pain	**Qi Stagnation** - indigestion, abdominal pain and fullness and pain, belching, flatulence, joint pain, fatigue, purple tongue, wiry pulse	gastroenteritis, peptic ulcer, intestinal obstruction, cholecystitis, hepatitis, mastitis, intercostal neuralgia

FORMULA	INGREDIENTS	ACTIONS	INDICATIONS	APPLICATIONS
Yang Xin Tang (Nourish the Heart Decoction)	Chinese angelica, cooked rehmannia, spirit of poria 8g each, ginseng, ophiopogon 6g each, zizyphus, biota 4g each, schizandra, licorice 2g each	1. Nourish Heart and calm the Spirit 2. Tonify Qi	**Heart Qi and Blood Deficiency -** palpitations, insomnia, dream disturbed sleep, poor concentration and memory, fatigue, dizziness, anxiety, dry stool, pale face, shortness of breath, spontaneous sweating, low and weak voice, dislike of speaking, a pale tongue with thin white coat, weak or empty pulse ● A general heart tonic for weak and debilitated persons	heart disease, insomnia, neurasthenia, anemia, amnesia, neuralgia
Yu Zhu San (Jade Candle Powder)	cooked rehmannia, peony, Chinese angelica, cnidium, rhubarb, mirabilite 5g each, licorice 2g	1. Tonify and circulate Blood 2. Purge accumulation	**Blood Stagnation and Excess Heat or Blood Deficiency with Interior Heat -** amenorrhea, constipation, dry hard stool	amenorrhea, dysmenorrhea, irregular menstruation, uterine fibroid, constipation
Zhu Sha Liang Ge Wan (Cinnabar Cooling the Diaphragm Pill)	coptis, gardenia 38g each, ginseng, poria 19g each, cinnabar 11g, borneol 2g	1. Clear Heat and Detoxify 2. Calm spirit	**Heart Fire -** fever, irritability, thirst, heat sensation in chest, palpitation, dry mouth and throat, mouth and tongue sores, insomnia, dream disturbed sleep, red tongue, rapid pulse ● Contraindicated during pregnancy	febrile diseases, stomatitis, neurasthenia, palpitations, depression, anxiety neurosis, panic attacks, amnesia, hysteria, psychosis, heart disease, menopausal syndrome, furuncles
Zi Yin Jiang Huo Tang (Nourish Yin and Descend Fire Decoction)	peony, Chinese angelica, 5g each, cooked rehmannia, ophiopogon, atractylodes 4g each, raw rehmannia, tangerine peel, anemarrhena, phellodendron, baked licorice 2g each, fresh	1. Tonify Kidney Yin 2. Sedate Fire	**Kidney Yin Deficiency with False Heat -** tidal fever, night sweats, dry cough, coughing up blood, spitting blood, fatigue, emaciation, low back and knee pain and weakness, steaming heat sensation in palms and soles, irritability, easily angered, malar flush steaming heat sensation in bones, dry mouth and throat, constipation, scanty urination, a red tongue with no coat, thready and rapid or large pulse	tuberculosis, menopausal syndrome, hypertension, diabetes, spermatorrhea, nocturnal emission, metrorrhagia, lumbago, infertility, chronic bronchitis

	ginger 3 pieces, date 2 pieces			• A commonly used formula for pulmonary tuberculosis and menopause
Zuo Gui Yin (Restore the Left/ Kidney Decoction)	lycium 9g, cooked rehmannia 15g, cornus, dioscorea, poria 9g each, baked licorice 2g	1. Tonify Kidney Yin	**Kidney Yin Deficiency** - irritability, dry mouth and throat, thirst with desire to drink, dizziness, low back and knee soreness and weakness, night sweats, insomnia, malar flush, spontaneous emission, a red peeled tongue, thready and rapid pulse	diabetes, tuberculosis, Addison's disease, spermatorrhea, amenorrhea, metrorrhagia, infertility, lumbago

BIBLIOGRAPHY

BOOKS IN ENGLISH

Bensky, Dan, and Andrew Gamble. *Chinese Herbal Medicine, Materia Medica.* Seattle, WA: Eastland, 1993.

Bensky, Dan, and Randall Barolet. *Chinese Herbal Medicine, Formulas & Strategies.* Seattle, WA: Eastland, 1990.

Cheng, Xi Nong. *Chinese Acupuncture and Moxibustion.* China: Foreign Language Press, 1987.

Hole, Jr., John. *Human Anatomy and Physiology.* Dubuque, Iowa: Wm. C. Brown Publishers, 1984.

Hsu, Hong Yen. *Commonly Used Chinese Herb Formulas with Illustrations.* Long Beach, CA: Oriental Healing Arts Institute, 1980.

Kaptchuk, Ted. *The Web That Has No Weaver.* New York, N.Y.: Congdon and Weed, 1983.

Monte, Tom. *World Medicine: The East West Guide to Healing Your Body.* New York, N.Y.: G.P. Putnam's Sons, 1993.

Luo, Xi Wen. *Treatise on Febrile Diseases Caused by Cold.* China: New World Press, 1986.

Sunu, Ki. *The Canon of Acupuncture.* Los Angeles, CA: Yuin University Press, 1985.

Yeung, Him Che. *Handbook of Chinese Herbs and Formulas, Vol. I & II.* Los Angeles, CA: Institute of Chinese Medicine, 1985.

BOOKS IN CHINESE & KOREAN

Cha, In Sik. *Annotations on Shang Han Lun.* Korea: Ko Mun Press, 1971.

Hong, Won Sik. *Interpretation of the Yellow Emperor's Inner Classic.* Korea: Ko Mun Press, 1971.

Hur, Jun. *Precious Mirror of Oriental Medicine*, originally published in 1613. Korea: Nam San Press, 1969.

Hwang, Do Yun. *Compendium of Formulas*, originally published in 1869. Korea: Nam San Press, 1977.

Lee, Jong Hwa. *Annotations on Shang Han Lun.* Seoul: Kae Cheuk Cultural Press, 1981.

Lee, Sang In. *Explanation on the Precious Formulas.* Korea: Sung Bo Press, 1987.

Li, Cun. *Introduction to Oriental Medicine*, originally published in 1580. Korea: Nam San Press, 1974.

Li, Shi Zhen. *Compendium of Materia Medica*. Taiwan: Wen Guang Press, 1982.

Shin, Jae Yong. *Explanation on the Compendium of Formulas*. Korea: Sung Bo Press, 1988.

Zhang, Jing Yue. *The Complete Works of Jing Yue*, originally published in 1624. China: Shanghai Science and Technology Press, 1960.

ABOUT THE TRANSLATOR

Dr. Kihyon Kim, OMD, Ph.D. is currently an Associate Professor of Oriental Medicine at Emperor's College of Traditional Oriental Medicine and is also a faculty member at Yuin University, School of Oriental Medicine. He holds a B.A. degree in psychology from UCLA and received a Master's degree from Emperor's College and Ph.D. from Yuin University. Dr. Kim is a third generation doctor of Oriental medicine and his father was also a Western medical doctor. In addition to receiving training from his father, he received advanced training both in China and Korea. Dr. Kim also has trained in several styles of martial arts and served as team doctor for the United States Tae Kwon Do team (ITF) in 1988. Currently, he serves as Vice President of the Korean Acupuncture and Oriental Medicine Association in California and maintains a private practice in Encino, California.

HERB INDEX

FORMULA INDEX

GENERAL INDEX